Principles and Foundations of Health Promotion and Education

SIXTH EDITION

Randall R. Cottrell, D.ED., MCHES
University of North Carolina Wilmington

James T. Girvan, PH.D., M.P.H.
Professor Emeritus, Boise State University

James F. McKenzie, PH.D., M.P.H., MCHES
Professor Emeritus, Ball State University

Denise Seabert, PH.D., MCHES
Ball State University

PEARSON

Boston Columbus Indianapolis New York San Francisco Upper Saddle River
Amsterdam Cape Town Dubai London Madrid Milan Munich Paris Montréal Toronto
Delhi Mexico City São Paulo Sydney Hong Kong Seoul Singapore Taipei Tokyo

Executive Editor: *Sandra Lindelof*
Program Manager: *Susan Malloy*
Editorial Assistant: *Tu-Anh Dang-Tran*
Text Permissions Project Manager: *Alison Bruckner*
Text Permissions Specialist: *Mark Schaefer, PreMediaGlobal*
Production Project Managers: *Michael Penne and Lauren Beebe*
Production Management, Composition, and Illustration: *Integra*
Copyeditor: *Claudia Gravier Frigo*
Design Manager: *Marilyn Perry*
Cover Designer: *Tandem Creative, Inc.*
Photo Permissions Management: *Maya Melenchuk*
Photo Researcher: *Carly Bergey, PreMediaGlobal*
Manufacturing Buyer: *Stacey Weinberger*
Executive Marketing Manager: *Neena Bali*
Cover Photo Credit: *Getty Images/Robert Churchill*

Credits and acknowledgments for materials borrowed from other sources and reproduced, with permission, in this textbook appear on the appropriate page within the text and on p. 369.

Many of the designations used by manufacturers and sellers to distinguish their products are claimed as trademarks. Where those designations appear in this book, and the publisher was aware of a trademark claim, the designations have been printed in initial caps or all caps.

Library of Congress Control Number: 2014930854

3 4 5 6 7 8 9 10—DOC—16 15 14

www.pearsonhighered.com

ISBN 10:   0-321-92714-1
ISBN 13: 978-0-321-92714-9

CONTENTS

Chapter 3 Philosophical Foundations 76

Chapter 4 Theories and Planning Models 96

This is an exciting time to be studying and/or entering the field of health education/ health promotion. There is now unparalleled interest in health as evidenced by the growing numbers of products and services that address health issues, and the dramatic growth in information and information-seeking related to health. Yet we are facing problems that are dramatic with the aging of the population, the shifting demographics of populations, the continuing challenges that come from new biological and social threats to health, and the explosive growth of social media and apps that are related to health issues. In Burke's preface to the second edition of *Connections*, he refers to: "the radical changes that lay ahead, caused by developments in communications and information technology, and of the urgent need to understand the process of scientific and technological change, the better to manage its increasingly unexpected ripple effects" (Burke, 2007).

Therein lies the challenge to crafting a book to serve as the foundational introduction to the field of health education/health promotion. Most would agree that change is the only constant in our world today—and that change is happening more rapidly and with greater consequence with each passing year. How then do Cottrell, Girvan, McKenzie, and Seabert provide a foundation for a profession as complex and changing as health education/health promotion? Let me give you two illustrations of that challenge. First, in my lifetime there have been incredible changes in our thinking about subjects such as nutrition. In that time we've gone from a basic seven, to a basic four, to a daily food guide with five groups, then a food wheel providing a platter for daily food choices, then a food guide pyramid followed by MyPyramid, and now MyPlate (U.S. Department of Agriculture, 2013). Certainly nutrition is not the only health-related content that changes so rapidly with changes in science and technology.

Second, as I write this foreword in 2013 and look back one decade to 2003, no one then knew what SARS was, Facebook and Twitter did not exist, the Human Genome Project has just been completed, iPhones and iPads were four years away from being introduced, and this country had not yet had an African American president. Think about the implications of this kind of rapid change in the field of health education/health promotion. Those responsible for the training of health education specialists/health promoters must train our students to be able to practice 10 years from now in a world that does not yet exist, to address problems that are as yet unknown, and to be able to use tools that do not yet exist.

The best definition of education I've ever heard has been attributed to Albert Einstein but its origin is unclear. However, I believe that "education is what's left over after you forget everything you've been taught." If you agree, you realize that we need to put into place not content related to fields of study such as health education/health promotion, but the building blocks that let aspiring professionals and others continue to grow in their understanding and professional practice. Cottrell and colleagues come as close as I've seen among the "foundations" books to achieving this.

Here's what the sixth edition of *Principles and Foundations of Health Promotion and Education* does to address the theme of change. The authors provide foundational history and philosophical guidelines allowing for consideration, thought, application, and adaptation. They don't prescribe, they provide building blocks. They do this in the context of applying multiple pedagogies in their chapters. I am particularly appreciative of their Practitioner's Perspective, A Day in the Career, Case Studies, and Critical Thinking Questions and Activities.

I am especially pleased to say that consistent with the theme of change, Chapter 10 on future trends in health education/promotion captures the essence of the forces driving these changes, and it is an interesting look at the implications for the profession and practice of health education/health promotion. Because of the overall tenor of the book and each of the elements I've discussed, it is critically important that a book such as this is available to those beginning their study of the field of health education/health promotion.

Welcome to the future.

Robert S. Gold, PhD, DrPH, FASHA, FAAHB
University of Maryland

References

Burke, James (2012-02-21). *Connections* (Kindle Locations 93-95). Simon & Schuster. Kindle Edition.

U.S. Department of Agriculture. A brief history of USDA food guides. Retrieved September 1, 2013, from http://www.choosemyplate.gov/food-groups/downloads/MyPlate/ABriefHistoryOfUSDAFoodGuides.pdf.

Many students enter the profession of health education/promotion knowing only that they are interested in health and wish to help others improve their health status. Typically, students' interest in health education/promotion is derived from their own desire to live a healthy lifestyle and not from an in-depth understanding of the historical, theoretical, and philosophical foundations of this profession. Other than perhaps a high school health education teacher, many students do not know any health education specialists. In fact, most beginning students are unaware of employment opportunities, the skills needed to practice health education/promotion, and what it would be like to work in a given health education/promotion setting.

This text is written for such students. The contents will be of value to students who are undecided as to whether health education/promotion is the major they want to pursue, as well as for new health education/promotion majors who need information about what health education/promotion is and where health education specialists can be employed. The text is designed for use in an entry-level health education/promotion course in which the major goal is to introduce students to health education/promotion. In addition, it may have value in introducing new health education graduate students, who have undergraduate degrees in fields other than health education/promotion, to the health education/promotion profession.

▷ New to the Sixth Edition

- All chapters have been updated for currency including tables, figures, references, terminology, end-of-chapter materials, Weblinks, and appendices.
- Many of the Practitioner's Perspective boxes have been replaced, offering fresh insights from practitioners in such diverse fields as community health education/promotion; health and wellness center education/promotion; wellness peer education/promotion in a higher education setting; health education/promotion for a governmental agency; and local school and community-based injury prevention programs, among others.

Important new issues and trends covered include

- the impact of healthcare reform on health education/promotion;
- Health Educator Job Analysis (HEJA) 2010;

- Health Education Specialist Practice Analysis (HESPA);
- *Healthy People 2020*;
- updated responsibilities, competencies, and sub-competencies of a health education specialist;
- Master Certified Health Education Specialists (MCHES);
- program accreditation for free-standing undergraduate public/community health programs; and
- The Patient Protection and Affordable Care Act's implications for public/community health education

▷ Chapter Overview

Chapter 1, "A Background for the Profession," provides an overview of health education/promotion and sets the stage for the remaining chapters. Chapter 2, "The History of Health and Health Education/Promotion," examines the history of health and health care, as well as the history of health education/promotion. This chapter was written to help students understand the tremendous advances that have been made in keeping people healthy, and it provides perspective on the role of health education/promotion in that effort. One cannot appreciate the present without understanding the past. The chapter will bring students up to date with the most recent happenings in the profession, such as the new Patient Protection and Affordable Care Act. Chapters 3, 4, and 5 provide what might best be called the basic foundations. All professions, such as law, medicine, business, and teacher education, must provide students with information related to the philosophy, theory, and ethics inherent in the field.

Chapter 6, "The Health Education Specialist: Roles, Responsibilities, Certifications, and Advanced Study," is designed to acquaint new students with the skills that are needed to practice in the field of health education/promotion. It also explains the certification process to students and encourages them to begin thinking of graduate study early in their undergraduate programs. New information related to changes in the competencies and sub-competencies of a health education specialist based on the Health Education Job Analysis Study is incorporated into this chapter. Chapter 7, "The Settings for Health Education/Promotion," introduces students to the job responsibilities inherent in different types of health education/promotion positions and provides a discussion of the pros and cons of working in various health education/promotion settings. With its "A Day in the Career of…" sections and the "Practitioner's Perspective" boxes, this chapter is unique among introductory texts. A new section has been added, warning students to be careful about what they post to social networking websites, and information is included on landing one's first job and how to excel in a health education/promotion career. This chapter truly provides students with important insights into the various health education/promotion settings and the overall profession of health education/promotion.

Chapter 8, "Agencies, Associations, and Organizations Associated with Health Education/Promotion," introduces students to the many professional agencies, associations, and organizations that support health education/promotion. This is an extremely important chapter because all health education specialists need to know of these resources and allies. We believe that all introductory students should be encouraged to join one or more of the professional associations described in this chapter. For that reason, contact information for all of the professional associations discussed is included in the chapter. Chapter 9, "The Literature of Health Education/Promotion," directs students to the information and resources necessary to work in the field. Included in this chapter is basic information related to the Internet and the World Wide Web that should be especially helpful to new students. With the explosion of knowledge related to health, being able to locate needed resources is a critical skill for health education specialists. Finally, health education/promotion students need to consider what future changes in health knowledge, policy, and funding may mean to those working in health education/promotion. They must learn to project into the future and prepare themselves to meet these challenges. Chapter 10, "Future Trends in Health Education/Promotion," is an attempt to provide a window into the future for today's health education/promotion students.

As one reads the text, it will be apparent that certain standard features exist in all chapters. These are designed to help the student identify important information, guide the student's learning, and extend the student's understanding beyond the basic content information. Each chapter begins by identifying objectives. Before reading a chapter, students should carefully read the objectives because they will guide the student's learning of the information contained in that chapter. After reading a chapter, it may also be helpful to review the objectives to make certain major points were understood. Being able to respond to each objective and define each highlighted term in a chapter is typically of great value in understanding the material and preparing for examinations.

Throughout the book take note of the "Practitioner's Perspective" boxes. These are boxes by health education/promotion professionals who are currently working in the field. Some of the boxes relate to working in a particular setting, while others focus on such areas as ethics, certification, internships, hiring, and graduate study. There are a total of 18 "Practitioner's Perspectives" boxes, 8 of them new to this edition.

At the end of each chapter, the student will find a brief summary of the information contained in that chapter. Following the summary are review questions. Students are encouraged to answer these questions because they provide an additional method for targeting learning and reviewing the chapter's contents. A case study follows the review questions. Case studies allow readers to project themselves into realistic health education situations and problem solve how to handle such situations. Next, readers will find critical thinking questions designed to extend readers' learning beyond what is presented in the chapter. They require readers to apply what they have learned, contemplate major events, and project their learning into the future. A list of activities, designed to extend readers' knowledge beyond what can be obtained by reading the chapter, is also included. In some activities students are asked to apply or synthesize the chapter's information. In others, students are encouraged to get actively involved with experiences that will help integrate learning from the text with a practical, real-world setting. By completing these activities, students should have a better understanding of health education/promotion. The activities are followed by Weblinks, which have been updated and expanded for this edition. Weblinks are sites that students can access to read more about a topic, extend their learning, or obtain interesting resource materials. Each chapter ends with a list of references the authors used to develop the chapter. All references are cited in the chapter, and students can use the references to obtain more detailed information on a topic from an original source when they desire to do so.

▷ Supplements

The following instructor supplements are available with the sixth edition:

- An Instructor's Manual that includes a synopsis, an outline, teaching ideas, Web site activities, and video resources for each chapter.
- A Test Bank that includes multiple-choice, true/false, and essay questions for each chapter. A computerized Test Bank is also available.
- PowerPoint presentations that feature chapter outlines and key points from the text.

All of the supplements are available in electronic format only; they can be downloaded from Pearson's Instructor Resource Center at http://www.pearsonhighered.com/educator.

Many thanks to Farah Kauffman, Penn State College of Medicine, for her careful revision of these supplements.

This text is also available as a CourseSmart eTextbook (ISBN: 0-321-96303-2). CourseSmart eTextbooks are an exciting new choice for students looking to save money. As an alternative to purchasing the printed textbook, students can subscribe to the same content online and save 40 percent off the suggested list price of the printed text. Access the CourseSmart eText at www.coursesmart.com.

We readily acknowledge that the information contained in this text represents our bias regarding what material should be taught in an introductory course. There may be important introductory information we have not included, or we may have included information that may not be considered introductory by all users. We welcome and encourage comments and feedback, both positive and negative, from all users of this text. Only with such feedback can we make improvements and include the most appropriate information in future editions.

Randall R. Cottrell
James T. Girvan
James F. McKenzie
Denise M. Seabert

ACKNOWLEDGMENTS

First, we would like to thank all of the health education faculty who have adopted our text and all of the students who have used the text with each new edition. The response we have received has been truly gratifying. Without you, we would not be writing the sixth edition.

We would also like to thank Pearson/Benjamin Cummings for producing the book. We would especially like to thank Meghan Zolnay and Susan Malloy for their editorial guidance as well as Michael Penne and Lauren Beebe for their hard work on this project.

We would like to express our sincere appreciation to those health education/promotion professionals who served as reviewers for the sixth edition. They had many good ideas that we tried to incorporate whenever possible. The reviewers were John Batacan, Idaho State University; Jerome Kotecki, Ball State University; Erin Largo-Wight, University of North Florida; Sarah Rush, University of Alabama; Erica Sosa, University of Texas at San Antonio; Lori Turner, University of Alabama; and Linda Wray, Pennsylvania State University. We would also like to thank the reviewers of previous editions: John Batacan, Idaho State University; Holly Harring, University of South Carolina; Joanna Hayden, William Paterson University; Adriana Rascon-Lopez, University of Texas at El Paso; Manoj Sharma, University of Cincinnati; Erica Sosa, University of Texas at San Antonio; Georgia Polacek, University of Texas, San Antonio; Kathleen Allison, Lock Haven University; Gregg Kirchofer, Canisius College; Dawn Larsen, Minnesota State University, Mankato; Sharon Thompson, the University of Texas, El Paso; M. Allison Ford, Florida Atlantic University; Mike Perko, University of North Carolina Greensboro; Georgia Johnston, the University of Texas, San Antonio; Craig Huddy, Concord College; Whitney Boling, University of Houston; Virginia Noland, University of Florida; R. Morgan Pigg, Jr., University of Florida; Marilyn Morrow, Illinois State University; Steve Nagy, Western Kentucky University; Emily Tyler, University of North Carolina at Greensboro (with additional helpful feedback from Julie Orta, MPH student); and Marianne Frauenknecht, Western Michigan University.

Finally, we would like to dedicate this book to the people in our lives who mean the most to us: our spouses, Karen, Georgia, Bonnie, and Matt; our children, Kyle, Lisa, Kory, Jennifer, Erik, Becky, Erik, Anne, Greg, Clark, Nathan, and Elias; our grandchildren, Kaylee, Anna, Jonah, Rose, Aevan, Mitchell, and Julia; and our parents, Russell and Edith Cottrell, Terry and Margaret Girvan, Gordon and Betty McKenzie, and Paul and Judy Seabert.

A Background for the Profession

After reading this chapter and answering the questions at the end,
you should be able to:

- Define the terms *health, health education, health promotion, disease prevention, public health, community health, global health, population health, coordinated school health*, and *wellness*.
- Describe the current status of health education/promotion.
- Define *epidemiology*.
- Explain the means by which health or health status can be measured.
- List and explain the goals and objectives of health education/promotion.
- Identify the practice of health education/promotion.
- Explain the following concepts and principles:
  a. health field concept
  b. levels of prevention
  c. risk factors
  d. health risk reduction
  e. chain of infection
  f. communicable disease model
  g. multicausation disease model
  h. selected principles of health education/promotion—*participation, empowerment, advocacy, social media*, and *cultural competence*

Health education/promotion has come a long way since its early beginnings. Health education/promotion as we know it today dates back only about 80 years, but the progress in development has accelerated most rapidly in the past 30 years (Glanz & Rimer, 2008). As the profession has grown and changed, so have the roles and responsibilities of health education specialists. The purpose of this book is to provide those new to this profession with a sense of the past—how the profession was born and on what principles it was developed; a complete understanding of the present—what it is that health education specialists are expected to do, how they should do it, and what guides their work; and a look at the future—where the profession is headed, and how health education specialists can keep pace with the changes to be responsive to those whom they serve.

This first chapter provides a common background in the terminology, concepts, and principles of the profession. It defines many of the key words and terms used in the profession, briefly discusses why health education/promotion is referred to as an emerging profession, looks at the current state of the profession, shows how health and health status have been measured, outlines the goals and objectives of the profession, identifies the practice of health education/promotion, and discusses some of the basic, underlying concepts and principles of the profession.

▷ Key Words, Terms, and Definitions

Each chapter introduces new terminology that is either important to the specific content presented in the chapter or used frequently in the profession. This chapter discusses the more common terms that will be used throughout this text. Like the profession, these words and definitions have evolved over the years. The most recent effort occurred in 2011 (Joint Committee on Health Education and Promotion Terminology [Joint Committee], 2012). The 2011 Joint Committee was convened by the American Association for Health Education (AAHE) of the American Alliance for Health, Physical Education, Recreation, and Dance (AAHPERD) (see Chapter 8 for information on this and other professional associations). The Joint Committee is charged with reviewing and updating the terminology of the profession. The members of the 2011 Joint Committee were comprised of representatives from the member organizations in the Coalition of National Health Education Organizations (see Chapter 8), the National Commission for Health Education Credentialing, Inc. (see Chapter 6), as well as governmental agencies (Joint Committee, 2012). Before this meeting, there have been seven major terminology reports developed for the profession over the past 80 years with the first dating back to 1927 (Johns, 1973; Joint Committee on Health Education Terminology, 1991a, 1991b; Joint Committee, 2001; Moss, 1950; Rugen, 1972; Williams, 1934; Yoho, 1962).

Before presenting some of the key terms used in the profession, an in-depth discussion of the word *health* may be helpful. Health is a difficult concept to put into words, but it is one that most people intuitively understand. The World Health Organization (WHO) has defined health as "the state of complete mental, physical and social well being not merely the absence of disease or infirmity" (WHO, 1947, p. 1). This classic definition is important because it identifies the vital components of health and further implies that health is a holistic concept involving an interaction and interdependence among these various components. A number of years after the writing of the WHO definition, Hanlon (1974) defined health as "a functional state which makes possible the achievement of other goals and activities. Comfort, well-being, and the distinction between physical and mental health differ in social classes, cultures, and religious groups" (p. 73). And more recently, the WHO (1986) has stated that "To reach a state of complete physical, mental, and social well-being, an individual or group must be able to identify and to realize aspirations, to satisfy needs, and to change or cope with the environment. Health is, therefore, seen as a resource for everyday life, not the object of living. Health is a positive concept emphasizing social and personal resources, as well as physical capacities" (p. 5). In other words, good health should not be the goal of life, but rather a vehicle to reaching one's goals of life. We feel that these major concepts of health are captured in the definition that states that **health** "is a *dynamic state or condition that is multidimensional* (i.e., physical, emotional, social, intellectual, spiritual, and occupational) a resource for living, and results from a person's interactions with and adaptation to the environment" (Joint Committee, 2012, p. 10). As such, health can exist in varying degrees—ranging from good to poor and everywhere in between—and depends on each person's individual circumstances. "For example, a person can be healthy while dying, or a person who is quadriplegic can be healthy in the sense that his or her mental and social well-being is high and physical health is as good as it can be" (Hancock & Minkler, 2005, p. 144).

In addition to the word *health*, it is also important to have an understanding of the following key terms and definitions:

> **community health**—"the health status of a defined group of people and the actions and conditions to promote, protect and preserve their health" (Joint Committee, 2012, p. 15)
>
> **health education**—"any combination of planned learning experiences using evidence based practices and/or sound theories that provide the opportunity to acquire knowledge, attitudes, and skills needed adopt and maintain healthy behaviors" (Joint Committee, 2012, p. 17)
>
> **health promotion**—"any planned combination of educational, political, environmental, regulatory, or organizational mechanisms that support actions and conditions of living conducive to the health of individuals, groups, and communities" (Joint Committee, 2012, p. 18) (See **Figure 1.1** for the relationship between health education and health promotion.)

▶ **Figure 1.1** Relationship between health education and health promotion

Source: From J. F. McKenzie, B. L. Neiger, and R. Thackeray, *Planning, Implementing and Evaluating Health Promotion Programs: A Primer*. 6th ed., p. 5, Fig 1.1 © 2013 Reproduced by permission of Pearson Education, Inc., Upper Saddle River, NJ.

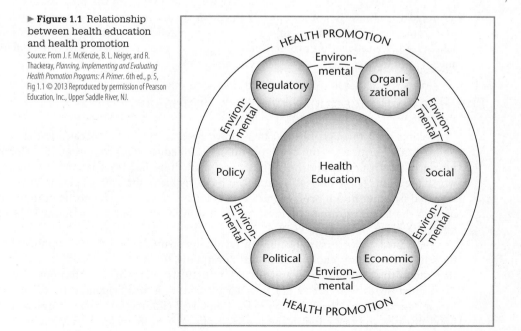

disease prevention—"the process of reducing risks and alleviating disease to promote, preserve, and restore health and minimize suffering and distress" (Joint Committee, 2001, p. 99)

public health—"is the science and the art of protecting and improving the health of communities through education, promotion of healthy lifestyles, and research for disease and injury prevention" (Association of Schools of Public Health, n. d., ¶1)

global health—"health problems, issues, and concerns that transcend national boundaries and are beyond the control of individual nations, and are best addressed by cooperative actions and solutions" (Joint Committee, 2012, p. 17)

population health—"the health status of people who are not organized and have no identity as a group or locality and the actions and conditions to promote, protect, and preserve their health" (McKenzie, Pinger, & Kotecki, 2012, p. 7)

coordinated school health—"an organized set of policies, procedures, and activities designed to protect, promote, and improve the health and well-being of pre-K through 12 students and staff, thus improving a student's ability to learn. It includes, but is not limited to, comprehensive school health education; school health services; a healthy school environment; school counseling; psychological and social services; physical education; school nutrition services; family and community involvement in school health; and school-site health promotion for staff" (Joint Committee, 2012, p. 16)

wellness—"an approach to health that focuses on balancing the many aspects, or dimensions, of a person's life through increasing the adoption of health enhancing conditions and behaviors rather than attempting to minimize conditions of illness" (Joint Committee, 2012, p. 10)

Before we leave the discussion about key words and terms of the profession, it should be noted that there is not complete agreement on terminology. We could easily have found another definition for each of the terms presented here written by either a respected scholar in health education/promotion or a legitimate professional or governmental health agency.

▷ The Health Education/Promotion Profession

In looking back through history, there have been a number of occasions that can be pointed to as "critical" to the development of health education/promotion. (See Chapter 2 for an in-depth presentation of the history.) But there has been no time in history in which the status of the profession has been more visible to the average person or as widely accepted by other health professionals as it is today. Much of this notoriety can be attributed to the health promotion era of public health history that began about 1974 in the United States.

The United States' first public health revolution spanned the late 19th century through the mid-20th century and was aimed at controlling the harm (morbidity and mortality) that came from infectious diseases. By the mid-1950s, many of the infectious diseases in the United States were pretty much under control. This was evidenced by the improved infant mortality rates, the reduction in the number of children who were contracting childhood diseases, the reduction in the overall death rates in the country, and the increase in

TABLE 1.1 **Life expectancy at birth, at 65 years of age, and at 75 years of age, according to sex: United States, selected years 1900–2010**

Year	At Birth			At 65 Years			At 75 Years		
	Both Sexes	Male	Female	Both Sexes	Male	Female	Both Sexes	Male	Female
1900	47.3	46.3	48.3	11.9	11.5	12.2	*	*	*
1950	68.2	65.6	71.1	13.9	12.8	15.0	*	*	*
1960	69.7	66.6	73.1	14.3	12.8	15.8	*	*	*
1970	70.8	67.1	74.7	15.2	13.1	17.0	*	*	*
1980	73.7	70.7	77.4	16.4	14.1	18.3	10.4	8.8	11.5
1990	75.4	71.8	78.8	17.2	15.1	18.9	10.9	9.4	12.0
2000	77.0	74.3	79.7	18.0	16.2	19.3	11.4	10.1	12.3
2010	78.7	76.2	81.0	19.1	17.7	20.3	12.1	11.0	12.9

* = Data not available

Source: Data from U.S. Department of Health and Human Services, National Center for Health Statistics (NCHS). (2013). *Health, United States, 2012: With Special Feature on Emergency Care.* Hyattsville, MD: Author

life expectancy (see **Table 1.1**). With the control of many communicable diseases, the focus moved to the major chronic diseases such as heart disease, cancer, and strokes—diseases that were, in large part, the result of the way people lived.

By the mid-1970s, it had become apparent that the greatest potential for reducing morbidity, saving lives, and reducing healthcare costs in the United States was to be achieved through health promotion and disease prevention. At the core of this approach was health education/promotion. In 1980, the U.S. Department of Health, Education, and Welfare (USDHEW) presented a blueprint of the health promotion and disease prevention strategy in its first set of health objectives in the document called *Promoting Health/Preventing Disease: Objectives for a Nation* (USDHEW, 1980). This document proposed a total of 226 objectives divided into three main areas—preventive services, health protection, and health promotion. This was the first time a comprehensive national agenda for prevention had been developed, with specific goals and objectives for anticipated gains (McGinnis, 1985). In 1985, it was apparent that only about one-half of the objectives established in 1980 would be reached by 1990, another one-fourth would not be reached, and progress on the others could not be judged because of the lack of data (Mason & McGinnis, 1990). Even though not all objectives were reached, the planning process involved in the 1980 report demonstrated the value of setting goals and listing specific objectives as a means of measuring progress in the nation's health and healthcare services. These goals and objectives published by the U.S. Department of Health and Human Services (USDHHS), now in their fourth generation as *Healthy People 2020*, have defined the nation's health agenda and guided its health policy since their inception. (See Chapter 2 for more on *Healthy People 2020*).

Now 10-plus years into the 21st century, the health of the people in the United States is better than any time in the past. "By every measure, we are healthier, live longer, and enjoy lives that are less likely to be marked by injuries, ill health, or premature death" (Institute of Medicine [IOM], 2002, p. 2). Yet, we could do better. "Four modifiable health risk behaviors—lack of physical activity, poor nutrition, tobacco use, and excessive alcohol consumption—are responsible for much of the illness, suffering, and early death related to chronic diseases" (Centers for Disease Control and Prevention [CDC], 2011a, ¶3). Thus, "behavior patterns represent the single most prominent domain of influence over health prospects in the United States" (McGinnis, Williams-Russo, & Knickman, 2002, p. 82).

As the health agenda has become more clearly defined, so has the health education/promotion profession. In 1998, the U.S. Department of Commerce and Labor formally recognized "health educator" as a distinct occupation, thus demonstrating that the health education/promotion profession is moving in the right direction. More recently a study titled "Marketing the Health Education Profession: Knowledge, Attitudes, and Hiring Practices of Employers" conducted by Hezel Associates (2007) was conducted. Through this study the term *health education specialist* has gained favor over the use of the term *health educator*. A **health education specialist** has been defined as "an individual who has met, at a minimum, baccalaureate-level required health education academic preparation qualifications, who serves in a variety of settings, and is able to use appropraite educational strategies and methods to facilitate the development of policies, procedures, interventions, and systems conducive to the heatlh of indivdiuals, groups, and communities" (Joint Committee, 2012, p. 18). Thus the term *health education specialist* will be used throughout the remainder of this book.

Clearly, there is a need for health education/promotion interventions provided by health education specialists in the United States both today and in the future.

▷ Measuring Health or Health Status

Though the definition of health is easy to state, trying to quantify the amount of health an individual or a population possesses is not easy. Therefore, most measures of health are expressed using health statistics based on the traditional medical model of describing ill health (injury, disease, and death) instead of well health. Thus, the higher the presence of injury, disease, and death indicators, the lower the level of health; the lower the presence of injury, disease, and death indicators, the higher the level of health. Out of necessity we have defined the level of health with just the opposite—ill health (McKenzie et al., 2012).

The information gathered when measuring health is referred to as **epidemiological data.** These data are gathered at the local, state, and national levels to assist with the prevention of disease outbreaks or control those in progress and to plan and assess health education/promotion programs. Epidemiology is one of those disciplines that helps provide the foundation for the health education/promotion profession. **Epidemiology** is defined as "the study of the distribution and determinants of health-related states or events (including disease), and the application of this study to the control of diseases and other health problems" (World Health Organization, 2013). In the following sections, several of the more common epidemiological means by which health, or lack thereof, are described and quantified.

EPIDEMIOLOGY Jaime Harding, MHS, CHES

CURRENT POSITION: Health Promotion Program Manager

EMPLOYER: Central District Health Department, Boise, Idaho

DEGREE/INSTITUTION/YEAR: Master of Health Science, Boise State University, August 2006; Bachelor of Science, Athletic Training and Bachelor of Science, Health Promotion, Boise State University, May 2001.

MAJOR: Health Science—Health Policy emphasis (graduate); Athletic Training (undergraduate); Health Promotion (undergraduate)

Describe your past and current professional positions and how you came to hold the job you now hold (How did you obtain the position?): During my senior year of undergraduate work, I interned at Saint Alphonsus Regional Medical Center in the Marketing Department. Upon my graduation, the internship position led into a full-time employment opportunity within the same department. I worked in this capacity for approximately one year when I obtained a promotional opportunity to work for the Idaho Department of Health and Welfare (IDHW). I worked in several capacities for the IDHW for ten years. Specifically, my positions were in the Division of Medicaid in the Regional Medicaid Services office as a Health Resources Coordinator in Medicaid's managed care program, Healthy Connections; in the Diabetes Prevention and Control Program; in the Physical Activity and Nutrition Program as a Health Program Specialist and finally as a Physical Activity and Nutrition Program Manager. These experiences honed my skills in grant writing to agencies such as the CDC and the U.S. Administration of Aging, negotiating and managing contracts, supervising employees, facilitating statewide networks for prevention activities, and creating and overseeing program budgets. Having these skills helped me obtain the Health Promotion Program Manager position at Central District Health Department in April 2012, where I helped guide the local health department's shift away from working on individual behavior change activities to that of broad-based population impact to increase access to physical activity and healthy eating opportunities.

Describe the duties of your current position: Within the Office of Health Promotion, my staff and I primarily focus on increasing access to physical activity and healthy eating along with reducing tobacco initiation and use. I also oversee the implementation of a senior fall prevention program and an agency worksite wellness program. Additionally, I conduct semi-annual and annual performance reviews along with providing regular coaching and mentoring to staff. I lead staff in strategic and policy agenda planning utilizing a policy, systems and environmental change approach to influence broad-based population impact, and negotiate and manage contracts with multiple agencies such as IDHW and non-profit organizations are major position duties. I'm also involved with staff in providing technical assistance and training to community partners; participating on state and local coalitions, alliances and advisory boards with a physical activity, nutrition, tobacco prevention and healthy aging emphasis.

Describe what you like most about this position: After having worked for ten years at a state agency, I've enjoyed gaining local-level experience. I appreciate the opportunity to work in each community to spend time developing and fostering relationships while gaining an understanding of the specific needs of that community. I have noticed I spend more time fostering partnerships through face-to-face meetings and phone calls than through email communication.

Describe what you like least about this position: Stable and ongoing funding for primary prevention has been problematic for public health. In the past, most funding opportunities came to us in a categorical manner or with a disease-specific focus.

BOX

1.1

continued

Recently, we are starting to see a shift to funding primary prevention work that is focused on mitigating chronic disease risk factors through broad-based population work. Public health funding continues to be inadequate and inconsistently funded so this is an ongoing challenge. Because we are often underfunded, we are limited on available human resources, which results in a challenge to have adequate staff to meet the workload demands.

In addition, we often have problems with programmatic siloes in public health resulting in duplication of effort. Programs tend to work independently of each other, often using the same community-based partners. Unfortunately, in a small state like Idaho, many community-based partners are serving on multiple coalitions and alliances. It is not uncommon for me to attend two different coalition meetings within a short period of time and usually the same core group of people is in attendance. We talk about integration and streamlining efforts among programs and community partners but it is difficult to put this into practice.

How do you use health data/epidemiology in your current position? We use health data to inform us on the current and changed state of our communities. These data help us determine the priority needs in each community for addressing access to physical activity, healthy eating and tobacco use prevention. Within our four-county jurisdiction, we are working with several communities to implement the CDC-developed Community Health Assessment and Group Evaluation (CHANGE) Tool. The CHANGE Tool community health assessment affords us an opportunity to assess community strengths, identify areas for improvement and assist the community with prioritizing community needs related to population-based strategies. Currently, we rely on state-collected data such as the CDC's Behavioral Risk

Factor Surveillance System (BRFSS) and Youth Risk Behavior Surveillance System (YRBSS) to assess health behaviors but we recognize there are health data gaps in Idaho. There are efforts underway to address these data gaps and develop a clearinghouse to store chronic disease risk factor data. We use best practice or evidence-based practices in our community-based work to create lasting, sustainable change. Our goal is to create an environment where the healthy choice is the default choice for all individuals.

What recommendations/advice do you have for current health education students desiring to become community health educators? I work with interns on a regular basis and am often interviewed by students seeking guidance for entering the public health field. I recommend developing skills to become a strong written and oral communicator. Much of our work is done through written documents and via oral presentations. I'm often asked to present to the Central District Health Department Board of Health or other groups within the community so being organized and comfortable with public speaking is key. Additionally, I write grant applications, reports, contracts, and communicate via email so strong written skills are a necessity. I recommend that students be nimble and flexible in their careers. Students need to know that an entry-level position may not be their dream job but it serves as an opportunity to develop skills and relationships with other individuals working in the field. It is a way to gain experience so when promotional opportunities are available, they can apply for them. It's also critical that students connect with working professionals through local, state and national societies and associations. Often times, networking opens the door for employment opportunities.

Rates

A **rate** "is a measure of some event, disease, or condition in relation to a unit of population, along with some specification of time" (National Center for Health Statistics [NCHS], 2013, p. 468). Rates are important because they provide an opportunity for comparison of events, diseases, or conditions that occur at different times or places. Some of the more commonly used rates are death rates, birth rates, and morbidity rates. **Death rates** (the number of deaths per 100,000 resident population), sometimes referred to as *mortality* or *fatality rates*, are probably the most frequently used means of quantifying the seriousness of injury or disease. (See **Table 1.2** for death rates and **Table 1.3** for an example of a formula used to tabulate rates.) "The transition from wellness to ill health is often gradual and poorly defined. Because death, in contrast, is a clearly defined event, it has continued to be the most reliable single indicator of health status of a population. Mortality statistics, however, describe only a part of the health status of a population, and often only the endpoint of an illness process" (USDHHS, 1991, p. 15). Rates can be expressed in three forms—(1) crude, (2) adjusted, and (3) specific. A **crude rate** is the rate expressed for a total population. An **adjusted rate** is also

TABLE 1.2 **Crude death rates for all causes and selected causes of death: United States, 2012**

Cause	Deaths per 100,000 Population
All causes	799.5
Diseases of the heart	193.6
Malignant neoplasms (cancer)	186.2
Cerebrovascular diseases (stroke)	41.9
Suicide	12.4
Motor vehicle–related injuries	11.4
Homicide	5.3

Source: Data from U.S. Department of Health and Human Services, National Center for Health Statistics (NCHS). (2013). *Health, United States, 2012: With Special Feature on Emergency Care.* Hyattsville, MD: Author.

TABLE 1.3 **Selected mortality rates and their formulas**

Rate	Definition	Example (U.S. 2012)
Crude death rate $= \dfrac{\text{Number of deaths (all causes)}}{\text{Estimated midyear population}} \times 100{,}000$		799.5/100,000
Age-specific death rate $= \dfrac{\text{Number of deaths, } 45-54}{\text{Estimated midyear population, } 45-54} \times 100{,}000$		407.1/100,000
Cause-specific mortality $= \dfrac{\text{Number of deaths, (HIV)}}{\text{Estimated midyear population}} \times 100{,}000$		2.7/100,000

Source: Data from U.S. Department of Health and Human Services, National Center for Health Statistics (NCHS). (2013). *Health, United States, 2012: With Special Feature on Emergency Care.* Hyattsville, MD: Author.

expressed for a total population but is statistically adjusted for a certain characteristic, such as age. A **specific rate** is a rate for a particular population subgroup such as for a particular disease (i.e., disease-specific) or for a particular age of people (i.e., age-specific). Examples include calculating the death rate for heart disease in the United States, or the age-specific death rate for 45- to 54-year-olds.

There are three other epidemiological terms that are used to describe the magnitude of a rate of some event, disease, or condition in a unit of population. They are: (1) **endemic**—occurs regularly in a population as a matter of course; (2) **epidemic**—an unexpectedly large number of cases of an illness, specific health-related behavior, or other health-related event in a population; and (3) **pandemic**—an outbreak over a wide geographical area, such as a continent. As you continue your preparation to become a health education specialist, you will be introduced to more and more epidemiological principles and terms.

Life Expectancy

Life expectancy is another means by which health or health status has been measured. It, too, however, is based on mortality. Even with this limitation, though, life expectancy has been described as "the most comprehensive indicator of patterns of health and disease, as well as living standards and social development" (CDC, 1994, pp. 2–8). **Life expectancy** "is the average number of years of life remaining to a person at a particular age and is based on a given set of age-specific death rates—generally the mortality conditions existing in the period mentioned. Life expectancy may be determined by sex, race and Hispanic origin, or other characteristics using age-specific death rates for the population with that characteristic" (NCHS, 2013, p. 452). The most frequently used times to state life expectancy are at birth, at the age of 65, and more recently at age 75 (see Table 1.1). It must be remembered that life expectancy is an average for an entire cohort (usually a single birth year) and is not necessarily a useful predictor for any one individual. In terms of evaluating the effect of chronic disease on a population, life expectancies calculated *after* birth have been found to be more useful measures than life expectancy *at* birth because life expectancy at birth reflects infant mortality rates.

Years of Potential Life Lost

A third means by which health or health status has been measured is **years of potential life lost (YPLL)**. YPLL "is a measure of premature mortality" (NCHS, 2013, p. 473) (see **Table 1.4**) and is calculated by subtracting a person's age at death from 75 years. For example, for a person who dies at age 30, the YPLL are 45. Until 1996, the U.S. government used age 65 in calculating YPLL, but because life expectancy in the United States has continued to increase and is greater than 75 years that age is now used (NCHS, 2013).

Disability-Adjusted Life Years

The three measures of health and health status noted previously are commonly used in the United States and other developed countries. However, because mortality does not express the burden of living with disability (for example, the resulting paralysis from an automobile crash or the depression that often follows a stroke), the WHO and the World Bank

TABLE 1.4 **Age-adjusted years of potential life lost (per 100,000 population) before age 75 for selected leading causes of death: United States, 1990 and 2006**

Cause	1990	2010
Malignant neoplasms	2,003.8	1395.8
Diseases of the heart	1,617.7	972.4
Unintentional injuries (accidents)	1,162.1	1025.2
Suicide	393.1	385.2
Homicide	417.4	239.0
Cerebrovascular diseases (stroke)	259.6	169.3
Chronic lower respiratory diseases	187.4	172.4
Diabetes mellitus	155.9	158.2
HIV	383.8	76.6
Chronic liver disease and cirrhosis	196.9	163.9
Influenza and pneumonia	141.5	71.4

Source: Data from U.S. Department of Health and Human Services, National Center for Health Statistics (NCHS). (2013). *Health, United States, 2011 with Special Feature on Emergency Care.* Hyattsville, MD: Author, p. 84.

developed a measure called **disability-adjusted life years (DALYs).** One DALY can be thought of as one lost year of "healthy" life as a result of being in states of poor health or disability (Murray & Lopez, 1996; WHO, 2008).

To calculate total DALYs for a given condition in a population, years of life lost (YLL) and years lived with disability (YLD) of known severity and duration for that condition must each be estimated, then the total summed. For example, to calculate DALYs incurred through road accidents in India in 1990, add the total years of life lost in fatal road accidents and the total years of life lived with disabilities by survivors of such accidents (Murray & Lopez, 1996, p. 7).

Figure 1.2 presents the DALYs for selected regions of the world. As noted, "DALYs in Africa are at least two times higher than in any other region" (WHO, 2008, p. 40).

Health-Adjusted Life Expectancy

One other measurement of health, which is used by the WHO and is based on disability and life expectancy rather than mortality, is **health-adjusted life expectancy (HALE).** Sometimes referred to as healthy life expectancy, HALE is the number of years of healthy life expected, on average, in a given population. Like life expectancy, HALE can be calculated at birth and at other ages. The methods used to calculate HALE are beyond the scope of this textbook (Mathers, Sdana, Salmon, Murray, & Lopez, 2001).

Health-Related Quality of Life

Even though DALYs and HALE go beyond measuring health in terms of just mortality, they really do not get at the quality of life (QOL). Although QOL refers to a person or group's general well-being, **health-related quality of life (HRQOL)** encompasses "those aspects of overall quality of life that can be clearly shown to affect health—either physical or mental" (CDC, 2011b, ¶3). Healthcare providers have often used HRQOL to measure the effects of

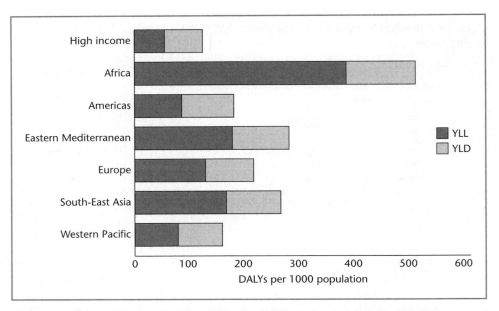

▲ **Figure 1.2** Burden of disease: Years of life lost as a result of premature mortality (YLL) and years of life lived with a disability (YLD) per thousand by region, 2004
Source: From "Burden of Disease: DALYs" in *The Global Burden of Disease: 2004 Update*. © World Health Organization, 2008. Reproduced by permission of the World Health Organization. http://www.who.int/healthinfo/global_burden_disease/GBD_report_2004update_part4.pdf
DALYs, disability-adjusted life years

chronic disease in their patients to better understand how a disease interferes with a person's daily life. Similarly, public health professionals have used HRQOL to measure the effects of numerous disorders, short- and long-term disabilities, and diseases in different populations. Tracking HRQOL in different populations can identify subgroups with poor physical or mental health and can help guide policies or other interventions to improve their health (CDC, 2011b).

In recent years, more and more health professionals have been using the concept of HRQOL to quantify and track the health status of people. Measures of HRQOL are now included on a number of different health surveys, including the Behavioral Risk Factor Surveillance Survey (BRFSS) and the National Health and Nutrition Examination Survey (NHANES) (see next section for discussion of these surveys). Both the BRFSS and the NHANES use the standard four-item "Healthy" Days core questions (CDC HRQOL-4) created by the Centers for Disease Control and Prevention (CDC) and presented in Box 1.2.

Health Surveys

Data collected through surveys conducted by governmental agencies are other means by which health or health status has been measured in the United States. Six examples are presented here. The first two, the National Health Interview Survey (NHIS) and the NHANES, are conducted by the National Center for Health Statistics (NCHS). The NHIS, which has been used for more than 50 years, is a telephone interview in which respondents are asked a number of questions about their health and health behavior. One of the questions, for

---

BOX 1.2

"Healthy" Days Core Questions (CDC HRQOL-4)

1. Would you say that in general your health is:
   a. Excellent
   b. Very good
   c. Good
   d. Fair
   e. Poor

2. Now thinking about your physical health, which includes physical illness and injury, for how many days during the past 30 days was your physical health not good?

3. Now thinking about your mental health, which includes stress, depression, and problems with emotions, for how many days during the past 30 days was your mental health not good?

4. During the past 30 days, approximately about how many days did poor physical or mental health keep you from doing your usual activities, such as self-care, work, or recreation?

Source: Centers for Disease Control and Prevention (CDC). (2011b). *Health-related Quality of Life.* Available from http://www.cdc.gov/hrqol/methods.htm.

---

example, asks the respondents to describe their health status using one of five categories: excellent, very good, good, fair, or poor.

The NHANES data are collected using a mobile examination center. Through direct physical examinations, clinical and laboratory testing, and related procedures, data are collected on a representative group of Americans. These examinations result in the most authoritative source of standardized clinical, physical, and physiological data on the U.S. population. Included in the data are the prevalence of specific conditions and diseases and data on blood pressure, blood cholesterol, body mass index, nutritional status and deficiencies, and exposure to environmental toxins (McKenzie et al., 2012).

The third example of data collected from surveys actually comes from a family of surveys called the National Health Care Surveys. These surveys are designed to "provide information about the organizations and providers that deliver health care, the services rendered, and the patients they serve across diverse settings" (CDC, 2012a, ¶2). The National Health Care Surveys are used to study resource use, including staffing; quality of care; clinical management of specific conditions; disparities in use; diffusion of certain healthcare technologies; and the effects of policy changes (CDC, 2012a).The fourth example of data collected through a survey is the data collected through the BRFSS. These data are collected by individual states, territories, and the District of Columbia through cooperative agreements with the CDC. Through the use of telephone survey techniques, each state selects a probability sample from the civilian, noninstitutionalized adult population (older than 18 years of age). Those selected are asked a set of standard core questions, developed by the CDC to produce data about health behaviors that can be compared across states (CDC, 2013a). In addition, states may include other questions that would be useful in monitoring health in that particular state.

Because of the success of the BRFSS a similar surveillance system was begun for youth. The Youth Risk Behavior Surveillance System (YRBSS) was developed in 1990 to monitor priority health-risk behaviors that contribute markedly to the leading causes of death, disability, and social problems among youth and adults in the United States. The six categories of priority health-risk behaviors include (1) tobacco use; (2) unhealthy dietary behaviors; (3) physical inactivity; (4) alcohol and other drug use; (5) sexual behaviors that contribute to HIV infection, other sexually transmitted diseases (STDs), and; and (6) behaviors that contribute to unintentional injuries and violence (CDC, 2013b).

The final survey presented, the National College Health Assessment (NCHA), is one that collects health data about college students. The NCHA is the only one presented here that is not conducted by a governmental agency. The NCHA is carried out by the professional organization American College Health Association (ACHA) (see Chapter 8 for more on this association). The ACHA developed the NCHA, which can be conducted as either a paper-pencil or online survey, to assist schools in collecting data about students' habits, behaviors, and perceptions about topics such as alcohol, tobacco, and other drug use; mental and physical health; weight, nutrition, and exercise; personal safety and violence; and sexual health. The ACHA charges schools for conducting the NCHA, but the schools have the flexibility to select the surveying method, sample size, priority population, and time it is offered (ACHA, 2013).

▷ Using Health Data in Health Education/Promotion

In the previous sections of this chapter we presented information on measuring health and health status, as well as where health education specialists may find health-related data that are collected by governmental and other organizations. Now we would like to give you an example of how health education specialists may use data. As you will soon learn, a major task of health education specialists is to assist those in the priority population (individuals, groups, and communities) in obtaining, maintaining and improving their health. Often this means planning some type of health education/promotion program that can be used by those in the priority population. These programs should be based on the needs of the priority population, and the needs are often described using data.

For example, let's say a health education specialist is working for a local (county) health department at a time when the state health department has just made funds available through a competitive grant process to deal with the high rates of cancer in the state. Because of some past concerns about cancer in the county, her supervisor has suggested she seek funding. Though she has heard some residents express concern about possible higher rates of cancer, she is really not sure about the type of cancer or whether there is a specific group of people affected. Therefore, she needs to be able to describe the potential problem and identify a priority population. One approach would be to determine if there are any health disparities associated with cancer in her county. It has long been "recognized that some individuals are healthier than others and that some live longer than others do, and that often these differences are closely associated with social characteristics such as race, ethnicity, gender, location, and socioeconomic status" (King, 2009, p. 339). These gaps between groups have been referred to as *health disparities* (also called health inequalities in some countries). More formally, **health disparity** has been defined as the difference in health between populations often caused by two health inequities—lack of access to care and lack of quality care (McKenzie et al., 2012).

One place to start looking for cancer health disparities would be the cancer mortality rates (i.e., crude and age-adjusted) for the state as a whole compared with the county where the health education specialist works. These data may be available from the NCHS or another center within the CDC, from the state department of health, or from a university research center. Similar comparisons could also be made based on the mortality rates for various types of cancer. If the health education specialist knew what types of cancers were of greatest concern in the county, she could then examine the data for the county on the basis of certain demographic characteristics that have been associated with certain cancers. So the health education specialist may be using sex-, age-, or race/ethnicity-specific rates to compare various subgroups while looking for disparities. Once the health education specialist identifies a subgroup problem with a type of cancer, she may turn to data from the BRFSS to look for risk behaviors that are known to contribute to or cause the type of cancer identified. Again, the health education specialist may find the needed data in a state or local agency or university as well. Using all of these different sources of data should help the health education specialist find the focus of her program for the priority population and put her in a position to compete for the grant money from the state department of health. Examples of what the health education specialist may have found through this process are higher rates of prostate cancer in African American men between the ages of 45 and 64 years or a higher prevalence of certain types of leukemia in children younger than 15 years of age.

In summary, to get to the point of being able to identify a priority population (i.e., a certain subgroup of people) and program focus (i.e., risk factors associated with a certain type of cancer) several different types of data were used. Initially, the health education specialist used cancer mortality data, then prevalence rates for various types of cancer and different subgroups, and finally risk factor data for various types of cancer.

▷ The Goal and Purpose of the Profession

The ultimate goal of all service professions, including health education/promotion, is to improve the quality of life, even though the quality of life is difficult to quantify (Raphael, Brown, Renwick, & Rootman, 1997). However, many professionals feel that there is a direct relationship between quality of life and health status. Quality of life is usually improved when health status is improved, or, as Ashley Montagu (1968, p. 206) has stated, "The highest goal in life is to die young, at as old an age as possible." To that end, "the goal of health education is to promote, maintain, and improve individual and community health. The teaching-learning process is the hallmark and social agenda that differentiates the practice of health education from that of other helping professions in achieving this goal" (National Commission for Health Education Credentialing, Inc. [NCHEC], 1996, pp. 2–3).

Because quality of life and health status are complex variables, they are not usually changed in a short period of time. To reach these goals, people usually work their way through a number of small steps over a period of time that equip them with all that is necessary to impact both their health status and, in turn, their quality of life. Thus, it is the work of health education specialists to create interventions (programs) that can assist people in working toward better health. This work is reflected in the purpose of health education that "is to positively influence the health behavior of individuals and communities as well as the living and working conditions that influence their health" (New York State as presented at Coalition for National Health Education Organizations [CNHEO], 2007, p. 1).

▷ The Practice of Health Education/Promotion

Although the specific practice of health education specialists is outlined in the responsibilities and competencies presented in Chapter 6, as noted in our discussion of the use of data previously, the primary role of health education specialists is to develop appropriate health education/promotion programs for the people they serve. The practice of health education/promotion is based on the assumption "that beneficial health behavior will result from a combination of planned, consistent, integrated learning opportunities. This assumption rests on the scientific evaluations of health education programs in schools, at worksites, in medical settings, and through mass media" (Green & Ottoson, 1999, pp. 93–94). The results of these *scientific evaluations*, referred to by Green and Ottoson, are one source of data that contribute to a body of data known as evidence. **Evidence** is data that can be used to make decisions about planning. When health education specialists practice in such a way that they systematically find, appraise, and use evidence as the basis for decision making when planning health education/promotion programs it is referred to as **evidence-based practice** (Cottrell & McKenzie, 2011).

Although the practice of health education specialists is easily stated, it is by no means easy to carry out. Much time, effort, practice, and on-the-job training are required to be successful. Even the most experienced health education specialists find program development challenging because of the constant changes in settings, resources, and priority populations (McKenzie, Neiger, & Thackeray, 2013).

The specific steps taken to develop a health education/promotion program vary depending on the planning model used (see Chapter 4); most models include the following steps (McKenzie et al., 2013) (see Figure 4.18):

1. Assessing the needs of the priority population
2. Setting goals and objectives
3. Developing an intervention that considers the peculiarities of the setting
4. Implementing the intervention
5. Evaluating the results

Therefore, it becomes the practice of health education specialists to be able to carry out all that is associated with these tasks.

Over the years, to be educated to serve as a health education specialist, indivdiuals have been trained in three different types of academic programs—community health education, public health education, and school health education. In recent years, mostly because of the profession's movement toward accreditation of all undergraduate programs in health education, there has been a movement to just two preparation tracks as opposed to three of the past. Community health education programs are increasingly switching over to public health education to meet accreditation requirements (see Chapter 6 for more on accreditation).

▷ Basic Underlying Concepts of the Profession

As is noted previously in this chapter and discussed in greater detail in Chapter 2, the profession of health education/promotion is one that has been built on the principles and concepts of a number of disciplines and professions. Within health education/promotion can be found pieces of community development and organizing, education, epidemiology, medicine, psychology, and sociology. In the sections that follow, we present some of the basic underlying concepts of the profession. Please note that we have not exhausted the discussion of each of these topics but, rather, present sufficient information to allow a basic understanding of each.

The Health Field Concept and the Determinants of Health

Shortly after the Canadian government implemented its national health plan that ensured health care for all Canadians, it began to look more closely at the health field as a way of improving Canadians' health. The **health field** is a term the government described as being far more encompassing than the "healthcare system." This term was much broader and included all matters that affected health (Lalonde, 1974). Because the health field was such a broad concept, it was felt that there was a need to develop a framework that would subdivide the concept into principal elements so that the elements could be studied. Such a framework was developed and called the **health field concept** (Laframboise, 1973).

The health field concept divided the health field into four elements: (1) human biology, (2) environment, (3) lifestyle, and (4) healthcare organization. "These four elements were identified through an examination of the causes and underlying factors of sickness and death in Canada, and from an assessment of the parts the elements play in affecting the level of health in Canada" (Lalonde, 1974, p. 31). **Human biology** "includes all those aspects of health, both physical and mental, which are developed within the human body as a consequence of the basic biology of man [sic] and the organic make-up of an individual" (Lalonde, 1974, p. 31). This includes not only the genetic inheritance of an individual but also the processes of maturation and aging and the complex interaction of the various systems of the human body (Lalonde, 1974). The element of **environment** "includes all those matters related to health which are external to the human body and over which the individual has little or no control" (Lalonde, 1974, p. 32). Some examples of things often included in the element of environment are geography, climate, community size, industrial development, economy, and social norms.

The element of **lifestyle** comprises the "aggregation of decisions by individuals which affect their health and over which they more or less have control" (Lalonde, 1974, p. 32). In more recent times, lifestyle has been more commonly referred to as **health behavior** (those behaviors that impact a person's health). The fourth element in the health field concept is healthcare organization. **Healthcare organization** "consists of the quantity, quality, arrangement, nature and relationships of people and resources in the provision of health care" (Lalonde, 1974, p. 32). This fourth element is often referred to as the healthcare system.

The utility of the health field concept has proved to be helpful over the years, both in Canada and the United States. Its greatest importance may have been to bring attention to the concept of health promotion and disease prevention. Before this point in history, the primary focus of health care had been on the cure of disease, not the prevention of disease. In fact, it was stated that the health field concept put human biology, environment, and lifestyle on equal footing with healthcare organization (Lalonde, 1974). Since its development, studies using this concept in both Canada and the United States have provided a greater understanding of what contributes to morbidity and mortality, and what health professionals can do to help improve the health of those whom they serve.

Using a similar framework as that of the elements of the health field concept, it is now believed that the health of populations is shaped by five intersecting domains (i.e., the **determinants of health**): (1) genetics (e.g., sex, age, individual characteristics), (2) health behavior (e.g., diet, physical activity, alcohol use), (3) social circumstances (e.g., education, socioeconomic status, housing, crime), (4) environmental conditions (e.g., safe water, where a person lives and crowding conditions), and (5) health services (e.g., access to quality health care, having or not having insurance) (CDC, 2013c; IOM, 2001; McGinnis, 2001; USDHHS, 2000) (Also see the discussion of Multicausation Disease Model later in the chapter). These domains are dynamic and vary in impact depending on where one is in the life cycle (IOM, 2001).

In addition to understanding the determinants of health as they contribute to a person's current state of health, the **social determinants of health** also play a critical role in the health of people and communities. Social determinants of health are "conditions in the environments in which people are born, live, learn, work, play, worship, and age that affect a wide range of health, functioning, and quality-of-life outcomes and risks. Conditions (e.g., social, economic, and physical) in these various environments and settings (e.g., school, church, workplace, and neighborhood) have been referred to as "place" (USDHHS, 2013, ¶4). Like the determinants of health, the social determinants of health encompass five areas: (1) economic stability (e.g., poverty, access to employment, housing stability such as homelessness or foreclosure); (2) education (e.g., high school graduation rates, safe school environments, enrollment in higher education); (3) social and community context (e.g., family structure, perceptions of discrimination and equity, civic participation); (4) health and health care (e.g., access to health services, access to primary care, health technology; (5) neighborhood and build environment (e.g., quality of housing, environmental conditions, access to healthy foods) (USDHHS, 2013, ¶8). Addressing these social determinants of health can impact the health of large numbers of people in ways that can be sustained over time.

We know that genetics play a big part in late-onset diseases such as diabetes, cancer, and cardiovascular disease, whereas employment and income (social circumstances) have a significant influence on health and health care throughout life. Further, sidewalks in neighborhoods make it possible for families to exercise safely if neighborhoods are safe and free of crime and violence (neighborhood and build environment).

> On a population basis, using the best available estimates, the impacts of various domains on early deaths in the United States distribute roughly as follows: genetic predispositions, about 30%, social circumstances, 15%, environmental exposures, 5%, behavioral patterns, 40%; and shortfalls in medical care about 10%. But more important than these proportions is the nature of the influences in play where the domains intersect. Ultimately, the health fate of each of us is determined by factors acting not mostly in isolation but by our experience where domains interconnect. Whether a gene is expressed can be determined by environmental exposures or behavioral patterns. The nature and consequences of behavioral choices are affected by our social circumstances. Our genetic predispositions affect the health care we need, and our social circumstances affect the health care we receive. (McGinnis et al., 2002, p. 83)

The Levels and Limitations of Prevention

The word *prevention* has already been used several times in this chapter. We now want to formally define the term, present the different levels of prevention, and briefly discuss the limitations of prevention. **Prevention,** as it relates to health, has been defined as the planning for

► **Figure 1.3** Vaccination is an example of primary prevention.

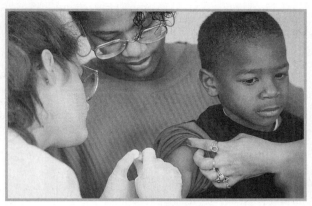

and the measures taken to forestall the onset of a disease or other health problem before the occurrence of undesirable health events. This definition presents three distinct levels of prevention: primary, secondary, and tertiary prevention. **Primary prevention** comprises those preventive measures that forestall the onset of illness or injury during the prepathogenesis period (before the disease process begins) (McKenzie et al., 2012). Examples of primary prevention measures include wearing a safety belt, using rubber gloves when there is potential for the spread of disease, immunizing against specific diseases (see **Figure 1.3**), exercising, and brushing one's teeth. Any health education/promotion program aimed specifically at forestalling the onset of illness or injury is also an example of primary prevention.

Illness and injury cannot always be prevented. In fact, many diseases, such as cancer and heart disease, can establish themselves in humans and cause considerable damage before they are detected and treated. In such cases, the sooner a condition is detected and medical personnel intervene, the greater the chances of limiting disability and preventing death. Such identification and intervention are known as secondary prevention. More specifically, **secondary prevention** includes the preventive measures that lead to an early diagnosis and prompt treatment of a disease or an injury to limit disability and prevent more serious pathogenesis. Good examples of secondary prevention include personal and clinical screenings and examinations such as blood pressure, blood cholesterol, and hemocult (hidden blood) screenings; breast self-examinations (BSEs); and testicle self-examinations (TSEs). The goal of such screenings and examinations is not to prevent the onset of the disease but rather to detect its presence during early pathogenesis, thus permitting early treatment and limiting disability (McKenzie et al., 2012).

The final level of prevention is **tertiary prevention.** It is at this level that health education specialists work to retrain, re-educate, and rehabilitate the individual who has already incurred disability, impairment, or dependency. Examples of some tertiary measures include educating a patient after lung cancer surgery or working with an individual who has diabetes to ensure that the daily insulin injections are taken. **Figure 1.4** provides a visual representation of the levels of prevention in relation to health status.

Though health education specialists can intervene at any of the three levels of prevention, and can have a great deal of success, it should be obvious from the previous discussion of the health field concept and the determinants of health that prevention is not the "magic bullet"

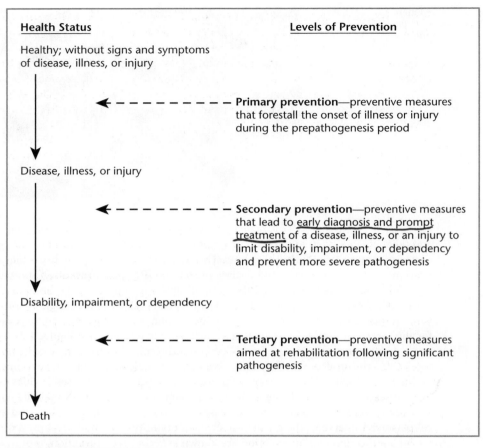

Health Status   **Levels of Prevention**

Healthy; without signs and symptoms
of disease, illness, or injury

Primary prevention—preventive measures
that forestall the onset of illness or injury
during the prepathogenesis period

Disease, illness, or injury

Secondary prevention—preventive measures
that lead to early diagnosis and prompt
treatment of a disease, illness, or an injury to
limit disability, impairment, or dependency
and prevent more severe pathogenesis

Disability, impairment, or dependency

Tertiary prevention—preventive measures
aimed at rehabilitation following significant
pathogenesis

Death

▲ **Figure 1.4** Levels of prevention
Source: Adapted from *Public Health: Administration and Practice*, 9th ed., by G. E. Pickett et al., eds. Copyright © Elsevier 1990. By permission of Elsevier Ltd.

for an endless life. Prevention does have its limits. McGinnis (1985) has noted four major categories of limitations: (1) biological, (2) technological, (3) ethical, and (4) economic. Biological limitations center on life span. How long should individuals expect to live healthy lives or, for that matter, how long should they expect to live at all? Even with the best inputs and a bit of luck, one should not expect to live longer than 80 to 110 years. Body parts will eventually wear out from use.

Technological advances also have their limitations. Today, healthcare workers have a vast array of technical equipment available to help them care for their patients, but technology still has not been able to eradicate AIDS or malaria or to explain the cause of Alzheimer's disease.

Prevention is also limited by ethical concerns (see Chapter 5). Even though helmets would increase the chances of survival in automobile crashes, is it ethical to have a law that says all drivers and passengers in automobiles must wear them? Or is it ethical to penalize people via fines, taxes, or surcharges for acting in unhealthy ways, such as driving an automobile without a safety belt on, buying and using tobacco products, or for not having a smoke detector and fire extinguisher in the home?

Finally, prevention has economic limitations. Prevention is limited by the amount of money that is put into it. Though the exact figures are difficult to determine, it is commonly understood that less than 5 percent of all dollars spent on health in the United States each year are spent on essential public heatlh services, government public health activity, and population-based public health activity (Turnock, 2012). Stated another way, approximately 95 percent of the two trillion plus dollars spent on health in the United States each year is spent on curing ill health, not on health promotion and disease prevention (Sultz & Young, 2011).

Risk Factors

The health field concept, the determinants of health, and the social determinants of health have provided those interested in health issues with a framework from which the health field can be studied. The levels of prevention and their limitations have provided this same group of people with a time frame from which to plan to help forestall the onset of, limit the spread of, and rehabilitate after pathogenesis or another health problem. What none of these concepts fully discloses is the focus at which health promotion and disease prevention programming should be aimed. The targets of such programming are **risk factors,** those inherited, environmental, and behavioral influences "which are known (or thought) to increase the likelihood of physical or mental problems" (Slee, Slee, & Schmidt, 2008, p. 510). Risk factors increase the probability of morbidity and premature mortality but do not guarantee that people with a risk factor will suffer the consequences.

Risk factors can be divided into two categories: (1) **modifiable risk factors** (changeable or controllable) and (2) **nonmodifiable risk factors** (nonchangeable or noncontrollable). The former include such factors as sedentary lifestyle, smoking, and poor dietary habits—things that individuals can change or control whereas the latter group includes factors such as age, sex, and inherited genes—things that individuals cannot change or do not have control over. Note that these two categories of risk factors are often interrelated. In fact, the combined potential for harm from a number of risk factors is greater than the sum of their individual potentials. For example, asbestos workers have an increased risk for cancer because of their exposure to this carcinogen. Further, if they smoke, they have a 30 times greater chance of developing lung cancer than do their nonsmoking coworkers and 90 times greater chance of getting lung cancer than do people who neither work with asbestos nor smoke. The risk increases further if they have an inherited respiratory disease.

Over the years, knowledge about the impact of risk behaviors has continued to grow. In looking back over the 20th century, we have seen disease prevention change "from focusing on reducing environmental exposures over which the individual had little control, such as providing potable water, to emphasizing behaviors such as avoiding use of tobacco, fatty foods, and a sedentary lifestyle" (Breslow, 1999, p. 1030). As noted previously, approximately 40 percent of the early deaths in the United States each year are caused by these behavior patterns that could be modified by preventive interventions (McGinnis et al., 2002). Therefore, much of the focus of the work of health education specialists has been to help individuals identify and control their modifiable risk factors.

Health Risk Reduction

To be able to take aim at specific risk factors, health education specialists must have a basic understanding of both communicable (infectious) and noncommunicable (noninfectious) diseases. **Communicable diseases** are those diseases for which biological agents or their products are the cause and that are transmissible from one individual to another (McKenzie et al., 2012), and **noncommunicable diseases** or illnesses are those that cannot be transmitted from an infected person to a susceptible, healthy one (McKenzie et al., 2012). Our intent in this section and the ones that follow is not to present information on all possible diseases and their related risk factors that a health education specialist may have to develop programs for, but rather to provide a general understanding of the spread and cause of disease. (See **Table 1.5** for leading causes of death and their risk factors.)

Before moving on, we would like to make a special note about one of the data presented in **Figure 1.5**. The term *leading causes of death* is used in this figure. That term refers to "the primary pathophysiological conditions identified at the time of death, as opposed to the root causes" (McGinnis & Foege, 1993, p. 2207). McGinnis and Foege (1993) conducted a study to see if they could identify the root causes of death. What they found was that the leading *actual causes of death* were modifiable behaviors; behaviors that people could change. The behavior that was the leading actual cause of death was tobacco use, accounting for some

TABLE 1.5 **Leading causes of death and associated risk factors for all ages: United States, 2010**

Rank	Cause	Risk Factors
1	Diseases of the heart	Tobacco use, high blood pressure, elevated serum cholesterol, diet, diabetes, obesity, lack of exercise, alcohol abuse, genetics
2	Malignant neoplasms (cancer)	Tobacco use, alcohol misuse, diet, solar radiation, ionizing radiation, worksite hazards, environmental pollution, genetics
3	Chronic lower respiratory diseases	Tobacco use, diseases
4	Cerebrovascular diseases (stroke)	Tobacco use, high blood pressure, elevated serum cholesterol, diabetes, obesity, genetics
5	Unintentional injuries (accidents)	Alcohol misuse, tobacco use (fires), product design, home hazards, handgun availability, lack of safety restraints, excessive speed, automobile design, roadway design
6	Alzheimer's disease	Age, family history, genetics, head injury, heart health, general healthy aging[a]
7	Diabetes mellitus	Obesity (for type II diabetes), diet, lack of exercise, genetics
8	Nephritis, nephrotic syndrome, and nephrosis	Infectious agents, drug hypersensitivity, genetics, trauma
9	Influenza and pneumonia	Tobacco use, infectious agents, biological factors
10	Suicide	Family history, previous suicide attempts, history of mental disorders, history of alcohol and substance abuse, cultural and religious beliefs, barriers to accessing mental health treatment[b]

Sources: [a]Alzheimer's Association. (2013). *Risk Factors*. Retrieved July 11, 2013, from http://www.alz.org/alzheimers_disease_causes_risk_factors.asp#riskfactors.
[b] Centers for Disease Control and Prevention. (2012). *Suicide: Risk and protective factors*. Retrieved July 11, 2013, from http://www.cdc.gov/violenceprevention/suicide/riskprotectivefactors.html.
Data from U.S. Department of Health and Human Services, National Center for Health Statistics (NCHS). (2013). *Health, United States, 2011 with Special Feature on Emergency Care*. Hyattsville, MD: Author.

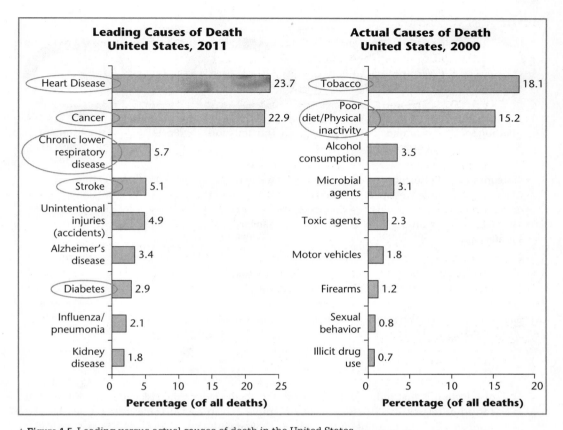

▲ Figure 1.5 Leading versus actual causes of death in the United States

Source: The 2011 data from Hoyert, D. L. & Xu, J. "Deaths: Preliminary Data for 2011." *National Vital Statistics Report 61*, 6 (October 2012): 4. The 2000 data from Mokdad, A. H., Marks, J. S., Stroup, D. F., and Gerberding, J. L. "Correction: Actual Causes of Death in the United States, 2000." *Journal of the American Medical Association 292*, 3 (2005): 293–294.

400,000, or 19 percent, of the mortality in 1990. A similar study to that of McGinnis and Foege was conducted by Mokdad, Marks, Stroup, and Gerberding in 2004 using 2000 mortality data. They also found tobacco to be the leading actual cause of death, but that poor diet and physical inactivity killed almost as many (see Figure 1.5). It is now estimated that tobacco is the primary cause of more than 440,000 deaths per year, about one in five deaths annually (CDC, 2013d). Figure 1.5 provides evidence that nearly half of all causes of death in the United States could be attributed to a number of largely preventable behaviors and that improving healthy behaviors, we can significantly reduce the consequences of chronic diseases. "These findings, along with escalating health care costs and aging population, argue persuasively that the need to establish a more preventive orientation in the U.S. health care and public health systems has become more urgent" (Mokdad et al., 2004, p. 1238).

THE CHAIN OF INFECTION

The **chain of infection** (see **Figure 1.6**) is a model used to explain the spread of a communicable disease from one host to another. The basic premise represented in the chain

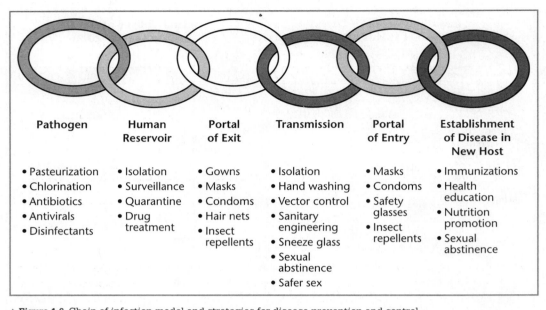

Pathogen	Human Reservoir	Portal of Exit	Transmission	Portal of Entry	Establishment of Disease in New Host
• Pasteurization • Chlorination • Antibiotics • Antivirals • Disinfectants	• Isolation • Surveillance • Quarantine • Drug treatment	• Gowns • Masks • Condoms • Hair nets • Insect repellents	• Isolation • Hand washing • Vector control • Sanitary engineering • Sneeze glass • Sexual abstinence • Safer sex	• Masks • Condoms • Safety glasses • Insect repellents	• Immunizations • Health education • Nutrition promotion • Sexual abstinence

▲ **Figure 1.6** Chain of infection model and strategies for disease prevention and control

Source: From J. F. McKenzie, R. R. Pinger, and J. E. Kotecki. *An Introduction to Community Health*. 7th ed. © 2012 Jones and Bartlett Publishers, Sudbury, MA. www.jbpub.com. Reprinted with permission.

of infection is that individuals can break the chain (reduce the risk) at any point; thus, the spread of disease can be stopped. For example, the spread of some waterborne diseases is stopped when the first link of the chain is broken with the chlorination of the water supply, thus killing the pathogens that cause a disease. The risk is reduced because the pathogen is destroyed before it is consumed. The chain can also be broken by placing a barrier between the means of transmission and the portal of entry, as when healthcare providers protect themselves with surgical masks and rubber gloves. In this case, the risk is reduced because individuals are not exposing themselves to the pathogen. With such information, health education specialists can help create programs that are aimed at "breaking" the chain and reducing the risks.

COMMUNICABLE DISEASE MODEL

A second model used to describe the spread of a communicable disease is the **communicable disease model. Figure 1.7** presents the elements of this model—agent, host, and environment. These three elements summarize the minimal requirements for the presence and spread of a communicable disease in a population. The agent is the element (or, using the chain of infection labels, the pathogen) that must be present for a disease to spread—for example, bacteria or a virus. The host is any susceptible organism that can be invaded by the agent. Examples include plants, animals, and humans. The environment includes all other factors that either prohibit or promote disease transmission. Thus, communicable disease transmission occurs when a susceptible host and a pathogenic agent exist in an environment conducive to disease transmission.

► **Figure 1.7** Communicable disease model
Source: From J. F. McKenzie, R. R. Pinger, and J. E. Kotecki. *An Introduction to Community Health*, 7th edition. © 2012 Jones and Bartlett Publishers, Sudbury, MA. www.jbpub.com. Reprinted with permission.

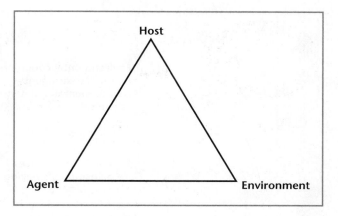

MULTICAUSATION DISEASE MODEL

Obviously, the chain of infection and communicable disease models are most helpful in trying to prevent disease caused by a pathogen. However, they are not applicable to noncommunicable diseases, which include many of the chronic diseases such as heart disease and cancer. Most of these diseases manifest themselves in people over a period of time and are not caused by a single factor but by combined factors. The concept of "caused by many factors" is referred to as the **multicausation disease model** (see **Figure 1.8**). For example, it is known that heart disease is more likely to manifest itself in individuals who are older, who smoke, who do not exercise, who are overweight, who have high blood pressure, who have high cholesterol, and who have immediate family members who have had heart disease. Note that within this list of factors there are both modifiable and nonmodifiable risk factors. As when using the chain of infection model, the work of health education specialists is to create programs to help people reduce the risk of disease and injury by helping those in the priority population identify and control as many of the multicausative factors as possible. This model should look familiar to you because it is made up of the five determinants of health discussed previously in this chapter.

Other Selected Principles

Several other principles of health education/promotion have been noted by Cleary and Neiger (1998). They have identified via the work of others that health education specialists must address the principles of participation, empowerment, and cultural competency if health education/promotion is to be successful. We would like to add two other principles to this list, socio-ecological approach and advocacy. **Participation** refers to the active involvement of those in the priority population in helping identify, plan, and implement programs to address the health problems they face. Without such participation, ethical issues associated with program development come into play, and the priority population probably will not support and feel **ownership** of (responsibility for) the program. For example, if the health education specialists for a large corporation are creating a health promotion program for all employees, they should not begin to plan without the participation of (or at least representation by) each of the segments (clerical, labor, and management) of the employee population.

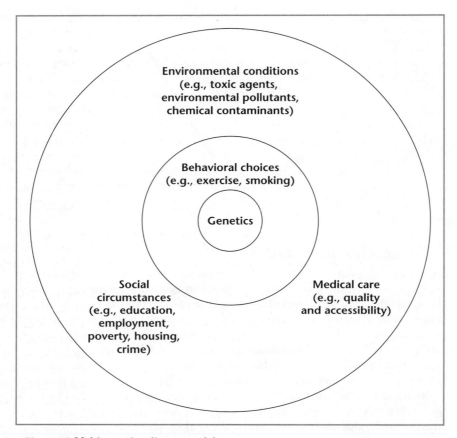

▲ **Figure 1.8** Multicausation disease model

In recent years, health education/promotion activities have placed more emphasis on socio-ecological approaches to improving health. The underlying concept of the **socio-ecological approach** (sometimes referred to as the *ecological perspective*) is that behavior has multiple levels of influences. This approach "emphasizes the interaction between, and the interdependence of factors within and across all levels of a health problem" (Rimer & Glanz, 2005, p. 10). That is to say, seldom does behavior change based on influence from a single level. People live in environments (i.e., physical, social, political, cultural, and economic) that shape behaviors and access to the resources they need to maintain good health (Pellmar, Brandt, & Baird, 2002). Scholars who study and write about the levels of influence have used various labels to describe them. However, commonly used labels include: individual and individual's characteristics (e.g., knowledge, attitudes, values, skills), social relationships, organizational influences, community characteristics, and public policy (McLeroy, Bibeau, Steckler, & Glanz, 1988). Physical environment and culture have recently been added to levels of influence (Simons-Morton, McLeroy, & Wendel, 2012). In practice, behavior change often involves influences on multiple levels. For example, to get a person to begin an exercise program it may take a conversation with his or her physician (i.e., social influence), a company policy (i.e., organizational-level influence), and also the county commissioners voting to put walking paths in the community (i.e., community-level influence). Thus, a central conclusion of the socio-ecological approach "is that it usually takes the combination of both individual-level and environmental/policy-level interventions to achieve substantial changes in health behavior" (Sallis, Owen, & Fisher, 2008, p. 467). Therefore, health education specialists must do more than just educate to help to change behavior. They must now work in new ways and develop new skills. As a group these new skills are often called **population-based approaches.** They include policy development, policy advocacy, organizational change, community development, empowerment of individuals, and economic supports.

To more clearly see how a population-based approach works, consider the following example. A state-level voluntary health organization was spending most of its time and resources helping individuals quit smoking or preventing others from starting to smoke. Recently the organization has developed a statewide advocacy network to respond to tobacco-related legislation. They are using a population-based approach to influence legislation and policy that will ultimately impact individual smoking behaviors. They still maintain the more individual approaches to dealing with the tobacco issue but have added the population-based approach.

Advocacy is another principle in which health education specialists have become more involved. **Advocacy** is defined "as the actions or endeavors individuals or groups engage in order to alter public opinion in favor or in opposition to a certain policy" (Pinzon-Perez & Perez, 1999, p. 29). Whereas, **health advocacy** has been defined as "the processes by which the actions of individuals or groups attempt to bring about social, environmental and/or organizational change on behalf of a particular health goal, program, interest, or population" (Joint Committee, 2012, p. 17). Professional associations encourage health education specialists to get more involved in advocacy for the profession and for health-related issues (Auld & Dixon-Terry, 2010). As an example, the Coalition of National Health Education Organizations (CNHEO) (see Chapter 8 for more on this organization) sponsors the Health Education Advocate Web site (see the Web link at the end of this chapter for the URL for this site). This site provides health education specialists with an easy link to contact their legislators whenever health education/promotion–related bills or concerns are considered by Congress.

If health education/promotion is going to create lasting change, then those in the priority population must be empowered as a result of the health education/promotion programming. **Empowerment** is a "social action process for people to gain mastery over their lives and the lives of their communities" (Minkler, Wallerstein, & Wilson, 2008, p. 294). Empowerment can take place at the individual, the organization or group, and the community level. Often, empowerment at one level can influence empowerment at the other levels. An example of empowerment occurred in Clatsop County, Oregon—a community with a significantly high rate of colorectal cancer. Six recognizable spokespeople from the community had been screened for colorectal cancer. These individuals shared their stories in radio ads, campaign materials, and on a Web site. Their stories focused on the ease and importance of being screened. The result was an increased number of individuals seeking screening and in many cases, preventing cancer (CDC, 2012b).Social media is one growing strategy being used by health education specialists to advocate and empower indivdiuals and communities. **Social media** is any type of "media that uses the Internet and other technologies to allow for social interaction (McKenzie et al., 2012, p. 448). Social media tools can include such things as online video sharing (e.g., YouTube), social networks (e.g., Facebook, Twitter), text messaging, podcasts, virtual worlds, blogs, and podcasts. The use of social media tools is a "powerful channel to reach target audiences with strategic, effective, and user-centric health interventions" (CDC, 2013e, ¶1). Because the Internet allows for a free flow of information, the CDC has developed guidelines, best practices, and toolkits for health education specialists using and developing social media materials (CDC, 2011c; CDC 2013e). Becoming familiar with these various social media tools during your preparation as a health education specialist will prove valuable as doctors' offices, hospitals, state and local health departments, and voluntary agencies are using these tools to communicate with patients, volunteers, employees, and the general public.

As you have probably gathered by now, there are many factors that impact the effectiveness of health education/promotion programming. Because of the health disparities that exist between and among the various subpopulations in the United States (Selig, Tropiano, & Greene-Moton, 2006) and because of the increasing diversification of the U.S. population (Pérez & Luquis, 2008), much more attention has been placed on understanding the impact of culture (i.e., values, beliefs, attitudes, traditions, and customs) on health and providing culturally appropriate programs (Davis & Rankin, 2006). Cultural factors arise from guidelines (both explicit and implicit) that individuals "inherit" from being a part of a particular society, racial or ethnic group, religious community, or other group. For health education specialists to be effective in a variety of communities, they need to strive to be culturally competent (Davis & Rankin, 2006; Luquis, Pérez, & Young, 2006; Selig et al., 2006). **Cultural competence** is "a developmental process defined as a set of values, principles, behaviors, attitudes, and policies that enable health professionals to work effectively across racial, ethnic and linguistically diverse populations" (Joint Committee, 2012, p. 16). Both health education specialists and the community health agencies providing health education/promotion programs need "to be able to communicate different communities and understand how culture influences health behaviors" (McKenzie & Pinger, 2013, p. 198).

▶ Summary

In this introductory chapter, many of the basic principles of the profession of health education/promotion were presented including definitions of many of the key words and terms used in the profession, including *health, health education, health promotion, disease prevention, community health, global health, population health, coordinated school health,* and *wellness*; a look at the current status of health education/promotion; an explanation of how health or health status has been measured, including mortality rates, life expectancy, YPLL, DALYs, HALE, HRQOL, and health surveys; an outline of the goal and purpose of the profession; the practice of health education/promotion, including planning, implementing, and evaluating programs; some of the basic underlying concepts and principles of the profession, including the health field concept, determinants of health, social determinants of health, levels of prevention, risk factors, health risk reduction via understanding disease; and the principles of participation, ecological approach, advocacy, empowerment, social media, and cultural competence.

Review Questions

1. Define—*health, health education, health promotion, disease prevention, public health, community health, global health, population health, coordinated school health,* and *wellness.*

2. What is the status of health education/promotion?

3. Explain each of the following means of measuring health or health status.
   - Mortality rates. What is the difference among crude, adjusted, and specific rates?
   - Life expectancy
   - Years of potential life lost (YPLL)
   - Disability-adjusted life years (DALYs)
   - Health-adjusted life expectancy (HALE)
   - Health-related quality of life (HRQOL)
   - Health surveys

4. Of all the different measures of health presented in this chapter, which one do you think is the best indicator of health? Why?

5. Why are health-related data and epidemiology such an important discipline for health education/promotion?

6. In a given community with a midyear population estimate of 50,000, there were 21 deaths as a result of strokes in the year. What is the rate of stroke deaths per 100,000 population?

7. What is the goal of health education/promotion? What is its purpose?

8. What constitutes the basic practice of health education/promotion?

9. What is the difference between the leading causes of death and the actual causes of death?

10. Briefly explain the following concepts and principles of health education/promotion.
    - Health field concept; determinants of health
    - Levels of prevention
    - Risk factors
    - Health risk reduction
    - Chain of infection
    - Communicable disease model
    - Multicausation disease model
    - Selected principles of health education/promotion—participation, socio-ecological approach, advocacy, empowerment, social media, and cultural competence.

Case Study

As a health education specialist with the Delaware County Health Department, Matt has been asked by a local religious leader to give a presentation on HIV and AIDS to the Christian youth group (9th to 12th graders) of the community. The request has taken Matt by surprise because for the past couple of years he has attempted to make similar presentations in the local schools but has been turned away because the superintendent said "the community was too conservative for such matters." Knowing that at least some of the people in the community think HIV and AIDS is too controversial to talk about, but also knowing the information is important for youth to have, Matt wants to make sure he prepares and delivers a program that is well received. This is finally the chance he has been waiting for to make his entry into the youth population of the community. Matt has decided to create a presentation on HIV and AIDS that incorporates information on both risk factors and the chain of infection. To make sure that his presentation is on target, he has asked several other employees of the health department to sit down with him and brainstorm some ideas for his presentation. He begins his session with his colleagues by asking them all to write down information they think he should include in his presentation. Assume that you are one of these other employees of the health department in this meeting. What would you include on your list for Matt? What would you advise Matt not to include? Why? He then asks his colleagues for ideas on how to present the information (e.g., lecture, video, role playing). What do you think would be the best method to use? Why did you select this method? How long do you think Matt's presentation should be? Why?

Critical Thinking Questions

1. In this chapter, the term *public health* was defined. To what extent do you think that the government, at any level, has the right to legislate good health? For example, do you think a governmental body has the responsibility (or right) to require all motorcycle drivers to wear helmets because statistics show that wearing helmets can save lives? Defend your answer.

2. If you were asked by the CDC to come up with a new measure to describe the health status of an individual, what would you include in such a measure and why?

3. If you had the opportunity to develop three new health education/promotion programs, one at each level of the three levels of prevention (primary, secondary, and tertiary) for the community in which you live, what would they be? Who would be the priority population? Why did you pick the three that you did?

Activities

1. If you have not already done so, access the government document *Healthy People: The Surgeon General's Report on Health Promotion and Disease Prevention*. It provides a good background on the health promotion era in the United States.

2. Write your own definitions for *health, health education*, and *health promotion* using the concepts presented in the chapter.

3. Write one paragraph for each of the following:
   - Why do you think the health field concept was so important in getting people to think about health promotion?
   - At what level of prevention do you think it would be most difficult to change health behavior? Why?

4. In a PowerPoint presentation, use the chain of infection to outline three different means for preventing the spread of HIV.

5. In a photo story, use the multicausation disease model to explain how a person develops heart disease.

 # Weblinks

1. http://www.cdc.gov/nchs/

National Center for Health Statistics (NCHS)

This site is a rich source of data about health in the United States and the instruments used to collect the data.

2. http://www.cdc.gov/brfss/

Behavioral Risk Factor Surveillance System (BRFSS)

The BRFSS, the world's largest telephone survey, tracks health risks in the United States. Information from the survey is used to improve the health of U.S. citizens. At this site, you will find general information about the BRFSS, data generated by the BRFSS, copies of the data collection instruments, and more.

3. http://www.cdc.gov/healthyyouth

Youth Risk Behavioral Surveillance System (YRBSS)

At this site, you will find general information about the YRBSS, data generated by the YRBSS, copies of the data collection instruments, and more.

4. http://www.iom.edu/

Institute of Medicine (IOM)

The IOM is a nonprofit organization specifically created to provide science-based advice on matters of biomedical science and medicine and health, as well as an honorific membership organization that was chartered in 1970 as a component of the National Academy of Sciences. The IOM's mission is to serve as adviser to the nation to improve health. The IOM provides unbiased, evidence-based, and authoritative information and advice concerning health and science for all. At this site you can find many of their reports cited in this chapter.

5. http://www.healtheducationadvocate.org

Health Education Advocate

The Health Education Advocate site is sponsored by the Coalition of National Health Education Organizations (CNHEO). The site was designed to provide a timely source of advocacy information related to the field of health education/promotion. Included on the site are a number of items to assist health planners with advocacy activities, as well as information about how to identify and contact senators and congressional representatives, the status of specific bills, health resolutions and policy statements of sponsoring agencies, and advocacy resources.

6. https://www.thinkculturalhealth.hhs.gov/

Think Cultural Health

This is a page at the U.S. Department of Health and Human Services, Office of Minority Health Web site that presents information on cultural competence for health professionals. The site has a tag line of "advancing health equity at every point of contact." Included at the site are educational programs, resources, and other materials.

7. **http://www.bls.gov/ooh/**

   Occupational Outlook Handbook, 2012–13: Health Educators

   This is a page at the U.S. Department of Labor, Bureau of Labor Statistics Web site that provides the occupational outlook for a wide range of professions. Search for "health educators" to see short explanations of: nature of the work; training, other qualifications, and advancement; employment; job outlook and projections; earnings; wages; and sources of additional information about health education specialists.

8. **http://www.countyhealthrankings.org/**

   County Health Rankings

   This Web site presents the *County Health Rankings*, which are a key component of the Mobilizing Action Toward Community Health (MATCH) project. MATCH is a collaboration between the Robert Wood Johnson Foundation and the University of Wisconsin Population Health Institute.

9. **http://www.teachepidemiology.org**

   Teach Epidemiology

   This is a Web site sponsored by the Robert Wood Johnson Foundation that provides middle and high school teachers with ideas about how to incorporate the teaching of epidemiology into their curriculum.

References

American College Health Association (ACHA). (2013). *About ACHA-NCHA*. Retrieved July 12, 2013, from http://www.acha-ncha.org/overview.html.

Association of Schools of Public Health. (n. d.). What is public health? Retrieved on July 8, 2013, from http://www.whatispublichealth.org/.

Auld, M. E., & Dixon-Terry, E. (2010). The role of health education associations in advocacy. In J. M. Black, S. Furney, H. M. Graf, & A. E. Nolte (Eds.), *Philosophical foundations of health education* (pp. 311–318). San Francisco: Jossey-Bass.

Breslow, L. (1999). From disease prevention to health promotion. *Journal of the American Medical Association, 281* (11), 1030–1033.

Centers for Disease Control and Prevention (CDC). (1994). *Chronic disease in minority populations*. Atlanta, GA: Author.

Centers for Disease Control and Prevention (CDC). (2011a). *Chronic diseases and health promotion*. Retrieved July 12, 2013, from http://www.cdc.gov/chronicdisease/overview.

Centers for Disease Control and Prevention (CDC). (2011b). *Health-related quality of life*. Retrieved July 12, 2013, from http://www.cdc.gov/hrqol/concept.htm.

Centers for Disease Control and Prevention (CDC). (2011c). *The health communicator's social media toolkit*. Retrieved July 14, 2013, from http://www.cdc.gov/socialmedia/tools/guidelines/pdf/socialmediatoolkit_bm.pdf.

Centers for Disease Control and Prevention (CDC). (2012a). *NCHS Fact Sheet*. Retrieved July 12, 2013, from http://www.cdc.gov/nchs/data/factsheets/factsheet_nhcs.htm.

Centers for Disease Control and Prevention (CDC). (2012b). *National Comprehensive Cancer Control Program (NCCCP): 2012 Success Stories*. Retreived July 13, 2013, from http://www.cdc.gov/cancer/ncccp/state.htm.

Centers for Disease Control and Prevention (CDC). (2013a). *Behavioral Risk Factor Surveillance System*. Retrieved July 12, 2013, from http://www.cdc.gov/brfss/.

Centers for Disease Control and Prevention (CDC). (2013b). *Youth Risk Behavior Surveillance System*. Retrieved July 12, 2013, from http://www.cdc.gov/healthyyouth/yrbs/index.htm.

Centers for Disease Control and Prevention (CDC). (2013c). *Social determinants: Frequently asked questions*. Retrieved July 13, 2013, from http://www.cdc.gov/socialdeterminants/FAQ.html.

Centers for Disease Control and Prevention (CDC). (2013d). *Smoking & tobacco use*. Retrieved July 13, 2013, from http://www.cdc.gov/tobacco/data_statistics/fact_sheets/fast_facts/index.htm.

Centers for Disease Control and Prevention (CDC). (2013e). *Social Media at CDC*. Retrieved July14, 2013, from http://www.cdc.gov/socialmedia/tools/guidelines/index.html.

Cleary, M. J., & Neiger, B. L. (1998). *The certified health education specialist: A self-study guide for professional competency* (3rd ed.). Allentown, PA: The National Commission for Health Education Credentialing.

Coalition for National Health Education Organizations (CNHEO). (2007). *Employer's guide*. Retrieved July 14, 2013, from http://www.cnheo.org/index.html.

Cottrell, R. R., & McKenzie, J. F. (2011). *Health promotion & education research methods: Using the five chapter thesis/dissertation model* (2nd ed.). Sudbury, MA: Jones and Bartlett Publishers.

Davis, P. C., & Rankin, L. L. (2006). Guidelines for making existing health education programs more culturally appropriate. *American Journal of Health Education, 37* (4), 250–252.

Glanz, K., & Rimer, B. K. (2008). Perspectives on using theory: Past, present, and future. In K. Glanz, B. K. Rimer, & K. Viswanath (Eds.), *Health behavior and health education: Theory, research, and practice* (pp. 509–517). San Francisco: Jossey-Bass.

Green, L. W., & Ottoson, J. M. (1999). *Community and population health* (8th ed.). Boston: WCB/McGraw-Hill.

Hancock, T., & Minkler, M. (2005). Community health assessment or healthy community assessment: Whose community? Whose health? Whose assessment? In M. Minkler (Ed.), *Community organizing and community building for health* (2nd ed., pp. 138–157). New Brunswick, NJ: Rutgers University Press.

Hanlon, J. J. (1974). *Public Health*. St. Louis: Mosby.

Hezel Associates. (2007). *Marketing the health education profession: Knowledge, attitudes, and hiring practices of employers*. Retrieved August 24, 2010, from http://www.cnheo.org/.

Institute of Medicine (IOM). (2001). *Health and behavior: The interplay of biological, behavioral, and societal influences*. Washington, DC: Academy Press.

Institute of Medicine (IOM). (2002). *Brief Report. The future of the public's health in the 21st century*. Retrieved March 25, 2004, from http://www.iom.edu/file.asp?id=4165.

Johns, E. B. (1973). Joint Committee on Health Education Terminology: Report of the Joint Committee on Health Education Terminology. *Health Education, 4* (6), 25.

Joint Committee on Health Education Terminology. (1991a). Report of the 1990 Joint Committee on Health Education Terminology. *Journal of Health Education, 22* (2), 105–106.

Joint Committee on Health Education Terminology. (1991b). Report of the 1990 Joint Committee on Health Education Terminology. *Journal of School Health, 61* (6), 251–254.

Joint Committee on Health Education and Health Promotion Terminology. (2001). Report of the 2000 Joint Committee on Health Education and Health Promotion Terminology. *American Journal of Health Education, 32* (2), 89–103.

Joint Committee on Health Education and Promotion Terminology. (2012). *Report of the 2011 joint committee on health education and promotion terminology*. Reston, VA: AAHE.

King, N. (2009). Health inequalities and health inequities. In E. E. Morrison (Ed.), *Health care ethics: Critical issues for the 21st century* (pp. 339–354). Sudbury, MA: Jones & Bartlett.

Laframboise, H. L. (1973). Health policy: Breaking it down into more manageable segments. *Journal of the Canadian Medical Association, 108* (Feb. 3), 388–393.

Lalonde, M. (1974). A *new perspective on the health of Canadians: A working document*. Ottawa, Canada: Ministry of National Health and Welfare.

Luquis, R., Pérez, M., & Young, K. (2006). Cultural competence development in health education professional preparation programs. *American Journal of Health Education, 37* (4), 233–241.

Mason, J. O., & McGinnis, J. M. (1990). Healthy people 2000: An overview of the national health promotion disease prevention objectives. *Public Health Reports, 105* (5), 441–446.

Mathers, C. D., Sdana, R., Salomon, J. A., Murray, C. J. L., & Lopez, A. D. (2001). Healthy life expectancies in 191 countries, 1999. *Lancet, 357*, 1685–1691.

McGinnis, J. M. (1985). The limits of prevention. *Public Health Reports, 100* (3), 255–260.

McGinnis, J. M. (2001). United States. In C. E. Koop (Ed.), *Critical issues in global health* (pp. 80–90). San Francisco: Jossey-Bass.

McGinnis, J. M., & Foege, W. H. (1993). Actual causes of death in the United States. *Journal of the American Medical Association, 270* (18), 2207–2212.

McGinnis, J. M., Williams-Russo, P., & Knickman, J. R. (2002). The case for more active policy attention to health promotion. *Health Affairs, 21* (2), 78–93.

McKenzie, J. F., Neiger, B. L., & Thackeray, R (2013). *Planning, implementing, and evaluating, health promotion programs: A primer* (6th ed.). San Francisco: Pearson.

McKenzie, J. F., & Pinger, R. R. (2013). *An introduction to community health: Brief edition.* Boston: Jones and Bartlett Publishers.

McKenzie, J. F., Pinger, R. R., & Kotecki, J. E. (2012). *An introduction to community health* (7th ed.). Boston: Jones and Bartlett Publishers.

McLeroy, K. R., Bibeau, D., Steckler, A., &. Glanz, K. (1988). An ecological perspective for health promotion programs. *Health Education Quarterly, 15* (4): 351–378.

Minkler, M., Wallerstein, N., & Wilson, N. (2008). Improving health through community organizing and community building. In K. Glanz, B. K. Rimer, & K. Viswanath (Eds.), *Health behavior and health education practice: Theory, research, and practice* (4th ed., pp. 287–312). San Francisco: Jossey-Bass.

Mokdad, A. H., Marks, J. S., Stroup, D. F., & Gerberding, J. L. (2004). Actual causes of death, in the United States, 2000. *Journal of the American Medical Association, 291* (10), 1238–1245.

Montagu, A. (1968). *Man observed.* New York: G. P. Putnam.

Moss, B. (1950). Joint Committee on Health Education Terminology. *Journal of Physical Education, 21,* 41.

Murray, C. J. L., & Lopez, A. D. (Eds.). (1996). *Summary of the global burden of disease: A comprehensive assessment of mortality and disability from diseases, injuries, and risk factors in 1990 and projected to 2020.* Geneva, Switzerland: World Health Organization.

National Center for Health Statistics (NCHS). (2013). *Health, United States, 2012: With special feature on emergency care.* Hyattsville, MD: Author.

National Commission for Health Education Credentialing, Inc. (NCHEC). (1996). *A competency-based framework for professional development of certified health education specialists.* Allentown, PA: Author.

Pellmar, T. C., Brandt, Jr., E. N., & Baird, M. (2002). Health and behavior: The interplay of biological, behavioral, and social influences: Summary of an Institute of Medicine Report. *American Journal of Health Promotion, 16* (4), 206–219.

Pérez, M. A., & Luquis, R. R. (2008). Changing U.S. demographics: Challenges and opportunities for health educators. In M. A. Perez & R. R. Luquis (Eds.) *Cultural competence in health education and health promotion* (pp. 1–21). San Francisco: Jossey-Bass.

Pinzon-Perez, H., & Perez, M. A. (1999). Advocacy groups for Hispanic/Latino health issues. *The Health Educator Monograph Series, 17* (2), 29–31.

Raphael, D., Brown, I., Renwick, R., & Rootman, I. (1997). Quality of life: What are the implications for health promotion? *American Journal of Health Behavior, 21* (2), 118–128.

Rimer, B. K., & Glanz, K. (2005). *Theory at a glance: A guide for health promotion practice* (2nd ed). NIH Pub. No. 05-3896. Washington, DC: National Cancer Institute.

Rugen, M. (1972). *A fifty year history of the public health section of American Public Health Association; 1922–1972.* Washington, DC: American Public Health Association, Inc.

Sallis, J. F., Owen, N., & Fisher, E. B. (2008). Ecological models of health behavior. In K. Glanz, B. K. Rimer, & K. Viswanath (Eds.), *Health behavior and health education practice: Theory, research, and practice* (4th ed., pp. 465–485). San Francisco: Jossey-Bass.

Selig, S., Tropiano, E., & Greene-Moton, E. (2006). Teaching cultural competence to reduce health disparities. *Health Promotion Practice, 7* (3), 247S–255S.

Simons-Morton, B. G., McLeroy, K. R., & Wendel, M. L. (2012). *Behavior theory in health promotion practice and research.* Burlington, MA: Jones & Bartlett Learning.

Slee, D. A., Slee, V. N., & Schmidt, H. J. (2008). *Slee's health care terms* (5th ed.). Sudbury, MA: Jones & Bartlett.

Sultz, H. A., & K. M. Young (2011). *Health Care USA: Understanding Its Organization and Delivery*, 7th ed. Sudbury, MA: Jones & Bartlett.

Turnock, B. J. (2012). *Public Health: What It Is and How It Works*, 5th ed. Burlington, MA: Jones & Bartlett Learning.

U.S. Department of Health, Education, and Welfare (USDHEW). (1980). *Promoting health/preventing disease: Objectives for the nation.* Washington, DC: U.S. Government Printing Office.

U.S. Department of Health and Human Services (USDHHS). (1991). *Health status of minorities and low-income groups* (3rd ed.). Washington, DC: U.S. Government Printing Office.

U.S. Department of Health and Human Services (USDHHS) (2000). *Healthy People 2010.* (Conference Edition, in Two Volumes). Washington, DC: U.S. Government Printing Office.

U.S. Department of Health and Human Services (USDHHS). (2013). *Healthy People 2020: Social Determinants of Health.* Retrieved July 12, 2013, from http://www.healthypeople.gov/2020/topicsobjectives2020/overview. aspx?topicid=39.

Williams, J. F. (1934). Report of the Health Education Section of the American Physical Education Association: Definitions of terms in health education. *Journal of Physical Education, 5* (16–17), 50–51.

World Health Organization (WHO). (1947). *Constitution of the World Health Organization.* Retrieved July 12, 2013, from http://apps.who.int/gb/bd/PDF/bd47/EN/constitution-en.pdf.

World Health Organization (WHO). (1986). *Health promotion sante: Ottawa charter.* Retrieved July 12, 2013, from http://www.euro.who.int/en/who-we-are/policy-documents/ ottawa-charter-for-health-promotion,-1986.

World Health Organization (WHO). (2008). *The global burden of disease: 2004 update.* Retrieved July 12, 2013, from http://www.who.int/healthinfo/global_burden_disease/GBD_report_2004update_full.pdf.

World Health Organization (WHO). (2013). "Epidemiology." Retrieved December 6, 2013, from http://www .who.int/topics/epidemiology/en/.

Yoho, R. (1962). Joint Committee on Health Education Terminology: Health education terminology. *Journal of Physical Education and Recreation, 33* (Nov.), 27–28.

The History of Health and Health Education/Promotion

Chapter Objectives

After reading this chapter and answering the questions at the end,
you should be able to:

- Discuss how health beliefs and practices have changed from the earliest humans to the present day.
- Identify the dual roots of modern health education/promotion.
- Explain why a need for professional health education specialists emerged.
- Trace the history of public health in the United States.
- Relate the history of school health from the mid-1800s to the present
- Identify important governmental publications from 1975 to the present and describe how these publications have impacted health promotion and education.

Although the history of health education/promotion as an emerging profession is slightly more than 100 years old, the concept of educating about health has been around since the dawn of humans. This chapter discusses the history of health, health care, and health education/promotion from the earliest human records to the present. The main focus is on Northern Africa and Europe. These areas had the greatest influence on the development of health knowledge and health care in the United States. Although other parts of the world—for example, the Far East, Africa, Central America, and South America—contributed to the history of health and health care, their accounts are not as directly relevant to the history of health in the United States.

It is important that students recognize the difference between "educating about health," which can be done by anyone who believes he or she has knowledge about health to share with someone else, and "health education/promotion," which is done by a professionally trained health education specialist. The need for professional health education specialists emerged as human knowledge of health and health care increased. This chapter emphasizes the health education/promotion profession during the past 150 years as it evolved from the dual roots of school health and public health. You cannot fully appreciate the health education/promotion profession without understanding its origin. History reveals how progress was made over time. It also depicts the obstacles faced by those who promoted health improvements throughout the years. "At the same time, historical study shows us that despite the difficulties, change is possible, given dedication, organization and persistence.... Historical case studies may be able to teach us useful lessons about successful strategies used by public health reformers in the past" (Fee & Brown, 1997, p. 1763).

▷ Early Humans

We assume that the earliest humans learned by trial and error to distinguish between things that were healthful and those that were harmful. They were able to observe how animals bathed to cool their bodies and remove external parasites, apply mud to calm insect bites, consume certain herbs to provide medicinal benefits and avoid other herbs that were poisonous (Goerke & Stebbins, 1968, p. 5).

It does not stretch the imagination too far to see how education about health first took place. Someone may have eaten a particular plant or herb and become ill. That person would then warn (educate) others against eating the same substance. Conversely, someone may have ingested a plant or an herb that produced a desired effect. That person would then encourage (educate) others to use this substance. Through observation, trial, and error, other types of health-related knowledge were discovered. Eventually, this knowledge was transformed into rules or taboos for a given society. Rules about preserving food and how to bury the dead may have been implemented. Perhaps taboos against defecation within the tribe's communal area or near sources of drinking water were established (McKenzie, Pinger, & Kotecki, 2012). The trial and error method, which undoubtedly produced serious illness and even death among some early humans, gradually became less needed. Knowledge was passed verbally from one generation to the next, preventing at least some of the potential ill effects of everyday life. As society progressed even further, this knowledge was written down and saved (see **Figure 2.1**).

▶ **Figure 2.1** Preparation of medicine from honey (the leaf from an Arabic translation of the *Materia Medica of Dioscorides*, dated 1224 Iraq, Baghdad School)

There was still much more unknown than known about protecting health. Disease and death were probably much more common than health and longevity. To early humans, it was puzzling when disease and death occurred for no apparent reason. In an attempt to make these events seem more rational, early man often attributed disease and accidents to magical spirits which were believed to live in trees, animals, the earth and air. When these spirits were angered they would punish individuals or communities with disease and death (Goerke & Stebbins, 1968). To prevent disease, sacrifices were made to the gods, taboos were obeyed, amulets were worn, and "haunted" places were avoided. Charms, spells, and chants were also used to protect from disease (Duncan, 1988). Again, it is likely that some form of rudimentary education about health was taking place to inform people how to keep from provoking the spirits and, thus, prevent disease.

▷ Early Efforts at Public Health

Evidence of broad-scale public health activity has been found in the earliest of civilizations. In India, sites excavated at Mohenjo-Daro and Harappa dating back 4,000 years indicate that bathrooms and drains were common. The streets were broad, paved, and drained by covered sewers (Rosen, 1958). Archeological evidence also shows that the Minoans (3000–1430 B.C.) and Myceneans (1430–1150 B.C.) built drainage systems, toilets, and water flushing systems (Pickett & Hanlon, 1990). The oldest written documents related to health care are the **Smith Papyri**, dating from 1600 B.C., which describe various surgical techniques. The earliest written record concerning public health is the **Code of Hammurabi** (see **Box 2.1**), named after the king of Babylon. It contained laws pertaining to health practices and physicians, including the first known fee schedule (Rubinson & Alles, 1984).

▷ Early Cultures

The medical lore of the distant past was handed down from generation to generation. In virtually every culture for which there are documented historical accounts, people turned to some type of a physician or medicine man for health information (education about health), treatments, and cures (Green & Simons-Morton, 1990). In Egypt, as in many other cultures, this role was held by the priests. Eventually, the various incantations, spells, exorcisms, prescriptions, and clinical observations were compiled into written format, some of which survive in our museums and libraries (Libby, 1922).

The Egyptians made substantial progress in the area of public health. They possessed a strong sense of personal cleanliness and were considered to be the healthiest people of their time (see **Figure 2.2**). They used numerous pharmaceutic preparations and constructed earth privies for sewage, as well as public drainage pipes (Pickett & Hanlon, 1990). Nevertheless, they relied primarily on priests for their health information and used remedies such as "dung of the gazelle and the crocodile, the fat of a serpent, mammalian entrails and other excreta, tissues and organs" (Libby, 1922, p. 6).

BOX 2.1

The Rights and Duties of the Surgeon of 2080 B.C.: From the *Code of Hammurabi*

"If a physician operate on a man for a severe wound (or make a severe wound upon a man), with a bronze lancet, and save the man's life; or if he open an abscess (in the eye) of a man, with a bronze lancet, and save the man's eye, he shall receive ten shekels of silver (as his fee)."

"If he be a freeman,* he shall receive five shekels."

"If it be a man's slave, the owner of the slave shall give two shekels of silver to the physician."

"If a physician operate on a man for a severe wound, with a bronze lancet, and cause the man's death; or open an abscess (in the eye) of a man with a bronze lancet, and destroy the man's eye, they shall cut off his hands."

"If a physician operate on a slave of a freeman for a severe wound, with a bronze lancet, and cause his death, he shall restore a slave of equal value."

"If he open an abscess (in his eye), with a bronze lancet, and destroy his eye, he shall pay silver to the extent of one half of his price."

"If a physician set a broken bone for a man or cure his diseased bowels, the patient shall give five shekels of silver to the physician."

"If he be a freeman, he shall give three shekels."

"If it be a man's slave, the owner of the slave shall give two shekels of silver to the physician."

"If a veterinary physician operate on an ox or ass for a severe wound and save its life, the owner of the ox or ass shall give the physician, as his fee, one sixth of a shekel of silver."

"If he operate on an ox or an ass for a severe wound, and cause its death, he shall give to the owner of the ox or ass one fourth its value."

*Freeman indicates a rank intermediate between that of "man" (or gentleman) and that of "slave."

Source: From R. F. Harper, *The Code of Hammurabi*, 1904, Chicago.

► **Figure 2.2** The Egyptians were known for their cleanliness and were considered the healthiest people of the time.

In approximately 1500 B.C., the Hebrews extended Egyptian hygienic thought and formulated (in the biblical book of Leviticus) what is probably the world's first written hygienic code. It dealt with a variety of personal and community responsibilities, including cleanliness of the body, protection against the spread of contagious diseases, isolation of lepers, disinfection of dwellings after illness, sanitation of campsites, disposal of excreta and refuse, protection of water and food supplies, and specific hygiene rules for menstruating women and women who had recently delivered a child.

The history of health and health care in the Greek culture (1000–400 B.C.) is intriguing as well as relevant to modern healthcare philosophy. The Greeks were perhaps the first people to put as much emphasis on disease prevention as they did on the treatment of disease conditions. Balance among the physical, mental, and spiritual aspects of the person was emphasized. Among the early Greeks, religion played an important role in health care. However, the role of physician began to take on a more defined shape, and a more scientific view of medicine emerged.

In the early stages of Greek culture, as represented in the *Iliad* and the *Odyssey*, the priesthood played a role in the healing arts. In the *Iliad*, **Asclepius** was a Thessalian chief who had received instruction in the use of drugs. By the beginning of the eighth century B.C., tradition had enshrined him as the god of medicine. He had two daughters who also had health-related powers. **Hygeia** was given the power to prevent disease, whereas **Panacea** was given the ability to treat disease. Hygeia was the more prominent figure and was often pictured with her father in sculptures and illustrations of the time (Schouten, 1967) (see **Figure 2.3**).

▶ **Figure 2.3** Asclepius and Hygeia

▶ **Figure 2.4** Illustration of a caduceus, a symbol that shows two snakes braided around a staff. It is representative of the medical profession and has its earliest association with Asclepius, the Greek healer.

The words *hygiene* and *panacea* can be traced back to these daughters of Asclepius (Libby, 1922).

Eventually, hundreds of elaborate temples were built throughout Greece to worship Asclepius. These temples were typically on beautiful sites overlooking the sea or beside healing fountains. The temple priests practiced their healing arts, which often involved fraud. The temple priests should not be confused with the **Asclepiads**. The Asclepiads were a brotherhood of men present at the temples who initially claimed descent from Asclepius. Although some of the Asclepiads probably helped the priests with their trickery, others broke away from the priests and began to practice medicine based on more rational principles. These ancient temples of Asclepius left their symbol as a permanent reminder of the past—the staff and serpent of the physician, known as the **caduceus** (Rubinson & Alles, 1984) (see **Figure 2.4**).

The famous Greek physician **Hippocrates** came from the Asclepian tradition. He lived from about 460 B.C. until 377 B.C. (See **Figure 2.5**.) Hippocrates developed a theory of disease causation consistent with the philosophy of nature held by leading philosophers of his day. Hippocrates taught that health was the result of balance, and disease was the result of an imbalance. To the Greeks, the ideal person was perfectly balanced in mind, body, and spirit. Thus, study and practice related to philosophy, athletics, and theology were all important to maintain balance. To do this, however, took a tremendous commitment of time and energy. Each day required physical activity, study, and philosophical discussion while maintaining proper nutrition and rest. Few people could afford to lead such a life. Those who did were the aristocratic upper class leading a life of leisure supported by a slave economy (Rosen, 1958). The ideal Greek human being that is so often mentioned was, in fact, a small percentage of the Greek population.

Hippocrates holds an important place in the history of medicine. His theory of health and disease was still being taught in medical schools as a valid theory of disease causation as recently as the first quarter of the 20th century. Hippocrates, however, did more than

▶ **Figure 2.5** Hippocrates, 460–359 B.C., "Father of Western Medicine"

just theorize about disease. He carefully observed and recorded associations between certain diseases and such factors as geography, climate, diet, and living conditions. Duncan (1988) noted, "One of his [Hippocrates's] most noteworthy contributions is the distinction between 'endemic' diseases, which vary in prevalence from place to place, and 'epidemic' diseases, which vary in prevalence over time" (p. 12). The traditional Hippocratic Oath is still used today and is the basis for medical ethics. Hippocrates and the Asclepiads moved health care away from religion and priests and attempted to establish a more rational basis to explain health and disease. Hippocrates's concept of balance in life is still promoted today as the best means for maintaining health and well-being.

Hippocrates has been credited as being the first epidemiologist and the father of modern medicine (Duncan, 1988). It is not hard to imagine that he was also a health educator. One can easily see Hippocrates educating his friends and patients about diet, exercise, rest, and the importance of balance in preventing disease and promoting health.

The Romans conquered the Mediterranean world, including the Greeks. In doing so, however, the Romans did not destroy the cultures they conquered but learned from them. The Romans accepted many Greek ideas, including those related to health and medicine. "As clinicians, the Romans were hardly more than imitators of the Greeks, but as engineers and administrators, as builders of sewerage systems and baths, and as providers of water supplies and other health facilities, they set the world a great example and left their mark in history" (Rosen, 1958, p. 38). (See **Figure 2.6**.)

The Roman Empire (500 B.C.–A.D. 500) built an extensive and efficient aqueduct system. "Evidence of some 200 Roman aqueducts remains today, from Spain to Syria and from Northern Europe to North Africa" (McKenzie, Pinger, & Kotecki, 2008, p. 12). The total capacity of the 13 aqueducts delivering water to the city of Rome has been estimated

▲ **Figure 2.6** Roman aqueducts

at 222 million gallons every 24 hours. At the height of the empire, this would have been enough to provide each citizen of Rome with at least 40 gallons of fresh water per day. Additionally, attention was paid to water purity. At specific points along the aqueduct, generally near the middle and end, settling basins were located, in which sediment might be deposited (Rosen, 1958).

The Romans also developed an extensive system of underground sewers. These served to carry off both surface water and sewage. The main sewer in Rome that emptied into the Tiber River was 10 feet wide and 12 feet high; it was still part of the Roman sewer system during the 20th century.

The Romans made other health advancements. They observed the effect of occupational hazards on health, and they were the first to build hospitals. By the second century A.D., a public medical service was set up whereby physicians were appointed to various towns and institutions. A system of private medical practice also developed during the Roman era (Rosen, 1958).

The Romans furthered the work of the Greeks in the study of human anatomy and the practice of surgery. Some Roman anatomists even dissected living human beings to further their knowledge of anatomy (Libby, 1922). In quoting the Latin writer Cornelius, Libby noted that these anatomists "procured criminals out of prison, by royal permission, and dissecting them alive, contemplated, while they were still breathing, the parts which nature had before concealed, considering their position, color, figure, size, order, hardness, softness, smoothness, and asperity" (Libby, 1922, p. 54). Although some opposed this hideous practice, others supported it, holding "it is by no means cruel as most people represent it, by the tortures of a few guilty, to search after remedies for the whole innocent race of mankind in all ages" (Libby, 1922, p. 54).

▷ Middle Ages

The era from the collapse of the Roman Empire to about A.D. 1500 is known as the Middle Ages or Dark Ages. This was a time of political and social unrest, when many health advancements of previous cultures were lost. Rosen (1958) notes that "the problem that confronted the medieval world was to weld together the culture of the barbarian invaders with the classical heritage of the defunct [Roman] Empire and with the beliefs and teachings of the Christian religion" (p. 52). This proved to be no easy task.

With the Roman Empire no longer able to protect settlements, each city had to defend itself against its enemies. For safety, people lived within city walls along with their domesticated animals. As the population grew, expansion was difficult and overcrowding common (Rosen, 1958). Lack of fresh water and sewage removal were major problems for many medieval cities; Roman public health advancements were lost.

To make matters worse, there was little emphasis on cleanliness or hygiene. The new religion, Christianity,

> found its disciples among the lower classes, where personal hygiene was not practiced, and as a consequence, an entirely different attitude toward the human body developed. Excessive care of the body, that is, man's earthly and mutable part, was unimportant in the Christian dualistic concept, which separated body from soul. For some Eastern churchmen and holy men, living in filth was regarded as evidence of sanctity: cleanliness was thought to betoken pride, and filthiness humility. (Goerke & Stebbins, 1968, p. 9)

Fortunately, as Christianity matured so did its concept of the human body. Eventually, Christians came to believe that the body is the soul's earthly dwelling, permitting better care of it.

Early Christians also reinforced the notion that disease was caused by sin or disobeying God. This propelled priests and religious leaders back into the position of preventing and treating disease. The health-related advancements of the Greco-Roman era were abandoned and shunned. Entire libraries were burned, and knowledge about the human body was seen as sinful.

The Middle Ages were characterized by great epidemics. Perhaps the cruelest of these was leprosy, a disease characterized by severe facial and extremity disfigurement. A highly contagious and virulent disease, all Western countries issued edicts against anyone suspected of having leprosy and regulated every aspect of the sufferer's life. In some communities, lepers were given the last rites of the church, forced to leave the city, made to wear identifying clothing, and required to carry a rod identifying them as lepers. Other lepers were forced to wear a bell around their necks and to ring it as a warning when other people came near. Such isolation usually brought about a relatively quick death resulting from hunger and exposure (Goerke & Stebbins, 1968). Eventually, leprosy hospitals were founded to treat the inflicted. It has been estimated that by A.D. 1200, there were 1,900 leper houses and leprosaria in Europe (Rosen, 1958).

The bubonic plague, known as the Black Death, may have been the most severe epidemic the world has ever known. The death toll was higher and the disruption of society greater than from any war, famine, or natural disaster in history. "At Constantinople, the plague raged with such violence that 5,000, and even 10,000 persons are said to have died in a single day" (Donan, 1898, p. 94). Estimates of casualties vary from 20 to 35 million, with Europe losing one quarter to one third of its entire population. In Avignon, France, 60,000 people died. As a result, the pope was forced to consecrate the Rhone River so that bodies might be thrown into it, because the churchyards were filled (Goerke & Stebbins, 1968).

Imagine what it must have been like to live through the plague. Literally one out of every three or four people you knew contracted the disease and died. The cause of the disease was unknown, causing widespread fear and superstition. Often, religious leaders and doctors were some of the first victims. They were exposed to the disease early in the epidemic through their contact with infected sufferers. This left many communities with no religious or medical leadership.

People reacted to the plague in different ways. Some became extremely pious, turned away from earthly pleasures, and practiced extreme self denial in hopes of pleasing God. Others took the opposite approach, lost faith in God, and disregarded legal, moral, and sexual restraints (Goerke & Stebbins, 1968). The Brotherhood of the Flagellants was a group of religious zealots who believed the plague could be avoided by admitting to their sins and then ritualistically beating themselves in atonement. Today, such a group would most likely be labeled a religious cult. Members of this group marched in long, two-column lines from city to city. In each city, they would chant a litany and conduct their ritualistic ceremony. At a signal from the group's master, the Flagellants would strip to the waist and march in a circle until they received another signal from the master. Upon receiving the second signal, they would throw themselves to the ground with their body position indicating the specific sin they had committed. The master would move among the bodies, thrashing those who had committed certain sins or had offended the discipline of the Flagellants in some way. This would be followed by a collective flagellation in which the group members would rhythmically beat their own backs and breasts with a heavy scourge made of three or four leather thongs tipped with metal studs. According to eyewitness accounts, the Flagellants lashed themselves until their bodies became swollen and blue, and blood dripped to the ground. Further complicating the health consequences of such punishment was a rule prohibiting bathing, washing, or changing clothes. When joining the Brotherhood, group members had to pledge to scourge themselves three times daily for 33 days and eight hours, which represented one day for each year of Christ's earthly life (Ziegler, 1969).

Debate existed during the Middle Ages concerning the cause of the plague. In 1348, Jehan Jacme wrote that the disease was caused by five factors: (1) the wrath of God, (2) the corruption of dead bodies, (3) waters and vapors formed in the interior of the earth, (4) unnatural hot and humid winds, and (5) the conjunction of stars and planets (Winslow, 1944).

Another story concerning the origins of the disease had Italian merchants trapped in a city on the Black Sea that was under siege by a local Mongol prince. The prince was forced to call off the siege because large numbers of his army were dying of a strange disease. Before leaving, the prince ordered his army to catapult the dead, diseased bodies into the city. Within days, the people inside the city began to die. Afraid, the Italian merchants set sail for Italy, but not before infected rats had boarded the ship. Soon many of the sailors became sick. The ship tried to dock in several cities but was denied permission because of the illness. Finally permission was granted to dock in Sicily where the rats came on shore and the plague began (De'ath, 1995).

Despite the disagreement that existed on the cause of the disease, contemporaries believed that the disease was contagious. In other words, it was passed from person to person in some unknown way. Although this concept of contagion had been around for many years and was discussed in the Bible, it was not until the Middle Ages and the epidemics of leprosy and bubonic plague that it started to become more universally accepted. The contagion concept opened the door to new interest in science and severely weakened the argument of those promoting the sin-disease theory.

The Middle Ages also saw epidemics of other communicable diseases, including smallpox, diphtheria, measles, influenza, tuberculosis, anthrax, and trachoma. The last major epidemic disease of this period was syphilis, which appeared in 1492. As with other epidemics, syphilis killed thousands of people (McKenzie, Pinger, & Kotecki et al., 2012).

Although there were no professional health education specialists during the Middle Ages, education about health continued to exist. Priests, medical doctors, and community leaders attempted to "educate" anyone who would listen to their ideas about health and disease prevention. Given the rudimentary level of health knowledge and the lack of consensus on prevention and causation of disease, a professional health education specialist would probably have contributed little to the general population's health in the Middle Ages.

▷ Renaissance

The Renaissance, which means "rebirth," lasted roughly from A.D. 1500 to 1700. This time period was characterized by a gradual change in thinking. People began to view the world and humankind in a more naturalistic and holistic fashion. Although progress was slow, science again emerged as a legitimate field of inquiry, and numerous scientific advancements were made. The world did not change overnight from the superstitious and backward beliefs of the Dark Ages to a completely enlightened society in the Renaissance. Disease and plague still ravaged Europe and overall medical care was still rudimentary. Bloodletting was a major form of treatment for everything from the common cold to tuberculosis. Popular remedies included crabs' eyes, foxes' lungs, oil of anise, oil of spiders, and oil of earthworms. A major means of diagnosing a patient's condition consisted of examining the urine for changes in color. The inspection of a patient's urine by a true physician was known as "water casting." For many years, this was the principal occupation of the medical profession.

Much surgery and dentistry was performed by barbers because they had the best chairs and sharpest instruments available. Some barbers dispensed health information, as can be seen in the following example from a Danish barber-surgeon: "It is very good for persons to drink themselves intoxicated once a month for the excellent reasons that it frees their strength, furthers sound sleep, eases the passing of water, increases perspiration, and stimulates general well-being" (Durant, 1961, pp. 495–496). Unfortunately, few were probably moderate enough to restrict their binges to once a month.

Rosen (1958) notes that, although the Renaissance "is characterized by the rapid growth and spread of science in various fields, public health as a practiced activity received very little, if any, direct benefit from these advances" (p. 84). Evidence of the poor public health conditions can be seen in this note describing the average English household floor of the 16th century:

> As to floors, they are usually made with clay, covered with rushes that grow in the fens and which are so seldom removed that the lower part remains sometimes for twenty years and has in it a collection of spittle, vomit, urine of dogs and humans, beer, scraps of fish and other filthiness not to be named. (Pickett & Hanlon, 1990, p. 25)

Although living conditions among the English royalty were certainly better than for those of the laboring class, health-related problems still were prevalent. Disposal of human waste was a major problem. Those who lived in old castles located their latrines in large projections on the face of walls. The excrement was discharged from these projections into deep-walled pits, moats, or streams near the walls of the castle. Those less fortunate used chamber pots and simply tossed their contents out the nearest window. Even among royalty, basic hygiene left much to be desired. Few monarchs bathed more frequently than once a week. Much of the material used in royal apparel, such as silk, velvet, and ermine, could not be washed; thus, it simply accumulated dirt and perspiration. Cloaking scents were used to try to renew the clothing, but they were not effective (Hansen, 1980).

On the positive side, the Renaissance was a period of exploration and expanded trade. The search for knowledge, characteristic of the Greek and Roman eras, was revitalized. Superstitions of the Middle Ages were slowly replaced with a more systematic inquiry into cause and effect. In the middle of the 15th century, learning gained momentum as a result of Johannes Gutenberg's invention of the printing press with moveable type. This allowed the great classical works of Hippocrates and Galen to be reproduced and distributed to larger audiences (Gordon, 1959).

There were also scientific advancements during the Renaissance. The human body was again considered appropriate for study, and realistic anatomical drawings were produced. John Hunter, the father of modern surgery, undertook a more orderly exploration of the workings of the human body. Antonie van Leeuwenhoek discovered the microscope and proved there were life forms too small for the human eye to see. These life forms, however, were not yet associated with disease. John Graunt forwarded the fields of statistics and epidemiology. Through studying the *Bills of Mortality*, published weekly in London, Graunt found more males than females were born, higher death rates during the first years of life than later in life, and higher death rates among urban dwellers than rural dwellers (Goerke & Stebbins, 1968).

In Italy, many cities had instituted health boards to fight the plague. It did not take long, however, for their responsibilities to be expanded. By the middle of the 16th century, numerous matters had fallen under the control and jurisdiction of these health boards. These included "the marketing of meat, fish, shellfish, game, fruit, grain, sausages, oil, wine and water; the sewage system; the activity of the hospitals; beggars and prostitutes; burials, cemeteries, and pesthouses; the professional activity of physicians, surgeons and apothecaries; the preparation and sale of drugs; the activity of hostelries and the Jewish community" (Cipolla, 1976, p. 32).

▷ Age of Enlightenment

The 1700s were a period of revolution, industrialization, and growth of cities. Both the French and American Revolutions took place during this century. Plague and other epidemics continued to be a problem. Science had not yet discovered that these diseases were produced by microscopic organisms. The general belief was that disease was formed in filth and that epidemics were caused by some type of poison that developed in the putrefaction process. The vapors, or "miasmas," rising from this rotting refuse could travel through the air for great distances and were believed to result in disease when inhaled. This concept, known as the **miasmas theory**, remained popular throughout much of the 19th century. As preventive measures, herbs and incense were often used to perfume the air, supposedly filling the nose and crowding out any miasmas (Duncan, 1988). It was still not known that contaminated water could cause disease infection.

Scientific advancements continued throughout the period. Dr. James Lind, a Royal Navy surgeon, discovered that scurvy could be controlled on long sea voyages by having sailors consume lime juice. To this day, British sailors are known as "limeys." Edward Jenner discovered a vaccine procedure against smallpox. Bernardino Ramazzini wrote on trade and industrial diseases. Theorists of the time conceived of the mind and body not as separate entities, but as dependent on each other. Philosophers of the 18th century, such as Diderot, Locke, Rousseau, and Voltaire, all "promoted the worth of each human life and the importance of individual health for the well being of society" (Rubinson & Alles, 1984, p. 5).

Although progress was made during this time, health education/promotion in itself still did not emerge as a profession. With the rudimentary state of medical knowledge in the 16th, 17th, and 18th centuries, there would have been little for a health education specialist to do other than promote the misconceptions and half-truths that predominated during the time period. However, health boards, the forerunner of today's health departments, did develop as scientific and medical knowledge increased. The roots of modern health education/promotion were planted, and the first sprouts would soon emerge.

The 1800s

In the first half of the 1800s, little happened to improve the public's health. In England, the streets of London were filthy with animal and human waste. Overcrowding and industrialization added to the problem. These conditions, under which so many people lived and worked, had dire results. Smallpox, cholera, typhoid, tuberculosis, and many other diseases reached high endemic levels (Pickett & Hanlon, 1990).

In 1842, a momentous event occurred in the history of public health when Edwin Chadwick published his *Report on an Inquiry into the Sanitary Conditions of the Labouring Population of Great Britain*. In the report, he documented the deplorable living conditions of Britain's laboring class, made a strong case that these conditions were the cause of much disease and suffering, and called for government intervention. This report eventually led to the formation of a General Board of Health for England in 1848 (Goerke & Stebbins, 1968).

Extraordinary advancements in biology and bacteriology took place by the middle of the 19th century in England and throughout Europe. In 1849, Dr. John Snow, who laboriously studied epidemiological data related to a cholera epidemic in London, hypothesized that the disease was caused by microorganisms in the drinking water from one particular water pump located on Broad Street (see **Figure 2.7**). He removed the pump's handle to keep people from using the water source, and the epidemic abated. Snow's action was remarkable because it predated the discovery that microorganisms cause disease and was in opposition to the prevailing miasmas theory of the time (Johnson, 2006).

In 1862, Louis Pasteur of France proposed his germ theory of disease. After this, advancements in bacteriology greatly accelerated. Over the next 20 years, Pasteur discovered how microorganisms reproduce, introduced the first scientific approach to immunization, and developed a technique to pasteurize milk. Robert Koch, a German scientist, developed the

▶ **Figure 2.7** By removing the handle of this pump, which is still in place on Broad Street in London, John Snow interrupted a cholera epidemic.

criteria and procedures necessary to establish that a particular microbe, and no other, caused a particular disease. Joseph Lister, an English surgeon, developed the antiseptic method of treating wounds by using carbolic acid, and he introduced the principle of asepsis to surgery. These are just a few of the tremendous advancements in bacteriology made during the second half of the 19th century. As a result, the years from 1875 to 1900 became known as the **bacteriological period of public health** (McKenzie et al., 2012).

▷ Public Health in the United States

1700s

During the 1700s, health conditions in the United States were similar to those in Europe—deplorable. Diseases such as smallpox, cholera, and diphtheria were prevalent. Because of the slave trade, diseases such as yaws, yellow fever, and malaria were common in southern states (Marr, 1982). Large numbers of immigrants were entering the ports, cities were growing, overcrowding was common, and the Industrial Revolution was about to begin.

The primary means of controlling disease were quarantine and regulations on environmental cleanliness. For example, as early as 1647, the Massachusetts Bay Colony enacted regulations to prevent pollution of Boston Harbor. In 1701, Massachusetts passed laws allowing for the isolation of smallpox patients and for ship quarantine, as needed. However, there was no overseeing body or agency to enforce compliance.

In an attempt to address health problems, some cities formed local health boards (Pickett & Hanlon, 1990). Prominent citizens who advised elected officials on health-related matters made up these boards. They had no paid staff, no budget, and no authority to enforce regulations. According to tradition, the first health board was formed in Boston in 1799, with Paul Revere as chairman. This is contested, however, by other cities claiming earlier health boards, including Petersburg, Virginia (1780), Baltimore (1793), Philadelphia (1794), and New York (1796).

Life expectancy is one measure of health status for a given population. It is defined as "the average number of years a person from a specific cohort is projected to live from a given

TABLE 2.1 **Expectation of life according to Wigglesworth life table—1789**

Expectation	Years	Expectation	Years
At birth	28.15	At age 50	21.16
At age 5	40.87	At age 55	18.35
At age 10	39.23	At age 60	15.43
At age 15	36.16	At age 65	12.43
At age 20	34.21	At age 70	10.06
At age 25	32.32	At age 75	7.83
At age 30	30.24	At age 80	5.85
At age 35	28.22	At age 85	4.57
At age 40	26.04	At age 90	3.73
At age 45	23.92	At age 95	1.62

Source: Ravenel, M. P. (Ed.). (1970). *A Half Century of Public Health*. New York: Arno Press and *The New York Times*. Originally published in 1921 by American Public Health Association.

point in time" (McKenzie et al., 2012, p. 76). The first life expectancy tables were developed for the United States in 1789 by Dr. Edward Wigglesworth (Ravenel, 1970). **Table 2.1** shows Wigglesworth's table. It provides strong evidence of the prevailing health conditions. In 1789, life expectancy at birth was only 28.15 years. In 2006, life expectancy at birth was 77.7—the highest ever in the United States. By 2020, the projected life expectancy at birth in the United States will be 79.5 years (U.S. National Center for Health Statistics, 2009).

1800s

From 1800 to 1850, health status improved little. Conditions of overcrowding, poverty, and filth worsened as the Industrial Revolution encouraged more and more people to move to the cities. Epidemics of smallpox, yellow fever, cholera, typhoid, and typhus were common. Tuberculosis and malaria also reached exceptionally high levels. For example, in 1850, the Massachusetts tuberculosis death rate was 300 per 100,000 population, and the infant mortality was about 200 per 1,000 live births. Conditions were so bad that life expectancy actually decreased in some cities during this period of time. In Boston, the average age at death dropped from 27.85 years in 1820–1825 to 21.43 in 1840–1845. In New York during the same period, the average age of death decreased from 26.15 to 19.69 (Shattuck, 1850).

Public health reform in the United States was slow to begin. Interestingly, a major report helped jump-start the public health reform movement in the United States, just as Chadwick's landmark 1842 report stimulated public health reform in Britain. Lemuel Shattuck's 1850 *Report of the Sanitary Commission of Massachusetts* contained remarkable insights about the public health issues of Massachusetts, including how to approach and solve these problems. Shattuck was a bookseller and publisher from Boston. He retired early at age 46 and dedicated the remainder of his life to his interest in community affairs (American Public Health Association [APHA 1959]). His report is remarkable because no national or state public health programs existed at the time, and local health agencies that did exist were functioning at a minimal level. Shattuck visualized how to improve the public's health through the initiation of state and local level health departments. "Of the 50 recommendations which Shattuck listed, 36 have become accepted principles of public health practice" (Goerke &

Stebbins, 1968, p. 28). Among his many <u>recommendations</u> were the keeping of vital statistics, environmental sanitation, control of food and drugs, teaching prevention and sanitary science in medical schools, smoke control in cities, control of alcoholism, the supervision of mental disease, exposure of nostrums, preaching health from pulpits, routine physical exams, and the establishment of nurse training schools (APHA, 1959; Pickett & Hanlon, 1990).

The publication of Shattuck's report did not mean an end to the public health problems in the United States. In fact, <u>the report went unnoticed for 19 years until 1869,</u> when the Commonwealth of Massachusetts established a state board of health made up of physicians and laymen exactly as Shattuck had envisioned. One year later, Virginia and California formed their own state boards of health (Ravenel, 1970). By 1900, 38 states had established state boards of health. Today, every U.S. state has a state board or department of health.

Despite the formation of state boards of health, state-level health departments could not meet health needs on a more local level. With limited resources, there was simply too much to accomplish. As a result, the first full-time county health departments were formed in Guilford County, North Carolina, and Yakima County, Washington, in 1911. Some sources have cited Jefferson County, Kentucky, as the first county health department, set up in 1908 (Pickett & Hanlon, 1990).

As states initiated boards of health, board members had to interact, communicate, and develop their skills. These needs led to the founding of the American Public Health Association (APHA). (See Chapter 8 for more information on the APHA.) Following a series of national conventions on quarantine held from 1857 through 1860, "Stephen Smith invited a group of 'refined gentlemen' to discuss informally the possibility of a national sanitary association" (Bernstein, 1972, p. 2). Smith's suggestion of an association for health officials and interested citizens was well received. A decision was made to establish a committee to work on a permanent organization. One year later, in 1873, the first annual meeting was held in Cincinnati, Ohio, and 70 new members were elected. Smith remained active in the association throughout his life. At the age of 99, he walked to the podium unassisted to speak at the 50th anniversary celebration of the APHA.

The federal government started a public health service that dates back to 1798, when Congress passed the Marine Hospital Service Act. Previously, sailors in the merchant marine had nowhere to turn for health care. Because they paid no local or state taxes, ill or injured sailors generally were not welcomed in port cities. The Marine Hospital Service Act required the owners of every ship to pay the tax collector 20 cents per month for every seaman they employed. This money was used to build hospitals and provide medical services in all major seaport cities (see **Figure 2.8**). This act "represented the first prepaid medical and hospital insurance plan in the world, under the administrative supervision of what eventually became a public health agency" (Pickett & Hanlon, 1990, p. 34).

Successive legislation throughout the 19th century gradually expanded the scope of the Marine Hospital Service. In 1902, Congress retitled it the Public Health and Marine Hospital Service and gave it a definite organizational structure under the direction of the surgeon general. In 1912, "Marine Hospital" was dropped from the name, and the service became known as it is today, the U.S. Public Health Service. "The mission of the U.S. Public Health Service Commissioned Corps is to protect, promote, and advance the health and safety of our Nation" (U.S. Public Health Service, 2013).

In 1879, Congress created the National Board of Health. The board was comprised of seven members appointed by the president, including representatives of the army, navy,

▲ **Figure 2.8** Old Marine Hospital in Charleston, South Carolina, 1934

Marine Hospital Service, and Justice Department. Its functions were to obtain information on all matters related to public health, and provide grants-in-aid to state boards of health. The National Board also provided money to university scientists for health-related research. Unfortunately, the board was short-lived. In administering quarantine functions, the board incurred opposition from state agencies and private shipping concerns. Others in positions of power were not in favor of the research grant program and felt such expenditures were extravagant. Thus, in 1882, the board's appropriations were transferred to the Marine Hospital Service, which carried on with the quarantine functions but discontinued the grant program (U.S. Department of Health, Education, and Welfare [USDHEW], 1976).

1900 to Present

The period from 1900 to 1920 is known as the **reform phase of public health** (McKenzie et al., 2012). During this time, urban areas expanded, and many people lived and worked in deplorable conditions. To address these concerns, federal regulations were passed concerning the food industry, states passed workers' compensation laws, the U.S. Bureau of Mines, and the U.S. Department of Labor were created, and the first clinic for occupational diseases was established. By the end of the 1920s, the movement for healthier workplace conditions was well established, and the average life expectancy had risen to 59.7 years.

Also during this period, the first national voluntary agencies were formed. They were run primarily by volunteers along with a few paid staff. Each of these agencies was designed to address a specific health problem. For example, the National Association for the Study and Prevention of Tuberculosis was established in 1902, and the American Cancer Society was founded in 1913. Today, volunteer agencies continue to be important players in the prevention of disease and the promotion of health (McKenzie et al., 2012).

The 1920s were a relatively quiet period in public health. Progress continued, but at a slower pace. However, the Public Health Education Section of the APHA was founded in 1922 (Bernstein, 1972). This is the APHA section to which most health education specialists belong. It "promotes the advancement of the health promotion and education profession and provides a forum for public health educators and those involved in health promotion activities to discuss ideas, research, and training; promotes activities related to training public health professionals" (APHA, 2013).

The need for health education/promotion existed in the early 20th century. Moore's book about public health in the United States (1923) included two chapters on questionable and unreliable health activities. One of the most interesting examples involved a cure-all product known as Tanlac. The May 11, 1917, edition of the *Holyoke Daily Transcript* contained Fred Wicks' testimonial in a Tanlac advertisement, as well as his obituary (Moore, 1923, pp. 173–174).

Other examples of questionable health practices also abound. William Harvey Kellogg and his younger brother W. K., founders of the Kellogg cereal company, were best known in the early 1900s for the sanitarium they established and operated in Battle Creek, Michigan. The rich and famous came from all over the world to be treated at the sanitarium. Many of the treatment modalities, however, would be considered questionable and even quackery by today's standards. For example, they used some 200 different types of hydrotherapy along with therapeutic enemas, electric horses, vibrators, and cold air (Butler, Thornton, & Stoltz, 1994). However, the sanitarium did promote exercise and good nutrition as ways to prevent and treat disease. (See **Figure 2.9**.) The concept of prevention was beginning to take hold.

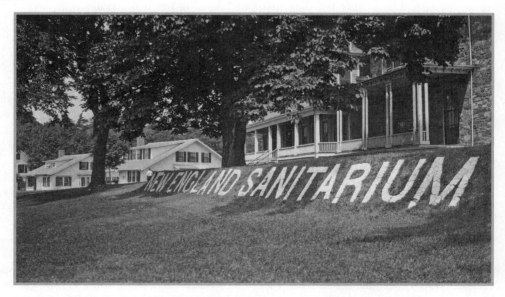

▲ **Figure 2.9** Sanitariums could be found throughout the United States in the early 1900s.

Tension between preventive medicine and curative medicine began to appear in the United States during the early 20th century. Moore (1923) related a story about a town in which public health work had banished malaria. A physician was asked how his profession had been affected by this public health advancement. He replied off-handedly, "If it hadn't been for the influenza, I'd have gone broke. That saved us" (p. 373).

In a more rational manner, Newsholme (1936) noted three reasons that treatment formed a larger part of public health efforts than prevention and why it would continue to do so in the future. First, the knowledge to prevent disease and death was only partial. Medical workers simply did not have the knowledge and skills to prevent many disease states. Second, even when knowledge to prevent disease did exist, many people did not know about it, and those that did found it difficult to make those changes necessary to prevent disease. Third, there were such a large number of sick people needing prompt medical treatment that it was difficult to focus attention on prevention. Many of the same arguments are used today to account for the emphasis on traditional medical interventions instead of prevention.

From 1930 through World War II, the role of federal government in social programs expanded. Prior to the Great Depression, medical services were provided by relatives and friends, as well as by religious organizations and some voluntary agencies. During the Depression, however, private resources could not meet the demands of those requiring assistance. In 1933, President Franklin D. Roosevelt created numerous agencies and programs as part of his New Deal, which improved the plight of the disadvantaged. Much of the money was used for public health efforts, including the control of malaria, the building of hospitals, and the construction of municipal water and sewage systems.

The Social Security Act of 1935 was a real milestone and the beginning of the federal government's involvement in social issues, including health. The act provided support for state health departments and their programs. Funding was made available to develop sanitary facilities and to improve maternal and child health.

Two major public health agencies were formed at this time. On May 26, 1930, the Ransdell Act converted the Hygienic Laboratory to the National Institute of Health, with a broad mandate to learn the cause, prevention, and cure of disease (USDHEW, 1976). The National Institutes of Health, as it is called today, is now one of the premiere—if not *the* premiere— medical research facilities in the world. In 1946, the Communicable Disease Center was established in Atlanta, Georgia. Now called the Centers for Disease Control and Prevention (CDC), it is one of the world's leading epidemiological centers. (See **Figure 2.10**.) The CDC is also a major training facility for health communications and educational methods (Pickett & Hanlon, 1990). The CDC's vision for the 21st century is "Health Protection…Health Equity" (CDC, 2013h). Its mission is "Collaborating to create the expertise, information, and tools that people and communities need to protect their health—through health promotion, prevention of disease, injury and disability, and preparedness for new health threats" (CDC, 2013h).

Following World War II, concern rose over the number of healthcare facilities and the adequacy of the care they provided. In 1946, Congress passed the National Hospital Survey and Construction Act, also known as the Hill-Burton Act, to improve the distribution and enhance the quality of hospitals. From the passage of the Hill-Burton Act through the 1960s, new hospital construction occurred rapidly. Little thought, however, was given to planning.

▶ **Figure 2.10** CDC's "Arlen Specter Headquarters and Emergency Operations Center" located on CDC's Roybal campus in Atlanta, Georgia

As a result, hospitals were built too close together and provided overlapping and unnecessary services (McKenzie et al., 2012).

In 1954, Dr. Mayhew Derryberry, the first chief of health education in the federal government, noted, "The health problems of greatest significance today are the chronic diseases.... The extent of chronic diseases, various disabling conditions, and the economic burden that they impose have been thoroughly documented" (*Voices From the Past,* 2004, p. 368). Before the 1950s, the major emphasis of public health had been on communicable or contagious diseases. However, through improved public health services, medical care, and immunization programs, many contagious diseases no longer threatened as they once had, and the focus shifted ever so slowly to the prevention of chronic diseases. Derryberry predicted how this change of focus would impact health education: "Health education and health educators will be expected to contribute to the reduction of the negative impact of such major health problems as heart disease, cancer, dental disease, mental illness and other neurological disturbances, obesity, accidents and the adjustments necessary to a productive old age" (*Voices From the Past,* 2004, p. 368). Although the seed may have been planted for health education specialists to play a greater role in the prevention of chronic diseases, it was not until the 1970s that the seed finally sprouted.

Public health prevention

In 1965, the federal government again passed major legislation designed to improve the health of the U.S. population. Although major improvements were made in health facilities and the quality of health care, there were still many underserved people. Most of these people were either poor or elderly. In response, Congress passed the Medicare and Medicaid bills as amendments to the Social Security Act of 1935. **Medicare** was created to assist in the payment of medical bills for the elderly, whereas **Medicaid** did the same for the poor. These bills provided medical care for millions of people who could not otherwise have obtained such services.

It was evident by the 1970s that disease prevention held the greatest potential for improving Americans' health and reducing healthcare costs. The first national effort to promote the health of citizens through a more preventive approach took place in Canada. In 1974, the Canadian Ministry of Health and Welfare released a publication titled *A New Perspective on the Health of Canadians* (Lalonde, 1974). This document, often called the *Lalonde Report,* presented epidemiological evidence that supported the importance of lifestyle and environmental factors. It called for numerous national health promotion strategies that encouraged Canadians to be more responsible for their own health. (See Chapter 1 for information on the Health Field Concept associated with this publication.) The Lalonde Report influenced many U.S. health professionals to rethink current assumptions that focused on high-technology, treatment-based medicine. So important was this report that Bates and Winder (1984) likened it to a re-emergence of Hygeia and the beginning of the second public health revolution (p. 24).

HEALTHY PEOPLE INITIATIVES AND PUBLIC HEALTH STANDARDS

In the United States, the government publication *Healthy People* was the first major recognition of the importance of lifestyle in promoting health and well-being (U.S. Public Health Service, 1979). This publication supported a shift from the traditional medical model toward lifestyle and environmental strategies that emphasized prevention.

In 1980, *Promoting Health/Preventing Disease: Objectives for the Nation* was released. This federal document contained 226 U.S. health objectives for the United States, divided into three areas: preventive services, health protection, and health promotion. These objectives provided the framework for public health efforts during the 1980s. They allowed public health professionals to focus on key areas while providing baseline data for measuring progress (U.S. Department of Health and Human Services [USDHHS], 1980). Although not all of these objectives were met, the planning and evaluation process used to develop them became a valuable way to measure progress in U.S. health and healthcare services. This led to the practice of developing U.S. health objectives each decade. In 1990, *Healthy People 2000: National Health Promotion and Disease Prevention Objectives* was released, and in 2000, *Healthy People 2010: Understanding and Improving Health* was released.

The Healthy People initiative has evolved into an important strategic planning tool for public health professionals at the federal, state, and local levels. Formal reviews measure the progress of these objectives at mid-course (halfway through the 10-year period) and again at the end of 10 years. The mid-course review provides an opportunity to update the document based on events that may impact the objectives. For example, in *Healthy People 2010,* a number of objectives were changed, updated, or deleted because of 9/11 and Hurricanes Katrina and Rita (2005). The results of both the mid-course and end reviews along with other available data are used to help create the next set of goals and objectives.

TABLE 2.2 *Healthy People 2020* Vision, Mission, and Goals

Vision

A society in which all people live long, healthy lives.

Mission

Healthy People 2020 strives to:

- Identify nationwide health improvement priorities;
- Increase public awareness and understanding of the determinants of health, disease, and disability and the opportunities for progress;
- Provide measurable objectives and goals that are applicable at the national, state, and local levels;
- Engage multiple sectors to take actions to strengthen policies and improve practices that are driven by the best available evidence and knowledge;
- Identify critical research, evaluation and data collection needs.

Overarching Goals

- Attain high quality, longer lives free of preventable disease, disability, injury, and premature death.
- Achieve health equity, eliminate disparities, and improve the health of all groups.
- Create social and physical environments that promote good health for all.
- Promote quality of life, healthy development and healthy behaviors across all life stages.

Source: U.S. Department of Health and Human Services. (2010). *Developing Healthy People 2020.*

Healthy People 2020 was released in December 2010 and will guide U.S. public health practice and health education specialists for the next 10 years. The Healthypeople.gov Web site has replaced the traditional hard copy of the report with a user friendly Web site where the entire report can be searched and accessed. The vision statement, mission statement, and four overarching goals of *Healthy People 2020* can be seen in **Table 2.2** (CDC, 2013a). The meat of the report includes numerous objectives spread over 42 different topic areas (see **Table 2.3**) (CDC, 2013g).

TABLE 2.3 *Healthy People 2020* Topic Areas

1. Access to Health Services
2. Adolescent Health
3. Arthritis, Osteoporosis, and Chronic Back
4. Blood Disorders and Blood Safety
5. Cancer
6. Chronic Kidney Diseases
7. Dementias, Including Alzheimer's Disease
8. Diabetes
9. Disability and Health
10. Early and Middle Childhood
11. Educational and Community-Based Programs
12. Environmental Health
13. Family Planning
14. Food Safety

continued

TABLE 2.3 *continued*

15. Genomics
16. Global Health
17. Healthcare Associated Infections
18. Health Communication and Health Information Technology
19. Health Related Quality of Life and Well-Being
20. Hearing and Other Sensory or Communication Disorders
21. Heart Disease and Stroke
22. HIV
23. Immunization and Infectious Diseases
24. Injury and Violence Prevention
25. Lesbian, Gay, Bisexual, and Transgender Health
26. Maternal, Infant, and Child Health
27. Medical Product Safety
28. Mental Health and Mental Disorders
29. Nutrition and Weight Status
30. Occupational Health
31. Older Adults
32. Oral Health
33. Physical Activity
34. Preparedness
35. Public Health Infrastructure
36. Respiratory Diseases
37. Sexually Transmitted Diseases
38. Sleep Health
39. Social Determinants of Health
40. Substance Abuse
41. Tobacco Use
42. Vision

Source: U.S. Department of Health and Human Services. (2013). *Healthy People 2020 Topic Areas.* Retrieved May 29, 2013, from www.cdc.gov/nchs/healthy_people/hp2020_topic_areas.htm.

For *Healthy People 2020* to be effective, programs must be developed and initiated to meet the established goals. This means that partner states, counties, communities, organizations, and individuals must get involved. The CDC uses a simple but powerful model to guide partners in establishing effective programs known as MAP-IT. (See **Figure 2.11**.) The MAP-IT model guides partners through five steps: mobilize, assess, plan, implement, and

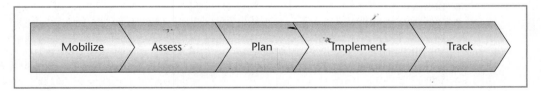

Mobilize ⟩ Assess ⟩ Plan ⟩ Implement ⟩ Track

▲ **Figure 2.11** MAP-IT
Source: http://healthypeople.gov/2020/implement/mapit.aspx

track (CDC, 2013e). It is important to note that the five MAP-IT steps are similar to four of the seven responsibilities of a health education specialist that you will learn more about later in this text (Chapter 6). The health education specialist responsibilities are to assess, plan, implement, and evaluate.

Another important initiative designed, in part, to improve the effectiveness of public health departments working on Healthy People objectives is the National Public Health Performance Standards Program (NPHPSP) (CDC, 2013f). This is a partnership initiative to develop performance standards; collect, monitor, and analyze data; and ultimately improve public health performance. It is the first time that a common, systematic strategy for measuring public health performance has been available. The goals of the program are to

- provide performance standards for public health systems and encouraging their widespread use;
- encourage and leverage national, state, and local partnerships to build a stronger foundation for public health preparedness;
- promote continuous quality improvement of public health systems;
- strengthen the science base for public health practice improvement (CDC, 2013f).

Local and state health departments are encouraged to use these performance standard assessments to conduct their own self-assessments. Through this process, weaknesses can be identified and improvements made to enhance the overall performance of public health departments (CDC, 2013f).

HEALTH EDUCATION/PROMOTION: A RECOGNIZED PROFESSION

One more important historical event for health education/promotion occurred on October 27, 1997, when the Standard Occupational Classification (SOC) Policy Review Committee approved the creation of a new, distinct classification for the occupation of health educator (Auld, 1997/1998). Health educators had pursued this goal for more than 25 years. Health educators were previously included in the category "Instructional Coordinator," a broad, primarily education-related category that failed to consider the many varied and unique responsibilities of health educators. Approval of health education as a separate occupational classification means that the Department of Labor's Bureau of Labor Statistics, the Department of Commerce's Bureau of the Census, and all other federal agencies that collect occupational data now collect data on health education specialists. Many state and local governments also maintain data on health education/promotion. For the first time, it is possible to determine the number of health education specialists employed and the outlook for future health education/promotion positions. This approval is one more sign that health education/promotion is gaining the respect and recognition it deserves.

In summary, tremendous advancements in public health and health education/promotion took place during the 20th century. It could reasonably be argued that the total number of advancements in public health during the 20th century were equal to or greater than the total number of public health advancements in all prior time. In reflecting on these great successes of public health, the Department of Health and Human Services identified 10 public health achievements they believed had the greatest impact on major causes of morbidity and mortality of the 20th century. **Box 2.2** lists these 10 achievements. Imagine what life would be like today if none of these achievements had been realized. Think of the role health education/promotion has played in these advancements.

School Health in the United States

Life in early America was hard, and there was little time for education. The labor of building homes, clearing forests, tilling fields, hunting, and preparing food filled the days. Most people lived under primitive conditions. Settlements were few and far apart. Travel and transportation were costly, slow, and limited to foot, horseback, boat, or wagon.

In the mid-1600s, as communities became more established, the call for education was soon heard. Religion had always been an important part of life in America, and it was the religious leaders who led the drive for education. They believed that Satan benefited when people were illiterate, because they could not read the scriptures. In 1647, Massachusetts passed the "Old Deluder" law to prevent Satan from deluding the people by keeping them from reading the Bible. The law specified that a town with 50 families should establish an elementary school, and a town with 100 households should set up a Latin grammar secondary school (Means, 1962).

The curriculum in these early schools was largely derived from the educational practices in England. Essentially, reading, as the avenue to religious understanding, was the primary subject. Writing, spelling, grammar, and arithmetic supplemented reading. Later, geography and history were added, but the teaching of health was not part of the early education system in the United States.

Because only boys attended these early schools, and working for the family was still a major concern, daily sessions were by necessity of short duration. The length of the school term was usually only a few months. Teachers were lacking in preparation, with their basic qualifications being only to (1) read, (2) know more of the Bible than the students, (3) work cheap, and (4) keep the students under control. Teachers were totally dependent on the rod for classroom management (Means, 1962).

School buildings typically were inadequate (see **Figure 2.12**). They were poorly built, inaccessible, and sometimes temporary structures. Their interiors were inadequately lighted, were furnished with uncomfortable seating, had no sanitary facilities, and were heated with wood-burning stoves. These schools were not even close to meeting modern standards for school construction (Means, 1962).

The schools and their curricula remained much the same until the 1800s. By the mid-1800s, most schools had become tax supported, and attendance was compulsory. Those concerned about public health pointed out the numerous health and safety problems in the

▶ **Figure 2.12** An old one-room schoolhouse

schools. These concerns helped bring attention to the conditions of the schools and ultimately paved the way for health instruction in the curriculum (Means, 1962).

Horace Mann, whose writings and speeches promoted the importance of education in general, was perhaps the first spokesperson for teaching health in schools. He was elected secretary of the Massachusetts State Board of Education in 1837. Beginning in 1837 with the publication of his *First Annual Report* and continuing through the publication of the *Sixth Annual Report* in 1843, Mann called for mandatory hygiene programs that would help students understand their bodies and the relationship between their behaviors and health (Rubinson & Alles, 1984).

Another momentous event in the development of school health occurred in 1850, when Lemuel Shattuck from Massachusetts wrote his *Report on the Sanitary Commission of Massachusetts* (1850). (This is the same report discussed previously in reference to public health.) Although the report has become a classic in the field of public health, it also provided strong support for school health (Means, 1975). In the report, Shattuck (1850) eloquently supports the teaching of physiology, as the term *health education* had yet to be coined:

> It has recently been recommended that the science of physiology be taught in the public schools; and the recommendation should be universally approved and carried into effect as soon as persons can be found capable of teaching it.... Every child should be taught early in life, that to preserve his own life and his own health and the lives and health of others, is one of the most important and constantly abiding duties. By obeying certain laws or performing certain acts, his life and health may be preserved; by disobedience, or performing certain other acts, they will both be destroyed. By knowing and avoiding the causes of disease, disease itself will be avoided, and he may enjoy health and live; by ignorance of these causes and exposure to them, he may contract disease, ruin his health, and die. Every thing connected with wealth, happiness and long life depend upon health; and even the great duties of morals and religion are performed more acceptably in a healthy than a sickly condition. (pp. 178–179)

Aside from local and state attempts to promote the teaching of health-related curricula in the schools, no concerted national effort existed until that of the Women's Christian Temperance Union. Originally founded in 1874, the union expounded on the evils of alcohol, narcotics, and tobacco through every conceivable means and was one of the most effective lobbying organizations ever (Means, 1962). Between 1880 and 1890, every state in the union passed a law requiring instruction concerning the effects of alcohol and narcotics due to stimulus from the Temperance Movement (Turner, Sellery, & Smith, 1957).

Other national movements soon followed. In 1915, the National Tuberculosis Association introduced the "Modern Health Crusade" as a device for promoting the health of school children. It was based on promotion to "knighthood" for those that followed certain health habits. The Child Health Organization of America encouraged the nation to adopt more functional health education/promotion programs. One of its active leaders, Sally Lucas Jean, was ultimately responsible for changing the name from hygiene education to health education (Means, 1962). With this name change, the focus of health education shifted from that of physiology and hygiene, which was factual and unrelated to everyday living, to an emphasis on healthy living and health behavior.

Despite these advancements, health education from 1900 to 1920 was generally characterized by inconsistency and awkward progress. World War I provided the impetus for widespread acceptance of school health education as a discipline in its own right (Turner, Sellery, & Smith, 1957). Out of 2,510,706 men examined as potential military draftees during World War I, 730,756 (29 percent) were rejected on physical grounds. A large portion of these physical deficiencies could have been prevented if the schools had been doing their part to train children concerning health and fitness (Andress & Bragg, 1922). In the immediate postwar years, 16 states required hygiene instruction in their public schools; 12 of these states made provisions for the preparation of health teachers in the teacher training schools supported by the state (Rogers, 1936).

Significant research and demonstration projects related to school health education were conducted in the 1920s and 1930s. Examples include the Malden, Massachusetts, project, done in cooperation with the Massachusetts Institute of Technology; the Mansfield, Ohio, project supported by the American Red Cross; the Fargo, North Dakota, project sponsored by the Commonwealth Fund; and the Cattaraugus County, New York, project financed by the Milband Memorial Fund. According to Turner, Sellery, and Smith (1957), "these programs showed that habits could be changed and health improved through health education" (p. 27).

In the 1930s, the drive for health education from the public slowed. Health education continued to address the major health issues of the time but without the enthusiasm brought on by World War I. Notable research studies supplemented authoritative opinion in helping to point out difficulties and offer solutions related to the teaching of health education. Several important conferences were held on health education and youth health at the national level (Means, 1962). The profession was moving forward.

Professional organizations emerged during the 1900s that still exist today. School health education, long associated with physical education, received official recognition in 1937, when the American Physical Education Association became the American Association for Health and Physical Education. One year later, recreation was added to the association, and the name changed to the American Association for Health, Physical Education and Recreation (AAHPER). In the 1970s, dance was added to the organization, making the acronym AAHPERD. In the 1990s AAHPERD changed from an association to an alliance of national and district associations, each representing one of the AAPHERD professions or all professions in a particular district of the United States. The national association that represented health education specialists was the American Association for Health Education

(AAHE). For many years AAHE was a major force in the health education field. At their 2013 National Convention, AAHPERD dropped the association structure and went back to one organization with a mission to, "advance professional practice and promote research related to health and physical education, physical activity, dance, and sport" (AAHPERD, 2013). This means that AAHE is no longer in existence. Although AAHPERD still intends to service those school health educators that also teach physical education, most health education specialists including those focused on school health will want to join another professional association such as the Society for Public Health Education, which represents all health education specialists, or the American School Health Association.

The American School Health Association evolved from the American Association of School Physicians, which was founded in 1927. Over the next 10 years this association of school physicians expanded its functions, interests, and scope of activity. As a result, it broadened its membership to include school health personnel other than physicians. In 1938, its name was changed to the American School Health Association to reflect these changes.

The American Public Health Association had long been an organization interested in and supportive of school health. In fact, many of the earliest supporters of health education in the schools had been leaders in public health. Appropriately, the organization established a separate section within its administrative structure to focus on school health interests. In 1942, the School Health Section of the American Public Health Association was formed. (Chapter 8 discusses in greater detail these professional associations.)

With the bombing of Pearl Harbor on December 7, 1941, the United States found itself at war. Once again, national focus turned to physical fitness and health. With no major threats of war in the previous 20 years, the physical status of young U.S. men had again degenerated. Of the approximately 2 million men examined for induction into the nation's armed forces, almost 50 percent were disqualified. Of those disqualified, 90 percent were found to be physically or mentally unfit (American Youth Commission, 1942). This unfortunate situation helped greatly to stimulate interest in the health of high school students and provided strong motivation for health education/promotion classes.

Following the war years, many demonstration projects and studies were again completed to examine the impact of school health education. The Massachusetts High School Study, the Astoria Study, the New York City Study, and the Denver Study were just a few of the efforts that provided valuable information on school health education (Means, 1975).

After World War II, school health education continued to grow as a profession. As Means (1975) observed, "This period from 1940 into the 1970s was one of appraisal, re-evaluation, and consolidation with respect to research accomplished in school health education. During this time leaders in the field attempted to look back, review, and take stock of what was known as a determinant of future action" (p. 107).

The **School Health Education Study** was a major study of significance to school health education. Directed by Dr. Elena M. Sliepcevich (1964), the study included 135 randomly selected school systems involving 1,460 schools and 840,832 students in 38 states. Health behavior inventories were administered to students in grades 6, 9, and 12. The results were appalling. Health misconceptions among students at all levels prevailed. Questionnaires were distributed to school administrators throughout the country to obtain data on organizational procedures and instructional practices related to school health education. Again the results indicated major problems in the organization and administration of health programs. Cortese (1993) noted, "...some health topics were omitted while others were repeated grade after grade at the same level of sophistication. No logical rationale placed learning exercises at various grade levels, and a need existed for a challenging and meaningful curriculum" (p. 21).

The second phase of the school Health Education Study established a curriculum writing team to develop a school health education curriculum based on needs identified from the first phase of the study. The team consisted of prominent names in school health education, including Gus T. Dalis, Edward B. Johns, Richard K. Means, Ann E. Nolte, Marion B. Pollock, and Robert D. Russell (Means, 1975). Over the next eight years, the writing team developed a comprehensive curriculum package that still influences school health curricula today.

The **School Health Education Evaluation Study** of the Los Angeles Area was one more important study. Its purpose was to evaluate the effectiveness of school health work in selected schools and colleges of the area. More specifically, the project aimed at the appraisal of the entire school health program, including administrative organization, school health services, health instruction, and healthful school environment. Further, it examined the students' health knowledge, attitudes, and behavior. The study resulted in 11 conclusions and 17 important recommendations for the field. Of equal importance, the study's planning, design, and operational process established a research pattern that has provided a model for the development of subsequent similar studies (Means, 1975).

School health programs have continued to evolve from the mid-1970s to the present. Several important events and trends have impacted school health education and overall school health programs. In 1978, the Office of Comprehensive School Health was established within the U.S. Department of Education. The primary purpose of the office was policy development for health issues that affected children and youth. Although the office held great promise for school health education efforts, unfortunately, it was never fully funded. A director was named, Peter Cortese, but the office was finally deactivated with the budget cuts during President Ronald Reagan's administration (Rubinson & Alles, 1984).

The 1980s saw the emergence of two important concepts: coordinated school health programs and comprehensive school health instruction. Based on the initial ideas of Turner, Sellery, and Smith (1957), and later refined by Allensworth and Kolbe (1987), a **coordinated school health program** consisting of eight interactive components that work together to enhance the health and well-being of the students, faculty, staff, and community was devised (see **Figure 2.13**). Leaders involved in each of these eight components work as an integrated team to coordinate the program (CDC, 2013c). Outside leadership is provided by a **school health advisory council (SHAC)**. The SHAC is formed by community members (such as parents; medical, health, and safety professionals; and political, religious, and corporate or business leaders) to assist with the planning and promotion of school health initiatives.

Comprehensive school health instruction is actually the curricular component of the coordinated school health program (see **Box 2.3**). It refers to the development and delivery of a planned, sequential, effective school health instruction program. Topics include, but are not limited to alcohol and other drugs, asthma, crisis preparedness, food safety, infectious diseases, injury and violence prevention, mental health, noise-induced hearing loss, sexual risk behaviors and pregnancy prevention, skin cancer, tobacco use, vaccines and immunizations (CDC, 2013d) The curriculum should be taught by a trained health education specialist and "designed to motivate and assist students to maintain and improve their health, prevent disease, and reduce health-related risk behaviors" (CDC, 2010b). Emphasis should be placed on six specific adolescent risk behaviors that are monitored by the Youth Risk Behavior Surveillance System (YRBSS) (CDC, 2013i). These six behaviors contribute to the leading causes of death and disability

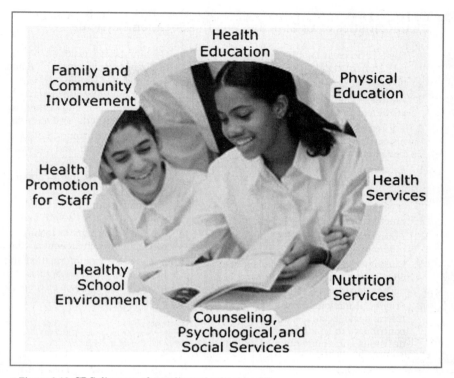

▲ **Figure 2.13** CDC diagram of coordinated school health
Source: CDC

among youth and adults. These behaviors usually are established during childhood, persist into adulthood, are inter-related, and are preventable. These risk behaviors are as follows:

- Behaviors that contribute to unintentional injuries and violence
- Sexual behaviors that contribute to unintended pregnancy and sexually transmitted diseases, including HIV infection
- Alcohol and other drug use
- Tobacco use
- Unhealthy dietary behaviors
- Inadequate physical activity (CDC, 2013i)

In 2006, the American Cancer Society released the second edition of the National Health Education Standards (see **Box 2.4**). The goal of the National Health Education Standards is improved educational achievement for students and improved health in the United States. The standards promote **health literacy**, the capacity of individuals to access, interpret, and understand basic health information and services, and the skills to use the information and services to promote health. The standards provide a foundation for curriculum development, instruction, and assessment of student performance. A rationale and numerous performance indicators, broken down by grade-level groupings, accompany each of the eight

BOX
2.3

Characteristics of an Effective Health Education Curricula

1. Focuses on clear health goals and related behavioral outcomes.
2. Is research based and theory-driven.
3. Addresses individual values, attitudes, and beliefs.
4. Addresses individual and group norms that support health-enhancing behaviors.
5. Focuses on reinforcing protective factors and increasing perceptions of personal risk and harmfulness of engaging in specific unhealthy practices and behaviors.
6. Addresses social pressures and influences.
7. Builds personal competence, social competence, and self-efficacy by addressing skills.
8. Provides functional health knowledge that is basic, accurate, and directly contributes to health-promoting decisions and behaviors.

9. Uses strategies designed to personalize information and engage students.
10. Provides age-appropriate and developmentally appropriate information, learning strategies, teaching methods, and materials.
11. Incorporates learning strategies, teaching methods and materials that are culturally inclusive.
12. Provides time for instruction and learning.
13. Provides opportunities to reinforce skills and positive health behaviors.
14. Provides opportunities to make positive connections with influential others.
15. Includes teacher information and plans for professional development and training that enhance effectiveness of instruction and student learning.

Source: Centers for Disease Control and Prevention (CDC). (2013). *Characteristics of an Effective Health Education Curricula* Available at: http://www.cdc.gov/healthyyouth/SHER/characteristics/index.htm

standards. The National Health Education Standards also provide an important guide for colleges and universities to enhance preprofessional preparation as well as the continuing education of health education/promotion teachers.

The National Board for Professional Teaching Standards, founded in 1987, developed national standards for school health education teachers. These standards go beyond the requirements for state teacher licensure. Since fall 2008, individuals with three years of full-time health education/promotion teaching experience and a valid state teacher's license for those three years may voluntarily complete a rigorous evaluation process to become a National Board Certified Health Education Teacher. This National Board Certification places school health education on an equal level with other teaching fields and allows highly qualified and dedicated health education teachers to be recognized for their work. Many states and districts provide salary bonuses for these highly qualified teachers who obtain National Board Certification (National Board for Professional Teaching Standards, 2010). It is expected that many exceptional and highly dedicated health education/promotion teachers will seek National Board Certification.

Since 1987, the concept of a coordinated school health program has dominated the school health arena. At first glance, it would seem that schools would be excited to initiate comprehensive school health programs. How could they not embrace a concept that would bring together multiple components of the school in an integrated attempt to improve the health of faculty, staff, students, and the community? A healthy child taught by a healthy teacher

National Health Education Standards

Health Education Standard 1—Students will comprehend concepts related to health promotion and disease prevention to enhance health.

Health Education Standard 2—Students will analyze the influence of family, peers, culture, media, technology, and other factors on health behaviors.

Health Education Standard 3—Students will demonstrate the ability to access valid information and products and services to enhance health.

Health Education Standard 4—Students will demonstrate the ability to use interpersonal communication skills to enhance health and avoid or reduce health risks.

Health Education Standard 5—Students will demonstrate the ability to use decision-making skills to enhance health.

Health Education Standard 6—Students will demonstrate the ability to use goal-setting skills to enhance health.

Health Education Standard 7—Students will demonstrate the ability to practice health-enhancing behaviors and avoid or reduce health risks.

Health Education Standard 8—Students will demonstrate the ability to advocate for personal, family, and community health.

Source: Reprinted with permission from the American Cancer Society. *National Health Education Standards Achieving Excellence, Second Edition.* (Atlanta, GA: American Cancer Society; 2007), 8, http://www.cancer.org/bookstore

in a health-conscious community should forward the school's overall mission to provide each child with the best education possible. Unfortunately, the full potential of coordinated school health programs has never been realized in most school districts. Factors may include the low priority placed on health by many school administrators; a lack of leadership to promote, coordinate, and oversee school health programs; and an overemphasis on competency testing. Another dynamic could be the adverse reactions from conservative groups that perceive coordinated school health as a means of incorporating sex education into the curriculum.

Despite the apparent lack of success with coordinated school health programs, schools still hold tremendous promise for health education/promotion efforts. With 55 million young people attending more than 132,700 schools (CDC, 2013a), health education specialists must remain diligent in their effort to bring health promotion and education programs to this population. Every health education specialist should be advocating for coordinated school health programs with national and state education agencies, federal and state government representatives, and local school boards.

▷ Patient Protection and Affordable Care Act

On March 23, 2010, amid both fanfare and criticism, President Barack Obama signed into law the Patient Protection and Affordable Care Act. Through a combination of cost controls, subsidies, and mandates, it expands healthcare coverage to 31 million uninsured Americans (Open Congress, 2010). Another important feature is the act's focus on prevention and prevention services (Koh & Sebelius, 2010; Society for Public Health Education [SOPHE], 2013). The bill provides better access to clinical prevention services by removing cost barriers. Further, the bill encourages and promotes worksite wellness programs, encourages evidence-based community prevention and wellness programs, and provides strong support for school-based health centers. (See **Table 2.4** for a summary of the act's prevention provisions.) This bill should create new and expanded opportunities for health education

TABLE 2.4 **Wellness and Prevention Provisions in the Patient Protection and Affordable Care Act (H.R. 3590)**

Immediate Effects 2010

- Establish the National Prevention, Health Promotion and Public Health Council
- Create a Prevention and Public Health Fund—500 million in FY 2010
- Create task forces on prevention services and community preventive services
- Establish a grant program to support the delivery of evidence-based and community-based prevention and wellness services
- Conduct a national worksite health policies and programs survey
- Award grants to support the operation of school-based health centers—50 million in FY 2010
- Eliminate cost sharing for tobacco cessation counseling and prescriptions for pregnant women in Medicaid and Medicare

2011

- National strategy to improve nation's health due March 2011
- Prevention & Public Health Fund receives up to $750 million
- School-based health centers receive another $50 million
- Improve access by eliminating cost sharing for prevention services in Medicare and Medicaid
- Provide grants to small employers to establish wellness programs
- Require chain restaurants and food from vending machines to disclose nutritional content

2012

- Worksite survey results due
- Prevention & Public Health Fund receives up to $1 billion
- School based health centers receive up to $50 million

2013

- Prevention & Public Health Fund receives up to $1.25 billion
- School-based health centers receive up to $50 million

2014

- Permit employers to offer employee rewards in the form of premium discounts, waivers of cost sharing, or other benefits for participating in a wellness program and meeting certain health-related standards
- Establish 10-state pilot program allowing states to apply similar rewards as noted above for employers
- Prevention & Public Health Fund receives up to $1.5 billion
- School-based health centers receive up to $50 million

2015 and Beyond

- Prevention & Public Health Fund receives up to $1.25 billion
- School-based health centers receive up to $50 million

Source: From Society for Public Health Education (SOPHE). 2010. What does health care reform do for prevention and wellness? http://www.sophe.org/advocacy_matters.cfm. Reprinted by permission.

specialists to promote health. More importantly, it is good for the health of Americans. As Koh and Sebelius (2010) state: "In short, to prevent disease and promote health and wellness, the Act breaks new ground…Moving prevention toward the mainstream of health may well be one of the most lasting legacies of this landmark legislation" (p. 5).

▷ Summary

The history of health and health education/promotion is important to the professional development of health education specialists. By understanding the past, you can appreciate the present and become a leader in this emerging profession.

Today's concept of health education/promotion is relatively new, dating back only to the middle to late 1800s. Since ancient times, however, humans have been searching for ways to keep themselves healthy and free of disease. Without knowledge of disease causation or medical treatment, it was only natural to rely on superstition and spiritualism for answers. The concept of prevention was intriguing, but the knowledge and skills to prevent disease were unknown.

Progress in preventing and treating disease is evident in the early civilizations of Egypt, Greece, and Rome. These cultures recognized a need for humans to maintain sound minds and bodies. Systems of rudimentary pharmacology, better waste disposal, and safer drinking water were among some of the most noteworthy improvements.

During the Middle Ages, much of what had been previously learned was lost. Society took a giant step backward. Science and knowledge were shunned, while religion gained new favor as the preferred means of preventing and treating disease. Great epidemics struck the European continent, and millions of people lost their lives.

The Renaissance witnessed a rebirth of interest in knowledge. Science again flourished, and healthcare advancements were made. Understanding of disease, however, was still rudimentary, and the effects of treatments were often worse than the diseases. Sanitary conditions were deplorable and would remain so through the 1800s. The emergence of health education/promotion as a profession was still more than a century away.

The Age of Enlightenment saw tremendous growth in cities as the Industrial Revolution got under way in both England and the United States. Unfortunately, this population growth compounded sanitation problems related to overcrowding. Epidemics were still prevalent. In addition, employment conditions of the working class were frequently unsafe and unhealthy.

By the mid-1850s, conditions were ripe for the birth of public health in the United States. The contagion theory of disease emerged, and early reformers called for the government to take control of environmental conditions that led to disease. Health departments at city, state, and county levels were established and began to monitor and regulate food safety, water safety, and waste disposal. Professional organizations for health personnel were created, and voluntary agencies were formed. Major pieces of legislation were passed as the government sought to improve working conditions and took greater responsibility for the poor and infirm. During the mid-1900s, emphasis was placed on building new medical facilities and enhancing the technology required to treat disease.

By the 1970s, the cost of medical treatment had escalated, and concern for prevention was enhanced. This set the stage for the development of national health objectives for the decades of the 1980s, 1990s, and 2000s. *Healthy People 2020* is now in place and identifies the objectives for the current decade. Health education/promotion has made and continues to make great strides as a profession.

In the mid-1800s, as public health was starting to make important strides, school health education was also budding. In addition to reading, writing, and arithmetic, early pioneers saw the need to educate students about health-related matters. In the early 1900s, groups such as the National Tuberculosis Association, the American Cancer Society, and the Women's Christian Temperance Union strongly supported educating school children about health. Both World War I and World War II provided important impetus for health-related instruction and physical training in the schools.

During the 1960s and 1970s, several important studies supported the need for school health education and documented its effectiveness. Coordinated school health programs, created in the 1980s and 1990s, are still important for today's schools. School Health Program Guidelines, national health education standards, and identifying the six leading causes of death and disability helped promote health education/promotion.

Although health and school health education have made great strides since the first humans contemplated how to treat and prevent disease, there is still a long way to go. Both in the United States and worldwide there are many people who do not have access to medical care or the important information and skills of professionally trained health education specialists. Heart disease, cancers, diabetes, obesity, and HIV are prevalent in both developed and developing countries, and traditional infectious diseases, parasitic infections, poor sanitation, unsafe water and malnutrition continue to affect people in developing countries.

As in the past, health professionals must envision what *can* be and strive to make that vision a reality. Turner, Sellery, and Smith (1957) noted,

> As society looks ahead, it can conceive the hope that some day almost every human being will be well, intelligent, physically vigorous, mentally alert, emotionally stable, socially reasonable and ethically sound. At least, society must concern itself with progress toward that goal. (p. 18)

Health education specialists must be important players in this process. The recent Affordable Health Care Act should expand opportunities for health education specialists to impact Americans' health through community, worksite, and school-based programs.

Review Questions

1. Describe the earliest efforts at health care and informal health education/promotion.

2. Compare and contrast the great societies of ancient Egypt, Greece, and Rome. How are these cultures similar in relation to health? How are they different?

3. What were the major epidemics of the Middle Ages? Why were they so feared? What factors contributed to their spread? What were some strategies people used to prevent these diseases?

4. Discuss the Renaissance and why it is important to the history of health and health care.

5. Who wrote the *Report of the Sanitary Commission of Massachusetts* (1850)? Explain how this report was important to the history of both school health and public health.

6. Identify at least five major groups or events that forwarded school health programs.

7. What Canadian publication and its U.S. counterpart helped focus attention on the importance of disease prevention and health promotion?

8. What are *national health objectives?* Where can they be found? Why are they so important?

9. Describe the initiatives that have shaped school health education programs over the past 10 years.

10. Explain how the Affordable Health Care Act may serve to improve the public's health and advance the health education/promotion profession in the United States.

Case Study

Angelita is a health education professor employed by a state university. The local newspaper wants to interview her about the Affordable Health Care Act's prevention components, including how the act may enhance the health of their readers. The newspaper reporter also wants her to talk about previous governmental initiatives designed to prevent disease and improve the public's health. In preparation for the interview, Angelita wants to develop an outline of important points she would like to make. Your task, as Angelita's graduate assistant, is to develop the first draft of these important points.

Critical Thinking Questions

1. If a health educator is simply considered as someone who educates others about health, who would be considered humanity's first health educators? Defend your answer.

2. If a health education specialist trained in the year 2013 could time-travel back to the Middle Ages, what impact could that person have on the health problems of that era? What positive factors would work in the health education specialist's favor? What negative factors would work against the health education specialist?

3. When the first schools were being started in Massachusetts, do you believe health education/promotion would have been accepted as an academic subject? Why or why not? Do you believe health education/promotion is accepted as an academic subject at the present time? Why or why not?

4. Go online and find a copy of the new *Healthy People 2020* objectives. Read the introduction and overview. Find the objectives for one of the topic areas and review them. Next, select one objective in that topic area that you feel strongly about, and explain why you feel it will or will not be met by the year 2020. What role might a health education specialist have in meeting the objective you selected?

Activities

1. Develop a timeline using 100-year increments from the early Egyptians to the current year. Mark all of the important health-related events as they occurred along the timeline. Next, continue your timeline 100 years into the future. Predict and mark important health-related events. Explain why you believe these predictions will come true.

2. Imagine what it would have been like to live through an outbreak of the Black Death in the Middle Ages. Write a 10-day personal diary, with daily entries depicting what you might have seen or heard and how you might have felt.

3. Interview several individuals who are at least 80 years old concerning the health care they received as young children. Ask them to describe any health education/promotion they can remember. When was it? Where did it take place? Who provided the education? Was it effective?

4. Contact your high school health teacher. Ask if he or she is aware of the new National Standards for Health Education and to what extent the curriculum in the school district has been based on these standards. Ask if the school district has a coordinated school health program. If so, how does the program function? Who coordinates the program? What programs or initiatives are a result of the program? If no program exists, ask why? Try to determine the barriers to initiating a coordinated school health program in the district.

▷ Weblinks

1. **http://www.cdc.gov**
   Centers for Disease Control and Prevention
   Search the CDC Web site for "timeline" to read about important events in the history of the CDC from its founding in 1946 to the present. Take note of the many important contributions to public health by this illustrious organization.

2. **http://history.nih.gov**
   National Institutes of Health, Office of History
   This National Institutes of Health (NIH) Web site provides a brief history of this organization, highlighting some of its more important accomplishments.

3. **http://www.library.vcu.edu**
   Virginia Commonwealth University
   Search the Tompkins-McCaw Library Web site for a list of "History of Health" science museums in the United States and around the world. These are fascinating places to visit, and they provide useful information for understanding how health knowledge has developed and been disseminated throughout history.

4. **http://www.healthypeople.gov/hp2020/**
   Healthy People 2020
   This is the home page for the *Healthy People 2020* goals and objectives. From this page you should be able to access the actual *Healthy People 2020* documents, as well as information on how the objectives are developed.

5. **http://www2.edc.org/MakingHealthAcademic**
   Education Development Center, Inc.
   This site provides additional detail on Coordinated School Health Program components and how they can be integrated into the school environment. This information is important for health education specialists who want to work in schools.

6. http://www.youtube.com

Kalaupapa, Molokai, A Story to Tell

This YouTube video provides information on the last leper colony still functioning in the United States.

References

Allensworth, D., & Kolbe, L. (1987). The comprehensive school health program: Exploring an expanded concept. *Journal of School Health, 57,* 409–412.

American Alliance for Health, Physical Education, Recreation and Dance (AAHPERD). (2013). *Mission.* Retrieved May 29, 2013, from http://www.aahperd.org/about/mission.cfm.

American Public Health Association. (May, 1959). Lemuel Shattuck (1793–1859): Prophet of American Public Health. *American Journal of Public Health Nations Health.* 49(5), 676–677.

American Public Health Association. (2013). APHA Sections. Retrieved May 29, 2013, from http://www.apha.org/membergroups/sections/aphasections/.

American Youth Commission. (1942). *"Health and fitness," youth and the future.* Washington, DC: American Council on Education.

Andress, M. J., & Bragg, M. C. (1922). *Suggestions for a program for health teaching in the elementary schools.* U.S. Department of the Interior, Bureau of Education, Health Education No. 10, Washington, DC: U.S. Government Printing Office.

Auld, E. (Winter 1997/1998). Executive edge. *SOPHE News&Views, 24* (4), 4.

Bates, I. J., & Winder, A. E. (1984). *Introduction to health education.* San Francisco: Mayfield.

Bernstein, N. R. (1972). *APHA: The first one hundred years.* Washington, DC: American Public Health Association.

Butler, M., Thornton, F., & Stoltz, D. (1994). *The Battle Creek idea.* Battle Creek, MI: Heritage Publications.

Centers for Disease Control and Prevention (CDC). (2013a). *About Healthy People.* Retrieved May 28, 2013, from http://www.healthypeople.gov/2020/about/default.aspx.

Centers for Disease Control and Prevention (CDC). (2013b). *About Us: Division of Adolescent and School Health.* Retrieved May 29, 2013, from http://www.cdc.gov/HealthyYouth/about/index.htm.

Centers for Disease Control and Prevention (CDC). (2013c). *Components of Coordinated School Health.* Retrieved May 29, 2013, from http://www.cdc.gov/healthyyouth/cshp/components.htm.

Centers for Disease Control and Prevention (CDC). (2013d). *Health Topics.* Retrieved May 29, 2013, from http://www.cdc.gov/healthyyouth/healthtopics/index.htm.

Centers for Disease Control and Prevention (CDC). (2013e). *Implementing Healthy People 2020.* Retrieved May 28, 2013, from http://healthypeople.gov/2020/implement/mapit.aspx.

Centers for Disease Control and Prevention (CDC). (2013f). *The National Public Health Performance Standards Program.* Retrieved May 28, 2013, from http://www.cdc.gov/nphpsp/index.html.

Centers for Disease Control and Prevention (CDC). (2013g). *Topic Areas at a Glance.* Retrieved May 28, 2013, from http://www.cdc.gov/nchs/healthy_people/hp2020/hp2020_topic_areas.htm.

Centers for Disease Control and Prevention (CDC). (2013h). *Vision, mission, core values, and pledge.* Retrieved May 29, 2013, from http://www.cdc.gov/about/organization/mission.htm.

Centers for Disease Control and Prevention (CDC). (2013i). *Youth Risk Behavior Surveillance System.* Retrieved May 29, 2013, from http://www.cdc.gov/healthyyouth/yrbs/index.htm.

Cipolla, C. M. (1976). *Public health and the medical profession in the Renaissance.* Cambridge, England: Cambridge University Press.

Cortese, P. A. (1993). Accomplishments in comprehensive school health education. *Journal of School Health, 63* (1), 21–23.

De'ath, E. (1995). *The Black Death—1347 AD.* [Film]. (Available from Ambrose Video Publishing Inc., 1290 Avenue of the Americas, Suite 2245, New York, NY 10104)

Donan, C. (1898). *The Dark Ages 476–918.* London: Rivingtons.

Duncan, D. (1988). *Epidemiology: Basis for disease prevention and health promotion.* New York: Macmillan.

Durant, W. (1961). *The Age of Reason begins.* Vol. 7. *The story of civilization.* New York: Simon and Schuster.

Fee, E., & Brown, T. M. (1997). Editorial: Why history? *American Journal of Public Health, 87* (11), 1763–1764.

Goerke, L. S., & Stebbins, E. L. (1968). *Mustard's introduction to public health* (5th ed.). New York: Macmillan.

Gordon, B. (1959). *Medieval and Renaissance medicine.* New York: Philosophical Library.

Green, W. H., & Simons-Morton, B. G. (1990). *Introduction to health education.* Prospect Heights, IL: Waveland Press.

Hansen, M. (1980). *The royal facts of life.* Metuchen, NJ: The Scarecrow Press.

Johnson, S. (2006). *The ghost map: The story of London's most terrifying epidemic—and how it changed science, cities, and the modern world.* New York: Penguin Books.

Koh, H. K., & Sebelius, K. G. (2010). Promoting prevention through the Affordable Care Act. *The New England Journal of Medicine.* Retrieved September 3, 2010, from http://healthpolicyandreform.nejm.org/?p=12171.

Lalonde, M. (1974). *A new perspective on the health of Canadians.* Ottawa: Government of Canada.

Libby, W. (1922). *The history of medicine in its salient features.* Boston: Houghton Mifflin.

Marr, J. (1982). Merchants of death: The role of the slave trade in the transmission of disease from Africa to the Americas. *Pharos, 31* (Winter; 45(1):31-5.

McKenzie, J. F., Pinger, R. R., & Kotecki, J. E. (2008). *An introduction to community health* (6th ed.). Boston: Jones and Bartlett.

McKenzie, J. F., Pinger, R. R., & Kotecki, J. E. (2012). *An introduction to community health* (7th ed.). Boston: Jones and Bartlett Learning.

Means, R. K. (1962). *A history of health education in the United States.* Philadelphia: Lea & Febiger.

Means, R. K. (1975). *Historical perspectives on school health.* Thorofare, NJ: Charles B. Slack.

Moore, H. H. (1923). *Public health in the United States.* New York: Harper & Brothers.

National Board for Professional Teaching Standards. (2010). *Eligibility and policies.* Retrieved September 5, 2010, from http://www.nbpts.org/become_a_candidate/eligibility_policies.

Newsholme, A. (1936). The last thirty years in public health. London: Arno Press & *New York Times.*

Open Congress. (2010). *H.R.3590—Patient Protection and Affordable Care Act: Open congress summary.* Retrieved September 3, 2010, from http://www.opencongress.org/bill/111-h3590/show#.

Pickett, G., & Hanlon, J. J. (1990). *Public health administration and practice* (9th ed.). St. Louis: Times Mirror/Mosby.

Ravenel, M. P. (Ed.). (1970). *A half century of public health.* New York: Arno Press & *New York Times.*

Rogers, J. F. (1936). *Training of elementary teachers for school health work.* U.S. Department of the Interior, Office of Education, Pamphlet No. 67. Washington, DC: U.S. Government Printing Office.

Rosen, G. (1958). *A history of public health.* New York: MD Publications.

Rubinson, L., & Alles, W. F. (1984). *Health education foundations for the future.* St. Louis: Times Mirror/Mosby.

Schouten, J. (1967). *The rod and serpent of Asclepius.* Amsterdam: Elsevier.

Shattuck, L. (1850). *Report of the Sanitary Commission of Massachusetts.* Boston: Dutton and Wentworth.

Sliepcevich, E. M. (1964). *School health education study: A summary report.* Washington, DC: SHES.

Society for Public Health Education (SOPHE). (2013). *What does health care reform do for prevention and wellness?* Retrieved May 29, 2013, from http://www.sophe.org/advocacy_matters.cfm.

Turner, C. E., Sellery, C. M., & Smith, S. A. (1957). *School health and health education* (3rd ed.). St. Louis: Mosby.

U.S. Department of Health and Human Services (USDHHS). (1980). *Promoting health/preventing disease: Objectives for the nation.* Washington, DC: U.S. Government Printing Office.

U.S. Department of Health and Human Services (USDHHS). (1999). Changes in the public health system. *Morbidity and Mortality Weekly Report, 48* (50), 1141.

U.S. Department of Health, Education, and Welfare (USDHEW). (1976). *Health in America: 1776–1976.* (DHEW Publication No. (HRA) 76–616). Washington, DC: U.S. Government Printing Office.

U.S. National Center for Health Statistics, National Vital Statistics Reports (NVSR). (2009). *Deaths: Final Data for 2006,* Vol. 57, No. 14, April 17, 2009.

U.S. Public Health Service. (1979). *Healthy people: The surgeon general's report on health promotion and disease prevention.* Washington, DC: U.S. Government Printing Office.

U.S. Public Health Service. (2013). *The mission of the Commissioned Corps.* Retrieved May 29, 2013, from http://www.usphs.gov/AboutUs/mission.aspx.

Voices From the Past. (2004). Today's health problems and health education. *American Journal of Public Health, 94* (3), 368–369.

Winslow, C. A. (1944). *The conquest of epidemic disease.* Princeton, NJ: Princeton University Press.

Ziegler, P. (1969). *The Black Death.* New York: Harper & Row.

Philosophical Foundations

Chapter Objectives

After reading this chapter and answering the questions at the end,
you should be able to:

- Define the terms *philosophy*, *philodoxy*, *wellness*, *holistic*, and *symmetry*, and explain the differences between them.

- Discuss the importance of developing a personal philosophy about life.

- Compare and contrast the advantages and disadvantages of having a life philosophy and an occupational philosophy that are similar.

- Formulate a statement that describes your personal philosophy of life and identify the influences that account for your philosophy.

- Identify and explain the differences between the following health education/promotion philosophies:

  a. behavior change philosophy
  b. cognitive-based philosophy
  c. decision-making philosophy
  d. freeing or functioning philosophy
  e. social change philosophy
  f. eclectic philosophy

- Explain how a health education specialist might use each of the five health education/promotion philosophies to address a situation in a scenario.

- Create and defend your own philosophy of health education/promotion.

Kristy has been exploring health-related careers and is interested in pursuing a major in health education/promotion. Her interest has been partially piqued by the fact that her parents' lives improved when they began to lower cholesterol and increase exercise by incorporating information and strategies presented to them by a health education specialist employed by their physician. The health education specialist worked with Kristy's parents on a regular basis for nearly six months, and they gave rave reviews on that specialist's method-ologies. As a result, her parents were able to reduce or eliminate several of the medications they had been taking. Kristy also had to admit that the entire family's health had benefited from her parents' "new" lifestyle.

In thinking about a career as a health education specialist, Kristy formulated several questions in her mind. A few of the questions involved the philosophies, styles, and methods of practice held or used by health education specialists. Others were related to the profession as a whole and how someone decides whether becoming a health education specialist is a good match for her or his philosophy of life.

This chapter addresses some of the same questions that Kristy contemplated in relation to the practice of health education/promotion and possibly becoming a health education specialist. To that end, we will explore questions such as

- What is a philosophy?
- Why does a person need a philosophy?
- What are some of the philosophies or philosophical principles associated with the notion of *health*?
- What philosophical viewpoints related to health education/promotion are held by some of the past and current leading health education specialists?
- How is a philosophy developed?
- What are the predominant philosophies used in the practice of health education/promotion today?
- How will adopting any of the health education/promotion philosophies impact the way health education specialists practice in their chosen setting?

The purpose of discussing the development of a health education/promotion philosophy is not to provide a treatise on "the nature of the world," so to speak, but to emphasize the importance of a guiding philosophy to the practice of any profession. Smith (2010) notes, "When a health educator identifies and organizes concepts deemed as valuable in relation to health outcomes, he or she can begin to form a philosophical framework for functioning comfortably and effectively" (p. 51).

The term *philosophy* may seem to some to describe an almost ethereal, esoteric academic exercise. In actuality, however, a well-considered philosophy provides the underpinnings that support the bridge between theory and practice.

▷ What Is a Philosophy?

The word *philosophy* comes from Greek and literally means "the love of wisdom" or "the love of learning." The term **philosophy** in this chapter means a statement summarizing the attitudes, principles, beliefs, values, and concepts held by an individual or a group. In an academic setting, a philosopher studies the topics of ethics, logic, politics, metaphysics, theology, or aesthetics. It is certainly not imperative that a person be an academic philosopher to have a philosophy. All of us have convictions, ideas, values, experiences, and attitudes about one or more of the areas listed as they apply to life. These are the building blocks (sometimes known as principles) that make up any philosophy. Dr. Buzz Pruitt, professor of health education at Texas A&M, has emphasized the difference between having a life guided by a grounded philosophy and one shaped by an approach termed **philodoxy**, literally the love of opinion (Pruitt, 2007). The person who has developed a philosophy often asks questions to

▲ **Figure 3.1** Young Man Contemplating the Tree of Life: What Will It Hold for Me?

discover what lies under the surface of issues; thus, the individual seeks answers in a quest for true meaning (reality) and lets that reality define opinion and practice (see **Figure 3.1**). The individual who rejects the possibility of alternative explanations is often practicing philodoxy—letting opinion define reality. Philodoxy presents problems for health education specialists largely because it stifles the incorporation of discovery and new knowledge, facts, or insight into the practice of health education/promotion.

Therefore, you most likely have already developed certain philosophical viewpoints or notions about what is real and true in the world as you know it. The manner in which you consistently act toward other people often reflects your philosophy concerning the importance of people in general. That you are studying to become a health education specialist says something about your philosophical leanings in terms of a career. For example, the profession of health education/promotion is considered a helping profession. Gambescia (2007) states that health education "is an enabling good that helps individuals and communities flourish" (p. 722). Those who work in the profession should value helping others.

In today's society there are many examples of the use of a philosophical position. Corporations, for example, create slogans espousing their purported philosophy. (Of course, they are also trying to sell a product or service at the same time.) Many of us recognize certain companies by phrases such as "Just Do It" (Nike), or "When you care enough to send the very best" (Hallmark Cards). The use of caring slogans and catchy phrases is meant to convey to the public that the company is in business solely because it is interested in the welfare of people everywhere and is responsive to their needs. If the company's actions match the slogan, the public is more likely to perceive the slogan as a true representation of the corporate philosophy.

Additionally, many not-for-profit and for-profit agencies and companies often have mission statements. A mission statement is meant to convey a philosophy and direction that form a framework for all actions taken by that organization. For example, the mission statement for the Central District Health Department in Boise, Idaho, is: "Healthy People in Healthy Communities."

After reading this statement there is little doubt that the overriding philosophy in this department is one of promoting prevention for both individuals and communities. For individuals who have a philosophy that emphasizes prevention and early intervention, this is likely to be a place where they might find employment that is personally rewarding and professionally fulfilling.

Just as often, insight into a person's philosophy can be gained by hearing, reading, or analyzing that person's quotes or sayings. For example, the following quote from actor Michael J. Fox embodies his philosophy of life in the face of an incurable disease: "Parkinson's demanded of me that I be a better man, a better husband, father, and citizen. I often refer to it as a gift. With a nod to those who find this hard to believe, especially my fellow patients who are facing great difficulties, I add this qualifier—it's the gift that keeps on taking...but it's a gift" (p. 89). As you will see later and as can be noted from Fox's statement, a philosophy is rarely stagnant, but rather continuous because it is formulated by considering values, beliefs, experiences, and consequences of actions. Composing a philosophy statement allows a person to reflect on what is important to him or her when viewing the world in its many manifestations.

The thoughts stated previously are well summarized by Loren Bensley (1993), one of the most influential health education specialists of the latter half of the 20th century:

> Philosophy can be defined as a state of mind based on your values and beliefs. This in turn is based on a variety of factors which include culture, religion, education, morals, environment, experiences, and family. It is also determined by people who have influenced you, how you feel about yourself and others, your spirit, your optimism or pessimism, your independence and your family. It is a synthesis of all learning that makes you who you are and what you believe. In other words, a philosophy reflects your values and beliefs which determine your mission and purpose for being, or basic theory, or viewpoint based on logical reasoning. (p. 2)

Please note that a philosophy does not have to be abstract. Pondering the reason for being gives people a chance to integrate their past, present, and future into a coherent whole that guides them through life.

▷ Why Does One Need a Philosophy?

The answer to the question "Why does one need a philosophy?" is both simple and complex. Each of us already has a view of the world and what is true for us. This image helps shape the way we experience our surroundings and act toward others in our environment. In other words, a person's philosophy helps form the basis of reality for her or him.

Of course, some philosophical change is probably inevitable. New experiences, new insights, and new learnings create the possibility that some of the tenets comprising the philosophy might need retooling. This is a normal part of growth. Most people's philosophical views are altered somewhat as they study, grow older, and experience the world in different ways.

Usually a person's philosophy (e.g., determining how to treat others, what actions are right or wrong, and what is important in life) needs to be synchronous in all aspects of life. This means that a person's philosophical viewpoint holds at home, at school, in the workplace, and at play. If incongruence develops between a person's philosophy and the philosophy of the leaders in the workplace, problems can occur.

As an example, consider the career of a public health education specialist working in HIV/AIDS prevention education who is employed by a state department of education. Assume that this individual has a philosophical view that all human life is sacred and education is the best source of prevention. Also assume that the person's work both on and off the job reflects consistency and a commitment to those ideals. In other words, the person's actions are synchronous with the aforementioned philosophy. As long as the administration in the state department of education and family and friends remain supportive of this health education specialist's role and philosophy, chances are that this person will do well. If, however, the state department leadership changes and the new superintendent is opposed to the idea that individuals infected with HIV are worth saving (because they chose their behaviors) or refuses to allow condoms to be mentioned as a secondary source of prevention, the specialist may have a difficult time remaining in that environment. The reason for this statement is that this educator is now not allowed to act according to his or her beliefs, ideals, and knowledge. There is a disharmony between the philosophical stance and the ability to act in concert with that stance.

Certainly, there are exceptions to this rule. Health education specialists might hold philosophies on how they personally live, yet they might have to educate those who have made choices that are opposed to their belief system. This situation begins to cross the bounds of a general philosophy and get into ethics (right behavior—see Chapter 5). Although a possible moral-philosophical conflict seems apparent in this situation, health education specialists need to remember that their primary concern is to protect and enhance the health of those they serve. Health is not a moral issue. The health of any one of us affects the health of all of us in some manner (legally, monetarily, physically, or emotionally). At the very least, the health education specialist should refer this situation to another trained individual who can fulfill the obligation to the public.

The late U.S. Surgeon General C. Everett Koop was confronted with the same dilemma when he was in office during the advent of the AIDS epidemic, 1981–1989. Although he was a strong conservative Christian leader and against the use of drugs and premarital sex, he championed the cause of HIV/AIDS education by stressing that the epidemic was a health problem that required a health-based prevention message. Through the power of his office, he insisted that HIV/AIDS prevention education include the merits of abstinence, the dissemination of needles to inner-city addicts, and the increased availability of condoms to individuals who choose to be sexually active or promiscuous.

A further example that illustrates the impact of a philosophy on the practice of a profession comes from an article by Governali, Hodges, and Videto (2005) in which they state, "philosophical thought is central to the delivery of health education. For a profession to stay vital and relevant, it is important to assess its activities, regularly evaluate its goals, and assess its philosophical direction" (p. 211). The emphasis the authors place on the influence of activities and goals related to philosophy is a direct reflection of their personal and professional philosophical foundation formed over the years. A well-reasoned philosophy often plays an important role in the choice of a career path.

▲ **Figure 3.2** The current U.S. Surgeon General, Regina Benjamin, is a strong supporter of the value of health education and promotion in creating a more prevention-focused approach to health.

A study identifying factors that influence career choices further validates that statement. Tamayose, Farzin, Schmieder-Ramirez, and Rice (2004) surveyed public health students enrolled at a west coast university to determine what major influences led them to pursue careers in public health. Researchers found that the top two items mentioned by the students were "enjoyment of the profession/commitment to health improvement" and "provide a health/community service to others." Both of these statements reflect a common philosophical thread that permeates the thinking of a majority of individuals currently practicing in the field of health education/promotion with whom we have come in contact.

In summary, the formation of a philosophy is one of the key determining factors behind the choice of an occupation, a spouse, a religious conviction, a political persuasion, and friends. A firm philosophical foundation serves as a beacon that lights the way and provides guidance for many of the major decisions in life.

▷ Principles and Philosophies Associated with Health

In Chapter 1, the meaning of the term *health* was discussed. Recall that, although the term *health* is elusive to define, nearly all definitions include the idea of a multidimensional construct that most people value, particularly when health deteriorates. Some see health as an end to itself; others see health as being important in large part because its presence enables the freedom to act as one wishes without major physical or mental impediments. Over the past 30 to 50 years, educators have identified several philosophies or philosophical principles that tend to be associated with the establishment and maintenance of health.

These philosophies provide a set of guiding principles that help create a framework to better understand the depth of the term *health.*

Rash (1985) mentions that, although health is often not an end in itself, good health does bring a richness and enjoyment to life that will make service to others more possible. He feels that those who seek to enhance the health of others through education should espouse a **philosophy of symmetry;** that is, health has physical, emotional, spiritual, and social components, and each is just as important as the others. Health education specialists should seek to motivate their students or clients toward symmetry (balance) among these components (see **Figure 3.3**).

Oberteufer (1953) rejected the notions of a dualistic (human = mind + body) or a triune (human = mind + body + spirit) nature for humanity. Instead, he embraced the ideal of a **holistic philosophy** of health when he stated, "The mind and body disappear as recognizable realities and in their stead comes the acknowledgment of a whole being…man is essentially a unified integrated organism" (p. 105). Thomas (1984) is convinced that the holistic view of health produces health professionals who are more passionate about creating a society in which the promotion of good health is seen as a positive goal.

Greenberg (1992), Donatelle (2011), Edlin and Golanty (2004), and Hales (2004), among others, have elevated the construct of wellness to the level of a philosophy. **Wellness,** always a positive quality (as opposed to illness being always a negative) is visualized as the integration of the spiritual, intellectual, physical, emotional, environmental, and social dimensions of health to form a whole "healthy person." Those who subscribe to this philosophy believe

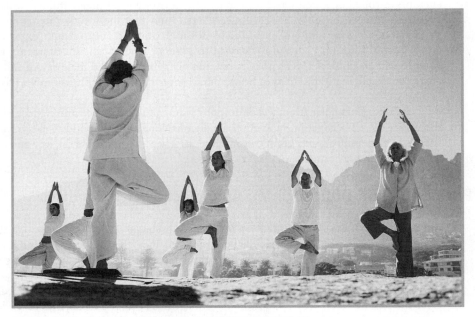

▲ **Figure 3.3** Total health allows people to function at their best.

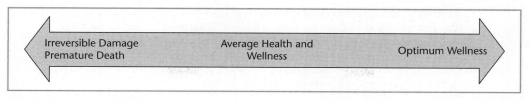

▲ **Figure 3.4** The Wellness Continuum

that all people can achieve some measure of wellness, no matter what limitations they have, and that achieving optimal health is an appropriate journey for everyone. The optimum state of wellness occurs when people have developed all six of the dimensions of health to the maximum of their ability. (See **Figure 3.4**.)

To be sure, there are those who differ in their philosophical view of health. For example, Balog (2005) believes that health must by nature be seen solely as a physical state because "health must reside in the person" (p. 269), and it is not possible for a person to be truly healthy if the systems of the body are not functioning in the way they were intended to operate. He argues that any other view of health is really not objective but introduces subjective views of what others value (the good life). In Balog's view, it is important for health educators to distinguish that which affects health from that which is health. In other words, he cautions against confusing "good life" with "good health."

The philosophies previously mentioned are not meant to be all inclusive. The purpose for discussing them is to help provide a framework to further assist the reader in developing a philosophy about health and, ultimately, health education/promotion.

▷ Leading Philosophical Viewpoints

Over the past 20 years, several publications and numerous articles have focused on recounting the philosophical positions of past and present leading health education specialists. To assist you in formulating your own health education/promotion philosophy, we present here a small sample of the philosophies expressed in these publications. As previously mentioned, one way a philosophical approach is developed is through the influence of role models, or mentors. The viewpoints that follow may help stimulate your thoughts and provide guidance as you consider a career in health education/promotion.

BECKY SMITH (2010)
Studying the definitions of health from the perspectives of scholars such as Dubos, Fromm, Maslow, Montagu, Tillich, and Tournier.
. . . helped me develop a personal understanding of how individuals express health and how the potential for health can manifest despite severe limitations in one or more dimension(s). . . . when internal and external elements that facilitate the development of human potential are available, individuals are more likely to experience optimal health. . . . I prefer to look for that expression of health as a starting point for professional interaction, education, and enhancement of health rather than focus on existing debilitation. (p. 52)

JOHN ALLEGRANTE (2006)
I have always believed that the goal of health education is to promote, maintain, and improve individual and community health through the educational process. I believe that there are

fundamental conceptual hallmarks and a social agenda that differentiate the practice of health education and that of medicine in achieving this goal. These hallmarks include the use of consensus strategies to identify health needs and problems, voluntary participation as an ethical requirement, and an obligation to foster social and political change. I also believe that our perspective and methodologies require that we enter into a social contract with people that engages them as partners, not merely as patients. (p. 306)

MARIAN HAMBURG (1993)
Eta Sigma Gamma has given me the chance to expound on a few of my beliefs about health education.

1. You can't plan everything. Unexpected opportunities appear and it is important to be ready to take advantage of them. (p. 68)
2. I believe in mentorship. Its power incorporated into health education programming has enormous strength for influencing positive health behaviors. (p. 70)
3. I believe that effective health education programming requires appropriate inter-sectoral cooperation, and that health educators, regardless of the source of their professional preparation, must be its facilitators. School-community can be one world. (p. 71)
4. I believe that we need to put more of our resources into joint efforts and coalition building. Much of health education's future as a profession depends upon the support that health educators, regardless of their specialized training, provide for the maintenance and expansion of certification. (p. 73)
5. It is not surprising to me that the concept of networking has become an important basis for health education practice. We bring together people with common problems to seek solutions through the sharing of feelings and information. (p. 73)

JOHN SEFFRIN (1993)
I believe the most fundamental outcome of health education is the enabling of individuals to achieve a level of personal freedom not very likely to be obtained otherwise. Freedom means being able to avoid any unnecessary encumbrance on one's ability to make an enlightened choice (p. 110). . . . We need to be resourceful and open to change. In doing so, however, we need to change in ways that do not violate certain basic principles:

1. appreciation for each individual's uniqueness;
2. respect for ethnic and cultural diversity;
3. protection for individual and group autonomy;
4. promotion and preservation of free choice; and
5. intervention strategies based on good science. (p. 114)

Philosophies are as individual as the people themselves, yet some common themes (development of individual potential, learning experiences that help in decision making, free choice, and enhancement of individual uniqueness) seem to emerge and hold true regardless of the health education specialist. Let us now examine how these philosophies are actually applied in the practice of health education/promotion.

▷ Developing a Philosophy

Now that it is clear that a philosophy is not some abstraction used only by individuals such as the Dalai Lama or Gandhi, let us explore the ways in which a philosophy is formed. In previous sections, it was noted that most practicing professionals and many organizations have developed certain philosophical stances that serve as a road map and guide for living and working in the world. What provides the basis for forming a philosophy?

Suppose you are searching through the Web sites of various health education/promotion programs, trying to determine which one might be best for you. In your search, you come across the Web site for the community health education program at the University of Wisconsin at La Crosse (see the Weblinks section at the end of the chapter for URL references). One of the prominent features of the site is a statement of the mission of the programs.

"The mission of the BS-CHE (Bachelor of Science—Community Health Education) program at the University of Wisconsin-La Crosse (UW-La Crosse) is to prepare professionals using entry-level (BS-CHE) health education competencies and public health core areas who will address quality of life enhancement through health education and health promotion, mindful of the holistic, dynamic and interdependent nature of humans and their interactions with and within the environment."

The process of developing this mission statement most likely involved at least several meetings of faculty, staff, students, and community leaders and administrators. During the meetings the core beliefs and principles regarding health education/promotion of those in attendance were probably assessed. After coupling the list of beliefs with the required list of core competencies, the mission statement was formulated. Notice that the statement concludes with "who will address quality of life enhancement . . . mindful of the holistic, dynamic and interdependent nature of humans and their interactions with and within the environment." This portion of the statement rises to the level of a philosophy.

In drafting your own philosophy statement, you should employ a similar process (without the committee, of course). Think about what a health education specialist does and what the result of his or her work should be. Construct lists of your thoughts under headings such as (1) personal values and beliefs (see the Weblinks section for examples of values), (2) what "health" means to you, (3) attributes of people you admire and trust, (4) results of health studies and readings that you find meaningful, and (5) outcomes you would like to see from the process of health education/promotion (e.g., better decision making, more community involvement, promotion of positive behaviors). From your lists, some common themes will emerge and the identification of these themes is a key to drafting your own health education/promotion philosophy statement. Exploring why you value the topics represented within these themes should enable you to compose your philosophy statement that will reflect a way of thinking, acting, and viewing the world that works for you.

Please note, however, that using this approach to formulate a philosophy is not a guarantee that the philosophy will remain stable. As a matter of fact, there is a strong likelihood that some changes will occur because of new learnings, activities, and experiences (e.g., working in a different culture, experiencing the premature death of a child or spouse, losing a job as a result of downsizing). A philosophy results from the sum of knowledge, experience, and principles from which it was formed.

As a further aid to formulating a philosophy statement about health and health education/promotion, we would like to reference a series of questions that Dr. Julie Dietz of Eastern Illinois University gives her students when they are assigned to write their personal philosophy of health education. These questions do a great job of capturing the interface between a personal philosophy of health and a professional philosophy of the profession of health education/promotion. They are:

Statement of Personal Health Philosophy

- What does it mean to be *healthy*?
- What are your health-related responsibilities and obligations to yourself?
- What are your health-related responsibilities and obligations to your community or society?
- What do you expect your community and society to do to keep you healthy?

Statement of Professional Health Education and Promotion Philosophy

- What is Health Education/Health Promotion, and what does it mean to be a professional in this field?
- What are your goals for yourself and your profession?
- What are your professional responsibilities to yourself, your community, and to your profession?
- How does community health education fit within these goals?

We conclude this section with a short vignette that illustrates several concepts or principles that need to be considered when formulating a philosophy statement about life, health, and health education/promotion practice.

The story, adapted from the book *Kamkwamba and Mealer* (2009), is about the amazing accomplishments of William Kamkwamba of the African nation of Malawi. William was curious about how things worked (particularly electricity) and had read a book titled *Using Energy*, which he accessed in a makeshift library in his town; so he was able to construct a functioning windmill from parts of engines and wrecked automobiles he found in a local junkyard. Most people around him said his dream of supplying his family and his community with reliable electricity for lighting homes and pumping water was "crazy." And like many youths in Africa, William's formal education was cut short by the inability of his family to pay the $80 annual tuition. Yet he maintained the initiative to keep on trying and learning despite his family's suffering through famine, disease, and government graft.

Although rudimentary, the windmill he constructed worked well enough to supply power to light four small light bulbs in his home. Eventually, educators and scientists throughout Africa and beyond learned of the accomplishments of this self-taught scholar. As a result, William has been a featured lecturer at several international conferences; he has completed high school at an international school in South Africa (as a result of a grant); and he began his freshman year at Yale in the fall of 2010. His refusal to abandon his dreams, fueled by his desire to make things better for his village and family, provided a stark contrast to many in his country (and around the world) who take for granted the educational opportunities they have or just give up and settle for the status quo.

All too often, in determining abilities, people set their sights and dreams too low. A personal philosophy needs to incorporate the realization that life sometimes dishes out bumps and bruises. Acknowledging this fact may well prevent any of us from excessively limiting our assessment of our place in the world. In addition, personal philosophy is often a reflection of an individual's perspective of the world and how and why it seems to work that way.

Remember, the formation of a philosophy, whether personal or occupational, requires several steps. First, individuals need to answer the following questions in reference to themselves: What is important? What is most valued? What beliefs are held? Second, they need to identify ways the answers to the first questions influence the way they believe and act. Third, after carefully considering and writing down the answers to these questions, a philosophy statement can be formulated. The statement (usually a paragraph or two in length—350 to 500 words) reflects and identifies the factors, principles, ideals, and influences that help shape reality for those individuals.

As previously mentioned, these steps can be used to formulate any type of philosophy statement. However, for those who are studying health education/promotion, there is one more important question to answer: Is this philosophy statement consistent with being a health education specialist? If the answer is "yes," then for that person health education/promotion is a profession worthy of further consideration.

▷ Predominant Health Education/Promotion Philosophies

Butler (1997) accurately points out that, even though there are several definitions of the phrase *health education/promotion*, recurring themes in many of the definitions allow for a general agreement as to its meaning. He notes, however, that the methods used to accomplish health education/promotion are less clear. The manner in which a person chooses to conduct health education/promotion can be demonstrated to be a direct reflection of that person's philosophy of health education/promotion. With that in mind, have any predominant philosophies of health education/promotion emerged? If so, what are they?

Welle, Russell, and Kittleson (1995) conducted a study to determine the philosophies favored by health education specialists. As part of the background for their study, they conducted a literature review and identified five dominant philosophies of health education/promotion that have emerged during the last 50 to 60 years. The philosophies identified were behavior change, cognitive-based, decision-making, freeing or functioning, and social change.

1. The **behavior change philosophy** involves a health education specialist using behavioral contracts, goal setting, and self-monitoring to try to foster a modification in an unhealthy habit in an individual with whom he or she is working. The nature of this approach allows for the establishment of easily measurable objectives, thus enhancing the ability to evaluate outcomes. (Example: setting up a contract to increase the number of hours of study each week)

2. A health education specialist who uses a **cognitive-based philosophy** focuses on the acquisition of content and factual information. The goal is to increase the knowledge of the individuals or groups so that they are better armed to make decisions about their health. (Example: simply posting statistics about the number of people killed or injured in automobile accidents who were not wearing seat belts)

3. In using the **decision-making philosophy,** a health education specialist presents simulated problems, case studies, or scenarios to students or clients. Each problem, case, or scenario requires decisions to be made in seeking a "best approach or answer." By creating and analyzing potential solutions, the students develop skills needed to address many health-related decisions they might face. An advantage of this approach is the

emphasis on critical thinking and lifelong learning. (Example: using a variety of case study examples of the Atkins Diet to see competing perspectives of effectiveness)

4. The **freeing or functioning philosophy** was proposed by Greenberg (1978) as a reaction to traditional approaches of health education/promotion that he felt ran the risk of blaming victims for practicing health behaviors that were often either out of their control or not seen as in their best interests. The health education specialist who uses this philosophical approach has the ultimate goal of freeing people to make the best health decisions possible based on their needs and interests—not necessarily the interests of society. Some health education specialists classify this as a subset of the decision-making philosophy discussed previously. (Example: lessons on the responsible use of alcohol)

5. The **social change philosophy** emphasizes the role of health education specialists in creating social, economic, and political change that benefits the health of individuals and groups. Health education specialists espousing this philosophy are often at the forefront of the adoption of policies or laws that will enhance the health of all. (Example: no smoking allowed in restaurants, or new housing developments with pedestrian-friendly areas such as sidewalks and parks)

The previously listed philosophies of health education/promotion are the products of more than 50 years of study, experimentation, and dialogue within the profession. The research conducted by Welle, Russell, and Kittleson (1995) found that the philosophy most preferred by both health education/promotion practitioners and academicians was decision making. Both groups listed behavior change as a second choice, and both agreed that their least favorite was cognitive based. The fact that health education specialists who are employed in the academic setting and those who are employed as practitioners in the field agreed on these choices as predominant philosophies speaks well for the interface between preparation programs and practice.

Another interesting finding from the study occurred when, as a part of the survey, the health education specialists were given health education/promotion vignettes to address or solve. In many cases, the respondents changed the philosophical approach they used depending on the setting (school, community, work site, medical). The responding health education specialists had earlier identified a specific health education/promotion philosophy they favored. These results indicate that health education specialists are adaptable and resourceful, and they will use any health education/promotion approach that seems appropriate to the situation or an **eclectic health education/promotion philosophy.**

In a thought-provoking essay, Buchanan (2006) introduces a different philosophical paradigm calling for health education specialists to "return to their roots" and reconsider the meaning of the word *education* in the practice of health education/promotion. He feels that the practice of health education/promotion buys into the medical model so often that health education specialists have lost their bearings and are now more often purveyors who almost demand that persons or the public adopt behaviors that "we know" will lead to a healthier life.

Instead he suggests that health education specialists should be "disseminators of factual information and facilitators of rational choice" (p. 301). Using this philosophy,

> The quality of a health educator's work would be evaluated not by its effectiveness in changing people's behavior but by whether their audiences find the dialogue valuable in helping them think about how they want to live their lives, the impact of their behaviors on the pursuit of their life goals, and the kinds of environmental conditions that community members find most conducive to living healthy and fulfilling lives. (p. 301)

In actuality, Buchanan's views seem to incorporate the use of the cognitive-based, the decision-making, and the freeing or functioning health education/promotion philosophies outlined previously. This is not surprising, because in any list of philosophies there is always the possibility of one philosophy overlapping with another, so in practice not all is as clean as it might seem. In making a similar argument as Buchanan, Governali, Hodges, and Videto (2005) call for an integrated behavioral ecological philosophy so that health education specialists use the multidimensional nature of the interaction of the individual and the environment. This approach also resembles the eclectic philosophical model.

BOX 3.1

Practitioner's Perspective

PHILOSOPHY OF HEALTH EDUCATION/PROMOTION Travis C. Leyva

CURRENT POSITION/TITLE: Disease Prevention Program Manager

EMPLOYER: New Mexico Department of Health

DEGREE/INSTITUTION/YEAR: Bachelor in Community Health, New Mexico State University, 2004

MAJOR: Community Health

MINOR: Environment Health

Describe your past and current professional positions and how you came to hold the job you now hold (How did you obtain the position?): A week prior to graduating with my Bachelor's in Community Health, I had come across a job posting online for a Disease Prevention Specialist (DPS)—Health Educator position that caught my interest. It was a position that would conduct surveillance and field investigations for all reportable Sexually Transmitted Diseases (STDs) in the region. I applied, interviewed and 3 months later I started my journey as a health educator.

After a year as a DPS, I was promoted to the Regional Emergency Preparedness Specialist where I coordinated responses to Public Health emergencies and bioterrorism threats. After 1 year in that position, I was promoted as the Border Infectious Disease Surveillance (BIDS) Officer Epidemiologist, where I coordinated with Mexican Health officials on Border Health Infectious Disease issues. Following 2 years in that position, I was promoted to Program Manager of Disease Prevention, where I now supervise all the positions I was in and more! I must say that all of my promotions started with a supervisor that encouraged and motivated me to work hard and promote myself to where I am today.

Describe the duties of your current position: I oversee 6 different program areas in my current position. They include; STD & TB Surveillance and Field Investigation, Hepatitis Surveillance and Field Investigation, HIV Prevention, HIV Medical Case Management, Harm Reduction Program, and Emergency Preparedness Program.

My job is to ensure that all deliverables are obtained by setting goals and objectives for our staff to follow. In separate intervals, I strategize, implement, and evaluate certain activities conducted by our staff to optimize the output of our services. An activity that I am most proud of is the creation of a small group, video based intervention titled, "iHEAL—Integrated Health Education for Addictive Lifestyles" This intervention educates and creates risk reduction plans for those who may be infected and/or affected by HIV, Hepatitis C, STDs, or Injection Drug Use. iHEAL is currently being presented at detention centers, state prisons, drug rehabilitation centers, probation and parole workshops, teen drug court programs, and some high schools. The intervention has now been requested to be presented throughout the state, and a DVD of the presentation is currently being made to distribute to health educators in the Disease Prevention field.

Describe what you like most about this position: The best thing about my position

BOX 3.1   *continued*

is the staff and clients I work with on a daily basis. All of the staff that I work with have a unique, non-judgmental attitude that focuses on helping people who may be infected or affected by a disease. Usually clients who we serve are unaware of how they became infected with a disease, or how they could transmit a disease to others, and after we as health educators work with them, it is quite rewarding that we have made a difference in one person's life, sometimes even saving it.

Describe what you like least about this position: There is always change in public health. Although it can be a good thing at times, sometimes change can be difficult and uncertain. Working with grant funded programs, there are always new deliverables that need to be met and at times it means to stop the processes that are in place and create new ones, usually without any new resources. Also, there is always a change in administration which means there may be new directives and new priorities.

How do you use your philosophy of health education/promotion in your position? My philosophy among my staff is to educate and promote healthy lifestyle choices to every individual as you would like for it to

be done to you. Being non-judgmental and courteous is key to being a successful health educator. A major component to my philosophy is that we as health educators cannot direct an individual to make healthier lifestyle choices, but rather we can provide them with options for them to choose how to make healthier lifestyle choices for themselves. Those who choose to make a change or difference usually succeed and maintain those choices.

What recommendations/advice do you have for current health education students? My advice to current health education students is to first find a niche in public health. Whether it be STDs, Children Medical Services, Family Planning, or Harm Reduction, once you find a niche, my best recommendation is to integrate all public health programs into your health education deliveries. Some of the best health educators I have seen and worked with are those who can educate on a topic, and also refer to other areas which can only benefit and support the topic area they are presenting on. People recognize when a health educator is an integrated subject matter expert.

▷ Impacting the Delivery of Health Education/Promotion

This section uses scenarios to help focus on the methods health education specialists might use, depending on their philosophical stance. The decision to use any philosophy involves understanding and accepting the foundation that helped create the philosophy in the first place. To this end, Welle, Russell, and Kittleson (1995) state,

> Health educators must remember that every single educational choice carries with it a philosophical principle or belief. Educational choices carry important philosophical assumptions about the purpose of health education, the teacher, and also the learner. Thus, health educators should take the time necessary for individual philosophical inquiry, in order to be able to clearly articulate what principles guide them professionally.... Different settings may produce the need for different philosophies. Every health educator should be aware of which elements of their individual philosophies they are willing to compromise. (p. 331)

At the outset, it is important to remember that one of the overriding goals of any health education/promotion intervention is the betterment of health for the person or the group involved. All of the philosophies have that goal. They differ, however, in how to approach that objective.

Consider the case of Julieta, a 30-year-old mother of two, who smokes, does not exercise regularly, eats many of her meals at fast-food restaurants, and has a family history of heart disease. Julieta is enrolled in a required health education course at a local university. She is going back to school to become a bilingual elementary school teacher. Because a health appraisal is a required part of the class, she has come in to visit the health education office. Three health education specialists (Javier, Nokomis, and Li Ming) are employed in the center. Each one has a different philosophy of health education/promotion. How will their approaches differ? Here is a possible intervention scenario.

Javier has adopted the philosophy of behavior change. As a proponent of this approach, he believes that all people are capable of adapting their health behavior if they can be shown the steps to success. He would use a behavior change contract method to get Julieta to try to eliminate one or two of her negative health behaviors. As a part of this process, some preliminary analysis would be done in an attempt to identify the triggers that cause her to practice the negative health behaviors. He would help her identify short-term and long-term goals. Together they would establish objectives to reach those goals, and strategies to reach the objectives. He would also try to ensure that she receives some appropriate reward for every objective and goal she accomplishes.

Nokomis, on the other hand, is an advocate of the health education/promotion philosophy known as decision making. This means that she believes in equipping her clients with problem-solving and coping skills, so that they make the best possible health choices. Initially, she might sit down with Julieta and hypothesize some situations that would necessitate Julieta thinking through the rationale behind the negative health behaviors she practices. Nokomis also would most likely try to encourage Julieta to see that some of her behaviors affect more people than just herself. The main goal is to move Julieta to a point where she admits that some of her health behaviors need to be changed and to help her identify the reasons that changing them would make her life better.

Finally, Li Ming advocates a freeing or functioning philosophy of health education/ promotion. She feels that, too often, health education specialists fail to find out the needs and desires of the client. They simply "barge in" and either overtly or covertly blame the client for any negative health behaviors. Li Ming would advocate change only if the behavior were infringing on the rights of others. In the beginning, Li Ming would confer with Julieta and find out "how her life was going." She would ask Julieta to identify any behaviors she wanted to change, making certain that Julieta had all of the information necessary to make an informed decision. Although Li Ming might believe that Julieta should stop smoking and start exercising, she would help Julieta change only those behaviors Julieta wanted to change.

One sidelight needs to be mentioned at this time. The fact that Julieta was required to take a health education course in her teacher preparation program and that the instructor required a health assessment illustrates the social change philosophy at work at a microlevel. If health were not a state requirement (legislation) in the first place, she might not have considered changing any of her negative health behaviors.

Julieta's situation demonstrates a point made previously—in practice, there often is a natural mixing of some of the philosophies. For example, all of the approaches mentioned used portions of the cognitive-based health education/promotion philosophy. To reiterate, this philosophy is based on the premise that persons need to be provided with the most current information that impacts their health behaviors, and the acquisition of that information should create a dissonance and cause change.

The fifth philosophy, social change, is probably not as well suited to addressing the health behaviors of individuals one on one. Proponents stress changes in social, economic, and political arenas to impact the health of populations. Of course, populations are made up of individuals, so changing the environment of a lower income neighborhood to be healthier (e.g., creating jobs, assuring adequate and safe housing and safe schools, providing healthcare coverage for all) ultimately impacts the health of people at the individual level as well.

▷ Summary

The term *philosophy* means a statement summarizing the attitudes, principles, beliefs, and concepts held by an individual or a group. Forming both a personal and an occupational philosophy requires reflection and the ability to identify the factors, principles, ideals, and influences that help shape your reality. The decision to use any philosophy involves understanding and accepting the foundation that helped create the philosophy in the first place. A sound philosophical foundation serves as a guidepost for many of the major decisions in life.

The five predominant philosophies of health education/promotion that were identified in the chapter are (1) behavior change, (2) cognitive based, (3) decision making, (4) freeing or functioning, and (5) social change. Health education specialists might disagree on which philosophy works best. They might even use an eclectic or multidimensional philosophical approach, depending on the setting or situation. However, it is important to remember that one of the overriding goals of any health education/promotion intervention is the betterment of health for the person or group involved. All of the philosophies have that goal. They simply differ in how to attain it.

▷ Review Questions

1. Define each of the following and explain their relationship to one another.
   - Philosophy
   - Wellness
   - Holistic
   - Symmetry

2. Why is it important to have a personal philosophy about life?

3. Compare and contrast the value of having a personal life philosophy and an occupational life philosophy that are similar.

4. Define and explain the differences between:
   - A behavior change philosophy and a cognitive-based philosophy
   - A decision-making philosophy and a social change philosophy
   - A freeing or functioning philosophy and an eclectic health education/promotion philosophy

5. Explain how a person might use each of the five major health education/promotion philosophies and the eclectic philosophy to address a societal problem that can be addressed by health education/promotion (e.g., smoking, seat belt use, air pollution, exercise, diet, medication compliance, cancer risk reduction).

▷ Case Study

You are entering the final semester of your senior year of study with a major in public health education. The health education/ promotion program at your university requires seniors in their last semester to intern a minimum of 25 hours per week at a state or nonprofit agency. For this capstone experience, you have been assigned to the mayor's office in a medium-size city near the campus.

During an orientation on the first day, you overhear that one of the tasks you will be assigned will involve meeting with the leaders of several community groups with the goal of creating smoke-free public parks in the city. The smoke-free park concept represents one of the mayor's main objectives in her second term in office. You also hear that the mayor is excited to have a health education student intern because she greatly respects the skills that a health education specialist possesses.

The second day you have the opportunity to meet with the mayor, and, in fact, she does introduce to you the idea of a smoke-free public park system. During this meeting you discover that she is quite knowledgeable about the negative health effects of second- and third-hand smoke in part because her son, a lifetime nonsmoker who worked in a pub in town (smoking was allowed in pubs), died last year from lung cancer at the age of 36. At the close of the meeting, the mayor asks you to submit to her your philosophy of health education/promotion so that she can see what approach you might take with the community groups.

Using the model outlined in this chapter, write out your health education/promotion philosophy. Based on your philosophy statement and given the project that you will be assigned, is the mayor's office a good place for you to intern to hone your skills? Why or why not?

▷ Critical Thinking Questions

1. Of the five basic health education/promotion philosophies identified by Welle, Russell, and Kittleson (1995), why do you think that the least favorite among health education specialists was the cognitive philosophy? Why do you think decision making was viewed as most popular?

2. What is the purpose of health education/promotion? How might the formulation of a purpose statement be reflected in your philosophy of health education/promotion?

3. You have been hired by a local pharmacy to provide health education/promotion services to customers and employees. Shortly after you begin work, however, you discover that much of your job is marketing nutritional supplements and nonpharmaceutical health-related services provided by the pharmacy and not the health education/promotion you had envisioned. How might this apparent conflict of interest have been avoided?

4. Suppose that you are a proponent of the social change health education/promotion philosophy. What advantage does this philosophy have for the health education specialist that might be a disadvantage for the consumer of health services and education? Defend your answer.

5. An article by Bruess (2003) in the *American Journal of Health Education* discusses the notion of "role modeling" for health education specialists. (The reference for the article can be found at the end of this chapter.) After reading the article, summarize Dr. Bruess's main points, and use your answer to determine which philosophical viewpoint(s) a health education specialist must hold to feel as Dr. Bruess does on the issue of role modeling. Finally, assess how you feel about the issue. Do you agree or disagree with him? Provide a rationale for your answer.

▷ Activities

1. Take a survey of your classmates to assess what predominant health education/promotion philosophy each of them might employ. Compare the results with those from the study by Welle, Russell, and Kittleson (1995) described in this chapter. What were the reasons for any differences? Similarities?

2. After re-examining the philosophies of health, write a paragraph that could be used to explain your philosophy of health to a friend or colleague.

3. Interview a school or community health educator in your city. Ask what his or her philosophy of health education/promotion is. Then ask about the influences that helped the educator form his or her philosophy. Summarize the interview in a one-page paper.

4. Use any three of the five philosophical approaches to health education/promotion discussed in the chapter and address the following situation: In the past week in your community, two teenagers have been killed in separate incidents while riding bicycles. In neither case was the teenager wearing a helmet. A local citizens group has asked you and two of your health education specialist colleagues to attend a meeting concerning what to do about this issue.

▷ Weblinks

1. http://www.uwlax.edu/

Mission statement of the Department of Health Education and Health Promotion program at the University of Wisconsin, La Crosse.

From the university's homepage, navigate to the Community Health Program. The program description provides a fine example of a mission and philosophy statement for health education and health promotion based on the seven responsibilities of community health educators.

2. http://www.mindtools.com

The Decision Making section of the Toolkit offers examples of terms that denote values and beliefs, thus, assisting students to identify possible values or beliefs they might hold. Having these terms delineated helps in the initial stages of the development of both a personal and a professional philosophy.

3. Login to your university library and find the online version of Dr. Stephen Gambescia's Presidential keynote address to the 2007 Society for Public Health Education (SOPHE) convention (see below in References list). It provides an excellent "tour" through the thought processes of the rationale for forming a philosophy of health education for the profession of health education.

References

Allegrante, J. P. (2006). Commentary: In search of the new ethics for health promotion. *Health Education and Behavior, 33* (3), 305–307.

Balog, J. E. (2005). The meaning of health. *American Journal of Health Education, 36* (5), 266–271.

Bensley, L. B. (1993). This I believe: A philosophy of health education. *The Eta Sigma Gamma Monograph Series, 11* (2), 1–7.

Bruess, C. E. (2003). This I believe: A philosophy of health education. *American Journal of Health Education, 34* (4), 237–239.

Buchanan, D. R. (2006). Perspective: A new ethic for health promotion: Reflections on a philosophy of health education for the 21st century. *Health Education and Behavior, 33* (3), 290–304.

Butler, J. T. (1997). *The principles and practices of health education and health promotion.* Englewood, CO: Morton.

Donatelle, R. J. (2011). *Health: The basics, green edition.* San Francisco: Pearson Education.

Edlin, G., & Golanty, E. (2004). *Health and wellness* (8th ed.). Sudbury, MA: Jones and Bartlett.

Fox, M.J. (2010). *A Funny Thing Happened on the Way to the Future: Twists and Turns and Lessons Learned.* New York: Harper-Collins.

Gambescia, S. F. (2007). 2007 SOPHE presidential address: Discovering a philosophy of health education. *Health Education and Behavior, 34* (5), 718–722.

Governali, J. F., Hodges, B. C., & Videto, D. M. (2005). *American Journal of Health Education, 36* (4), 210–214.

Greenberg, J. S. (1978). Health education as freeing. *Health Education, 9* (2), 20–21.

Greenberg, J. S. (1992). *Health education: Learner centered instructional strategies* (2nd ed.). Dubuque, IA: William C. Brown.

Hales, D. (2004). *An invitation to health* (3rd ed.). Belmont, CA: Thomson-Wadsworth.

Hamburg, M. V. (1993). Would I do it all over! *The Eta Sigma Gamma Monograph Series, 11* (2), 67–74.

Kamkwamba, W., & Mealer, B. (2009). *The boy who harnessed the wind.* New York: Harper-Collins.

Oberteufer, D. (1953). Philosophy and principles of school health education. *Journal of School Health, 23* (4), 103–109.

Pruitt, B. E. (2007). Paper presented for the annual American Association for Health Education Scholar Address, March 16, Baltimore, MD.

Rash, J. K. (1985). Philosophical bases for health education. *Health Education, 16* (3), 48–49.

Seffrin, J. R. (1993). Health education and the pursuit of personal freedom. *The Eta Sigma Gamma Monograph Series, 11* (2), 109–118.

Smith, B. J. (2010). Connecting a personal philosophy of health to the practice of health education. In J. M. Black, S. Furney, H. M. Graf, & A. E. Nolte, eds., *Philosophical foundations of health education* (pp. 49–54), San Francisco: Jossey-Bass.

Tamayose, T. S., Farzin, M., Schmieder-Ramirez, J., & Rice, G. T. (2004). Important issues when choosing a career in public health. *Californian Journal of Health Promotion, 2* (1), 65–73.

Thomas, S. B. (1984). The holistic philosophy and perspective of selected health educators. *Health Education, 15* (1), 15–20.

Welle, H. M., Russell, R. D., & Kittleson, M. J. (1995). Philosophical trends in health education: Implications for the 21st century. *Journal of Health Education, 26* (6), 326–333.

Theories and Planning Models

Chapter Objectives

After reading this chapter and answering the questions at the end,
you should be able to:

- Define and explain the difference among *theory, concept, construct, variable*, and *model*.

- Explain the importance of theory to health education/promotion.

- Explain what is meant by behavior change theories and planning models.

- Describe how the concept of socio-ecological approach applies to using theories.

- Explain the difference between continuum theories and stage theories.

- Identify and briefly explain the behavior change theories and their components used in health education/promotion:

  - Health Belief Model
  - Protection Motivation Theory
  - Theory of Planned Behavior
  - Elaboration Likelihood Model of Persuasion
  - Information-Motivation-Behavioral Skills Model
  - Transtheoretical Model of Change
  - Precaution Adoption Process Model
  - Social Cognitive Theory
  - Social Network Theory
  - Social Capital Theory
  - Diffusion Theory
  - Community Readiness Model

- Identify and briefly explain the planning models and their components used in health education/promotion:

  - PRECEDE-PROCEED
  - Multilevel Approach to Community Health (MATCH)
  - Intervention Mapping
  - CDCynergy
  - Social Marketing Assessment and Response Tool (SMART)
  - Mobilizing for Action through Planning and Partnerships (MAPP)
  - Generalized Model (GM)

A s noted in Chapter 1, the profession of health education/promotion evolved from other biological, behavioral, psychological, sociological, and health science disciplines. As this profession has grown, so has the number of theories and models used by health education specialists in their work. This chapter introduces the terms *theory, concept, construct, variable*, and *model*. It explains why theory is used in health education/promotion. It also presents an overview of theories that focus on behavior change, as well as the models associated with program planning. However, space does not permit comprehensive coverage of all theories and models used by health education specialists. For example, theories and models associated with implementation and evaluation processes are not covered in this chapter.

Because theories and models are dynamic, they change and evolve (Crosby, Kegler, & DiClemente, 2009). As a result, you will continually deal with both revised and new theories and models. Future courses and their books will likely expose you to more complete coverage of health education/promotion's theoretical base (e.g., DiClemente, Salazar, & Crosby, 2013; DiClemente, Crosby, & Kegler, 2009; Edberg, 2015; Glanz, Rimer, & Viswanath, 2008a; Goodson, 2010; Green & Kreuter, 2005; Hayden, 2014; Institute of Medicine [IOM], 2001; Sharma & Romas, 2012; Simons-Morton, McLeroy, & Wendel, 2012).

▷ Definitions

To understand the theoretical foundations presented in this chapter, you must be familiar with some key related terms. Let us begin with **theory**. One of the most frequently quoted definitions of this term was provided by Glanz, Lewis, and Viswanath (2008b), who modified a previous definition by Kerlinger (1986). It states: "A *theory* is a set of interrelated concepts, definitions, and propositions that presents a *systematic* view of events or situations by specifying relations among variables in order to *explain* and *predict* the events of the situations" (p. 26). Stated a little differently, "a theory is a systematic arrangement of fundamental principles that provide a basis for explaining certain happenings of life" (McKenzie, Neiger, & Thackeray, 2013, p. 163). Thus, "the role of theory is to untangle and simplify for human comprehension the complexities of nature" (Green et al., 1994, p. 398).

As applied to the profession of health education/promotion, a theory is a general explanation of why people act, or do not act, to maintain and/or promote the health of themselves, their families, organizations, and communities. The primary elements of theories are known as **concepts** (Glanz et al., 2008b). When a concept has been developed, created, or adopted for use with a specific theory, it is referred to as a **construct** (Kerlinger, 1986). In other words, "the key concepts of a theory are its constructs" (Rimer & Glanz, 2005, p. 4). The operational form (practical use) of a construct is known as a **variable**. A variable is a quantitative measurement of a construct.

A **model** "is a composite, a mixture of ideas or concepts taken from any number of theories and used together" (Hayden, 2014, p. 2). Stated a bit differently, "Models draw on a number of theories to help people understand a specific problem in a particular setting or context. They are not always as specific as theory" (Rimer & Glanz, 2005, p. 4). Unlike theories, models do "not attempt to explain the processes underlying learning, but only to represent them" (Chaplin & Krawiec, 1979, p. 68).

Consider how these terms are used in practical application. A personal belief is a *concept* related to various health behaviors. For example, people are more likely to behave in a healthy way—such as, exercise regularly—if they feel confident in their ability to actually engage in a healthy form of exercise. Such a concept is captured in a *construct* of the Social Cognitive Theory (SCT) called *self-efficacy*. (See the discussion of the SCT later in this chapter.) If health education specialists want to develop an intervention to assist people in exercising, the ability to measure the peoples' self-efficacy toward exercise will help create the intervention. The measurement may consist of a few questions that ask people to rate their confidence in their ability to exercise. This measurement, or operational form, of the self-efficacy construct is a *variable*. However, because of the complexity of getting a non-exerciser to become an exerciser, the health education specialist may need to use a *model*, composed of constructs from several theories, to plan the intervention.

In the health education/promotion profession, the adjective *theory-based* (as in theory-based planning, theory-based practice, or theory-based research) commonly refers to both theories and models. In fact, some of the best-known and often used theories use "model" in their title (e.g., Health Belief Model). Goodson (2010) explains why "model" and "theory" are used inconsistently. She indicates that when some models were created, they were properly titled as models. They were created using constructs from several theories to explain specific phenomena. They had little empirical testing to prove their worth. Over time, these models were tested and refined, gaining theory status. Goodson (2010) concludes, "because we tend to borrow the theories we employ from other disciplines and fields and because our concern usually centers in applying these theories (or models) to practice or research, it seems to matter little to us whether we deal with theories or with models; it seems to matter even less what labels we attach to them" (p. 228).

▷ The Importance of Using Theory in Health Education/Promotion

Using theory is important in all professions, not just in health education/promotion. Theory helps organize various forms of knowledge (e.g., data, facts, and information) so that they take on meaning that would not occur if the pieces of knowledge were presented in isolation. Such meaning helps to guide the work of a practitioner (Timmreck, Cole, James, & Butterworth, 2010).

Theory helps health education specialists plan, implement, and evaluate programs. More specifically, it: (1) indicates reasons why people are not behaving in healthy ways, (2) identifies information needed before developing an intervention, (3) provides a conceptual framework for selecting constructs to develop the intervention, (4) gives insights into how best to deliver the intervention, and (5) identifies measurements needed to evaluate the intervention's impact (Crosby et al., 2009; Glanz et al., 2008b; Salazar, Crosby, & DiClemente, 2013). Theory also "provides a useful reference point to help keep research and implementation activities clearly focused" (Crosby et al., 2009, p. 11), and it infuses ethics and social justice into practice (Goodson, 2010). In addition, "using theory as a foundation for program planning and development is consistent with the current emphasis on using evidence-based interventions in public health, behavioral medicine, and medicine" (Rimer & Glanz, 2005, p. 5).

In the rest of this chapter, some of the theories and models used by health education specialists are presented in two main groups. The first group contains theories that focus on behavior change. Through their constructs, these theories help explain how change might take place. The second group contains planning models, which give structure and organization to the program planning process. These models provide health education specialists with step-by-step procedures, "integrating multiple theories to explain and address health problems," (Rimer & Glanz, 2005, p. 36), as they plan, implement, and evaluate health education/promotion programs.

▷ Behavior Change Theories

There are a number of behavior change theories that can be used by health education specialists to design interventions to encourage behavior change. Each theory provides a distinct process for helping to explain and change health behavior (Crosby, Salazar, & DiClemente, 2013a), and each works better in some situations than in others, depending on which level of influence is used to plan a health education/promotion program.

"Levels of influence" are at the heart of the **socio-ecological approach** (also called the *ecological perspective*). This multilevel, interactive approach examines how physical, social, political, economic, and cultural dimensions influence behaviors and conditions. The socio-ecological approach "emphasizes the interaction between, and the interdependence of factors within and across all levels of a health problem" (Rimer & Glanz, 2005, p. 10). In other words, changes in health behavior do not take place in a vacuum. "Individuals influence and are influenced by their families, social networks, the organizations in which they participate (workplaces, schools, religious organizations), the communities of which they are a part, and the society in which they live" (IOM, 2001, p. 26).

The concept of the socio-ecological approach comes from Bronfenbrenner's (1974, 1979) ecological paradigm that was created to understand human development. Several authors applied his work to health promotion/education. Those most often cited in the literature are McLeroy, Bibeau, Steckler, and Glanz (1988) who identified five levels of influence: "(1) the individual and individual's characteristics, such as knowledge, attitudes, values, and skills; (2) social relationships, including family and friendship ties and connections; (3) organizational influences and factors; (4) community characteristics; and (5) public policy" (Simons-Morton et al., 2012, p. 45). Recently, Simons-Morton et al. (2012, p. 45) added two additional levels "(6) the physical environment and (7) culture." **Table 4.1** lists and defines each of the seven levels. **Figure 4.1** provides a visual representation of the socio-ecological framework. By examining a health problem using this multilevel approach health education specialists can get a better understanding of how to "attack" the problem.

Consider how the levels of influence can be applied to cigarette smoking in the United States. At the *intrapersonal* (or *individual*) *level,* a large majority of smokers know that smoking is bad for them, and a slightly smaller majority have indicated they would like to quit. Many have tried to quit—some have tried on many occasions. At the *interpersonal level,* many smokers are encouraged to quit by those in their social networks, such as their physician and/or family and friends. Some smokers may attempt to quit on their own, or they may join a formal smoking cessation group.

At the *institutional* (or *organizational*) *level,* institutions, such as churches and businesses, often have policies that regulate smoking. These institutions may offer smoking

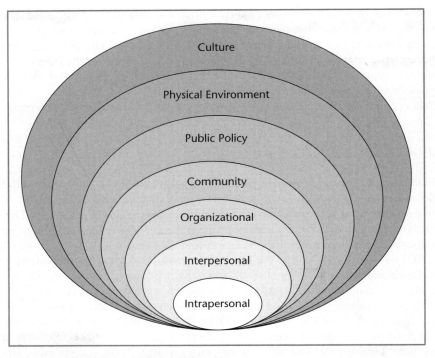

▲ **Figure 4.1** The socio-ecological model

Source: Simons-Morton, B. G., McLeroy, K. R., & Wendel, M. L. (2012). *Behavior theory in health promotion practice and research.* Burlington, MA: Jones & Bartlett Learning. p. 45

TABLE 4.1 **An ecological perspective: Levels of influence**

Ecological Level	Definition
Intrapersonal	Individual characteristics that influence behavior, such as knowledge, attitudes, beliefs, and personality traits
Interpersonal	Interpersonal processes and primary groups, including family, friends, and peers that provide social identity, support, and role definition
Organizational	Rules, regulations, policies, and informal structures, which may constrain or promote recommended behaviors
Community	Social networks and norms, or standards, which exist as formal or informal among individuals, groups, and organizations
Public Policy	Local, state, and federal policies and laws that regulate or support healthy actions and practices for disease prevention, early detection, control, and management
Physical Environment	Natural and built environment
Culture	Shared beliefs, values, behaviors and practices of a population

Sources: Rimer, B. K., & Glanz, K. (2005). *Theory at a Glance: A Guide for Health Promotion Practice,* 2nd ed. (NIH Pub. No. 05-3896). Washington, DC: National Cancer Institute. Simons-Morton, B. G., McLeroy, K. R., & Wendel, M. L. (2012). *Behavior theory in health promotion practice and research.* Burlington, MA: Jones & Bartlett Learning.

cessation classes or support groups to assist those who "belong" to the organization, to quit smoking. At the *community level*, some towns, cities, and counties have ordinances that prohibit smoking in public places. At the *public policy or population level*, many states have high cigarette taxes and/or laws that limit smoking. Also at this level, the federal government spends many dollars for public service announcements (PSAs) and other forms of media advertising the dangers of tobacco use.

The *physical environment* can also impact smoking behavior. Some of the laws that are written to prohibit indoor smoking are written in such a way that people are permitted to smoke in certain areas of a building if it has a separate ventilation system. And finally, culture can play a part in smoking behavior. "Tobacco use is no longer viewed and marketed as a positive, sexually appealing, adult behavior; rather, it is more frequently viewed as a deviant, negative behavior, practiced by individuals who lack the willpower to quit" (Simons-Morton et al., 2012, p. 61).

The following sections describe some of the theories and models that focus on behavior change. These theories/models are grouped according to the levels of influence where they may be most effective. To simplify the presentation of the socio-ecological model Glanz and Rimer (1995) combined the levels of institutional, community, and public policy factors into a single "community" level. We have used it here as well.

Intrapersonal (Individual) Theories

Intrapersonal theories focus on factors within individuals such as knowledge, attitudes, beliefs, self-concept, developmental history, past experiences, motivation, skills, and behavior (Rimer & Glanz, 2005). Several of the theories used by health education specialists to develop interventions at the intrapersonal level are the Health Belief Model (HBM), the Protection Motivation Theory (PMT), the Theory of Planned Behavior (TPB), the Elaboration Likelihood Model of Persuasion (ELM), the Information-Motivation-Behavioral Skills Model (IMB), the Transtheoretical Model of Change (TMC), and the Precaution Adoption Process Model (PAPM).

Although all of the theories listed above fall into the intrapersonal theories category, they can be divided further into continuum theories or stage theories. A **continuum theory** identifies variables that influence actions (i.e., beliefs, attitudes), quantifies the variables, and combines those variables into a single equation that predicts the likelihood of action (Weinstein, Rothman, & Sutton, 1998; Weinstein, Sandman, & Blalock, 2008). Thus, people can be "placed along a continuum of action likelihood" (Weinstein et al., 1998, p. 291). The HBM (Rosenstock, 1966), PMT (Rogers, 1975), TPB (Ajzen, 2006), ELM (Petty & Cacioppo, 1986), and IMB (Fisher & Fisher, 1992) are examples of continuum theories that are appropriate for use at the intrapersonal level.

A **stage theory** consists of an ordered set of categories into which people can be classified. It identifies factors that could induce movement from one category to the next (Weinstein & Sandman, 2002). More specifically, stage theories have four principal elements: (1) a category system to define the stages, (2) an ordering of stages, (3) barriers to change that are common to people in the same stage, and (4) different barriers to change, facing people in different stages (Weinstein et al., 1998). Advocates of stage theories "claim that there are *qualitative* differences among people and question whether changes in health behaviors can be described by a single prediction equation" (Weinstein et al., 2008, pp. 124–125). Some of the most commonly reported stage theories are the TMC (Prochaska, 1979; Prochaska & DiClemente, 1983), and PAPM (Weinstein, 1988; Weinstein et al., 1998).

HEALTH BELIEF MODEL (HBM)

The **Health Belief Model (HBM)** was developed in the 1950s by a group of psychologists to help explain why people would or would not use health services (Rosenstock, 1966). The HBM "addresses the individual's perceptions of the threat posed by a health problem (susceptibility, severity), the benefits of avoiding the threat, and factors influencing the decision to act (barriers, cues to action, and self-efficacy)" (Rimer & Glanz, 2005, p. 12). As you read the following example of why a person may or may not do self-screening for cancer, refer to the graphic representation of the HBM in **Figure 4.2**.

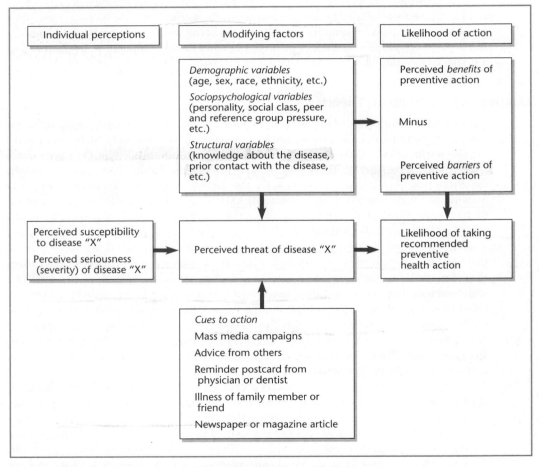

▲ **Figure 4.2** Health Belief Model as a predictor of preventive health behavior

Source: Becker, M. H., et al., from "A New Approach to Explaining Sick-Role Behavior in Low Income Populations," *American Journal of Public Health* 64, March 1974: 205–216, Fig 1. Used by permission of Sheridan Press.

▶ **Figure 4.3** A single billboard along a highway can serve as a cue to action for many people.

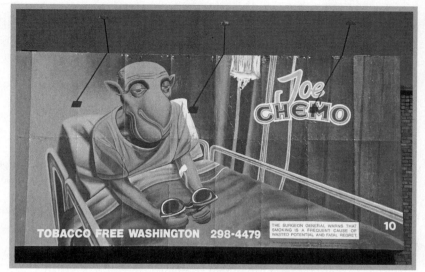

(handwritten in margin: HBM EXAMPLE:)

(handwritten in margin: DODGER WORLD SERIES 2017)

Suppose a person sees an advertisement about self-screening for cancer while reading a weekly news magazine. This is a **cue to action** that gets the person thinking about his possibility of getting cancer (see **Figure 4.3**). There may be some variables (demographic, socio-psychological, and structural) that cause the person to think about it a little more. The person remembers his college health course, which included information about self-screenings and cancer. This person knows he is at a higher than normal risk for cancer because of family history, age, and less than desirable health behavior. Therefore, he comes to the conclusion that he is susceptible to cancer (**perceived susceptibility**). The person also believes that, if he develops cancer, it can be serious (**perceived seriousness/ severity**).

Based on these factors, the person thinks that there is reason to be concerned about cancer (**perceived threat**). This person knows that self-screening can help detect cancer earlier and thus reduce the severity (**perceived benefits**). But self-screening takes time, and this person does not always remember to do it (**perceived barriers**). He must now analyze the difference between the benefits of self-screening and the barriers to self-screening (**reduction of threat**). For this person, the **likelihood of taking action** (self-screening) will be determined by weighing the perceived threat against the reduction of threat.

When the HBM was first conceived, **self-efficacy** (confidence in one's own ability to perform a certain task or function) was not part of the model. However, because evidence showed self-efficacy was a meaningful concept in the perceived barriers construct, it was recommended that self-efficacy be added to the HBM (Rosenstock, Strecher, & Becker, 1988). According to the HBM, if people are going to be successful in changing a behavior they must feel threatened by their current behavior (i.e., perceived susceptibility and severity), feel that a change in the behavior will result in an outcome they value (perceived benefit), and believe that they are competent (self-efficacy) to overcome perceived barriers (perceived cost) to engage in the new behavior (Champion & Skinner, 2008).

PROTECTION MOTIVATION THEORY (PMT)

The Protection Motivation Theory (PMT) (Rogers, 1975) was created to help explain the effects of fear appeals on health attitudes and behavior. Later (Rogers, 1983) it was revised and extended to a more general theory of persuasive communication. The PMT has some similarities to the HBM in that they are both premised on expectancy-value theory and they include some of the same constructs (Floyd, Prentice-Dunn, & Rogers, 2000; Prentice-Dunn & Rogers, 1986).

As explained by the PMT, inputs come from environmental sources of information such as verbal persuasion (i.e., a physician stressing the importance of exercise) and observational learning (i.e., seeing others exercise), and from intrapersonal sources such as one's personality and feedback from personal experiences associated with the targeted maladaptive and adaptive responses (Floyd et al., 2000) (see **Figure 4.4**). Based on these inputs people make a cognitive assessment of whether there is a threat to their health. This assessment can arouse two cognitive mediating processes: threat appraisal and coping appraisal (Floyd et al., 2000; McClendon & Prentice-Dunn, 2001). It is during these appraisals that the rewards and costs of a response are evaluated.

When the results of the threat appraisal and coping appraisal processes are combined it is the protective motivation that an individual possesses. Stated a bit differently, "The output of these appraisal-mediating processes is the decision (or intention) to initiate, continue, or inhibit the applicable adaptive responses (or coping modes)" (Floyd et al., 2000 p. 411). When using the PMT to design an intervention protection motivation has been measured using behavioral intentions (Floyd et al., 2000).

Prentice-Dunn and Rogers (1986, p. 156) offered the following summary of the PMT:

> PMT assumes that protection motivation is maximized when: (i) the threat to health is severe; (ii) the individual feels vulnerable; (iii) the adaptive response is believed to be an effective means for averting the threat; (iv) the person is confident in his or her abilities to complete successfully the adaptive response; (v) the rewards associated with the maladaptive behavior are small; and (vi) the costs associated with the adaptive response are small. Such factors produce protection motivation and, subsequently, the enactment of the adaptive, or coping, response.

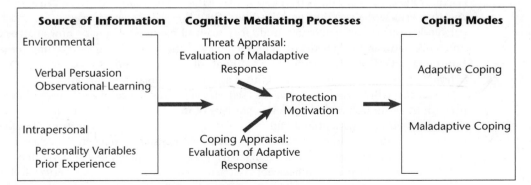

▲ **Figure 4.4** Overall Model of Protection Motivation Theory

Source: "A meta-Analysis on Protection Motivation Theory." Donna Floyd, Steven Prentice-Dunn, Ronald W. Rogers, from *Journal of Applied Social Psychology, Volume 30.* Copyright © 2000 by John Wiley & Sons, Inc.

THEORY OF PLANNED BEHAVIOR (TPB)

The Theory of Planned Behavior (TPB) (see **Figure 4.5**) is an extension of the Theory of Reasoned Action (Fishbein & Ajzen, 1975). According to the TPB, individuals' intention to perform a given behavior is a function of their attitude toward performing the behavior, their beliefs about what relevant others think they should do, and their perception of the ease or difficulty of performing the behavior. **Intention** "is an indication of a person's readiness to perform a given behavior, and it is considered to be the immediate antecedent of behavior" (Ajzen, 2006). Unlike the Theory of Reasoned Action, the TPB was developed to explain not just health behavior but all volitional behaviors ("behaviors that can be performed at will" [Luszczynski & Sutton, 2005, p. 73]). Using the example of the use of spit tobacco as a behavior not fully under volitional control, the TPB predicts that people intend to give up its use if they

- have a positive attitude toward quitting (**attitude toward the behavior**),
- think that others whom they value believe it would be good for them to quit (**subjective norm**) (see **Figure 4.6**),
- perceive that they have control over whether or not they quit (**perceived behavioral control**), and
- have the skills, resources, and other prerequisites needed to quit (**actual behavioral control**).

ELABORATION LIKELIHOOD MODEL OF PERSUASION (ELM)

The Elaboration Likelihood Model of Persuasion, or the Elaboration Likelihood Model (ELM) for short, was initially developed to help explain inconsistencies in research results

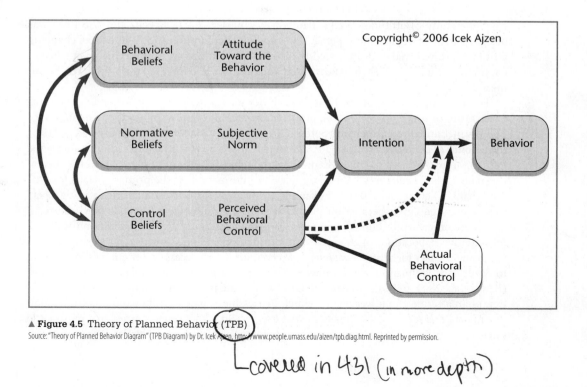

Copyright© 2006 Icek Ajzen

▲ **Figure 4.5** Theory of Planned Behavior (TPB)

Source: "Theory of Planned Behavior Diagram" (TPB Diagram) by Dr. Icek Ajzen, http://www.people.umass.edu/aizen/tpb.diag.html. Reprinted by permission.

Covered in 431 (in more depth)

▲ **Figure 4.6** Subjective norm is an important construct to be considered when planning programs for adolescents and young adults.

from the study of attitudes (Petty, Barden, & Wheeler, 2009). Specifically, the ELM was designed to help explain how persuasion messages (communication), aimed at changing attitudes, are received and processed by people. Though not created specifically for health communication, the ELM has been used to interpret and predict the impact of health messages.

The ELM does three things. First, it proposes that attitudes can be formed via two different types of routes to persuasion: peripheral routes and central routes (Petty et al., 2009). The distinction between the two routes is the amount of elaboration. **Elaboration** refers to the amount of cognitive processing (i.e., thought) that a person puts into receiving messages. Peripheral route processing involves minimal thought and relies on superficial cues or mental shortcuts (called *heuristics*) about issue-relevant information, as the primary means for attitude change (Petty et al., 2009). For example, people may form an attitude after hearing a persuasive message simply because the person delivering the message is someone they admire.

On the other hand, central route processing involves thoughtful consideration (or effortful cognitive elaboration) of issue-relevant information and one's own cognitive responses as the primary bases for attitude change: "Two conditions are necessary for effortful processing to occur—the recipient of the message must be both *motivated* and *able* to think carefully" (Petty et al., 2009, p. 188). An example of central route processing is a motorcyclist's formation of an attitude about wearing a helmet. Processing is based on thoughtful consideration of a message about the pros/cons of helmet use, recalling knowledge learned in a motorcycle safety class, and possibly the outcomes of a motorcycle crash in which a relative was involved.

Second, when using the ELM, the results of the two routes can be similar. However, the two routes usually lead to attitudes with different consequences. "Attitudes changed through central route processing are more enduring and have different effects on behavior than attitude change achieved through more peripheral processing, which is less resilient to counterarguments" (Simons-Morton et al., 2012, p. 285).

Third, "the model specifies how variables have an impact on persuasion" (Petty et al., 2009, p. 197). The variable can have an influence on people's motivation to think or ability to think, as well as the valence of people's thought or the confidence in the thoughts generated (Petty et al., 2009). For example, variables that have an impact on how a message is processed include the source of the message (e.g., friend, expert), the message itself (e.g., funny, serious), the context (e.g., delivered person-to-person, on the Internet), and various characteristics of the recipient (e.g., intelligence, age, attentiveness).

Keeping in mind these three things that the ELM provides, health education specialists can create health messages that are more meaningful to a priority population, and in turn, can be more successful in reaching program goals. **Figure 4.7** provides a diagram of the ELM as presented by Petty and colleagues (2009).

INFORMATION-MOTIVATION-BEHAVIORAL SKILLS MODEL (IMB)

The Information-Motivation-Behavioral Skills Model (IMB) (see **Figure 4.8**) was initially created to address the critical need for a strong theoretical basis for HIV/AIDS prevention efforts (Fisher & Fisher, 1992). Because of its success in dealing with HIV/AIDS prevention behavior, the IMB model has been applied to a number of other risk reduction behaviors (Fisher, Fisher, & Shuper, 2009). According to this model, the constructs of information, motivation, and behavioral skills are the fundamental determinants of preventive behavior. The information provided needs to be relevant, easily enacted based on the specific circumstances, and serve as a guide to personal preventive behavior. "In addition to facts that are easy to translate into behavior, the IMB model recognizes additional cognitive processes and content categories that significantly influence performance of preventive behavior" (Fisher et al., 2009, p. 27). An example is the following guideline that someone may use to make a decision: "If my best friend is willing to ride a motorcycle without a helmet, it must be okay."

Even though people are well informed about a particular health issue, they may not be motivated to act. According to the IMB model, prevention motivation includes both personal motivation to act (i.e., one's attitude toward a specific behavior) and social motivation to act (social support for the preventive behavior) (Fisher et al., 2009). Both types of motivation are necessary to act.

In addition to being well informed and motivated to act, the IMB model also indicates that people must possess behavioral skills to engage in the preventive behavior. The behavioral skills component of the IMB model includes an individual's objective ability and his or her perceived self-efficacy to perform the preventive behavior.

When applying the IMB model, health education specialists cannot just use their own judgment to determine what information to provide, how best to motivate, and what behavioral skills to teach to a given population. The process should begin by eliciting information from a subsample of the priority population to identify deficits in their health-relevant information, motivation, and behavioral skills. Next, health education specialists need to design and implement "*conceptually-based, empirically-targeted, population-specific*" (p. 29) interventions, constructed on the bases of the elicited findings (Fisher et al., 2009). Then, after the

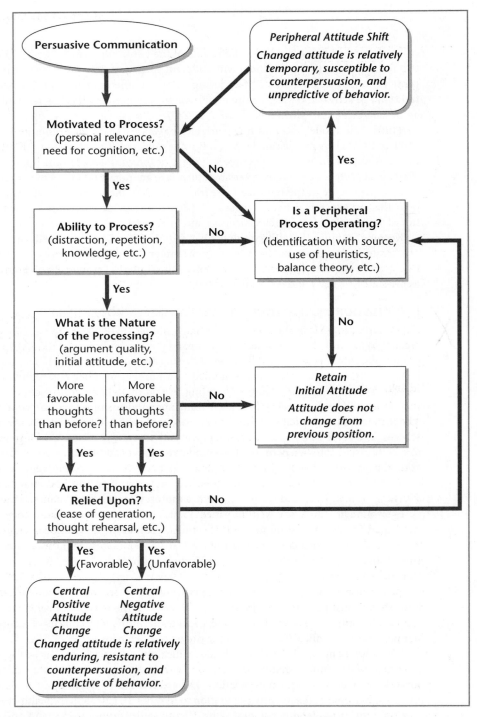

▲ **Figure 4.7** The Elaboration Likelihood Model of Persuasion (ELM)

Source: From Petty, R. E., Barden J., & Wheeler, S. C., "The Elaboration Likelihood Model of Persuasion: Developing Health Promotions for Sustained Behavioral Change" in *Emerging Theories in Health Promotion Practice and Research*, 2nd ed., DiClemente, R. J., Crosby, R. A., & Kegler, M. (Eds.), p. 196. Copyright © 2009 John Wiley & Sons, Inc. Reproduced with permission of John Wiley & Sons, Inc.

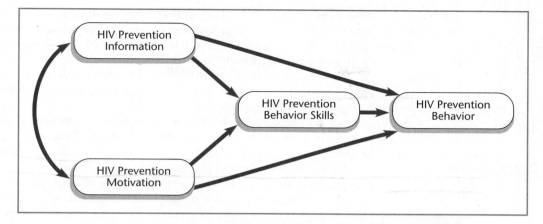

▲ **Figure 4.8** The Information-Motivation-Behavioral Skills Model of HIV Prevention Health Behavior

Source: From Fisher, J. D., & Fisher, W. A., "Changing AIDS Risk Behavior," *Psychological Bulletin 111*(3), 455–474, 1992. Published by American Psychological Association (APA). Reprinted by permission.

implementation of the intervention, health education specialists must evaluate the intervention to determine if it had significant and sustained effects on the information, motivation, and behavioral skill determinants of the preventive behavior and on the preventive behavior itself (Fisher et al., 2009).

TRANSTHEORETICAL MODEL OF CHANGE (TMC)

The TMC proposes that intentional behavior change "occurs in stages. As people attempt to change their behavior, they move through a variety of stages using different processes to help them get from one stage to the next until a desired behavior is attained" (Hayden, 2014, pp. 138–139). The **TMC** draws from the constructs of a number of theories, "hence the name 'Transtheoretical'" (Prochaska, Johnson, & Lee, 1998, p. 59).

Although each TMC construct is important, this model is best known for its stages of change. TMC suggests that "people move from *precontemplation*, not intending to change, to *contemplation*, intending to change within 6 months, to *preparation*, actively planning change, to *action*, overtly making changes, and into *maintenance*, taking steps to sustain change and resist temptation to relapse" (Prochaska, Redding, Harlow, Rossi, & Velicer, 1994, p. 473).

TMC was first used in psychotherapy. It was developed by Prochaska (1979) after he completed a comparative analysis of various therapy systems and many therapy studies. Since then, program planners have used TMC with a wide variety of topics ranging from alcohol abuse to weight control (Prochaska, Redding, & Evers, 2008; Spencer, Adams, Malone, Roy, & Yost, 2006).

Following is an example of TMC's stage construct applied to smoking cessation. In the **precontemplation stage**, smokers "have no intention to take action in the foreseeable future (usually defined as within the next 6 months)" (DiClemente, Redding, et al. 2013, p. 109). There are a number of reasons why people are in this stage. It may be because that they are discouraged from previous unsuccessful attempts at changing or it may be that they are either uninformed or under-informed about the consequences of their behavior (Prochaska et al., 2008).

In the **contemplation stage**, smokers know that smoking is bad for them and consider quitting. They "are intending to take action in the next six months" (Prochaska, 2005, p. 111). In the **preparation stage**, the smokers have combined intention and behavioral criteria. Often, during the past year, they have already taken a step toward changing their behavior. For example, they may have enrolled in an organized class to help them change, had a conversation with a physician or counselor, or purchased a self-help book or app for their smartphone to help guide their change (Prochaska et al., 2008).

In the **action stage**, smokers have overtly made changes in their behavior, experiences, or environment to stop smoking in the past six months. "Not all modifications of behavior count as action in this model" (Prochaska et al., 2008, p. 100). To be considered in this stage, people need to meet a level of behavior that scientists and professionals agree is sufficient to reduce the risk of disease. In our example, reducing the number of cigarettes smoked per day does not meet the necessary level for action; only total abstinence qualifies (Prochaska et al., 2008). As the smokers make these changes, they are moving toward the next stage, maintenance.

The focus of the **maintenance stage** is to prevent relapse. Thus, individuals who have quit smoking are working not to smoke again. People in this stage have changed their problem behavior for at least six months and are increasingly more confident that they can continue their change (Prochaska et al., 1998; Redding, Rossi, Rossi, Velicer, & Prochaska, 1999). In other words, their change is more of a habit, and their chance of relapse is lower, but their new behavior still requires some attention (Redding et al., 1999).

The final stage is **termination**. This stage is defined as the time when individuals who made a change now have zero temptation to return to their old behavior. They have 100 percent self-efficacy (a lifetime of maintenance). In our example, smokers have become non-smokers. No matter what their mood, they will not return to their old behavior (Prochaska et al., 2008). This is a stage that few people reach with certain behaviors (e.g., alcoholism).

PRECAUTION ADOPTION PROCESS MODEL (PAPM)

The Precaution Adoption Process Model (PAPM) tries to explain how people get to the point of making a decision about taking action and how they apply their decision to taking action (Weinstein et al., 2008). Although the Transtheoretical Model of Change and the PAPM are both stage models that appear similar, they are applied quite differently. The PAPM is most applicable for the adoption of a new precaution (e.g., getting a mammogram or a hepatitis B vaccination), or the abandonment of a risky behavior that requires a deliberate action (e.g., not wearing a safety belt). It can also be used to explain why and how people make deliberate changes in habitual patterns (e.g., flossing one's teeth two times a day instead of one). The PAPM is not applicable for actions that require the gradual development of habitual patterns of behavior, such as exercise and diet (Weinstein et al., 2008).

In the following example, the seven stages of the PAPM (see **Figure 4.9**) are applied to participating in a medical screening program. In Stage 1, Unaware of Issue, people are totally unaware of the need to be screened. When people first learn something about the screening, they are no longer unaware, but they are not necessarily engaged by it, either. This is Stage 2, Unengaged.

In Stage 3, Undecided about Acting, people have become engaged in thinking about the screening, and they are considering participation. Once people have reach this stage one of three things happen: 1) they suspend judgment and stay in this Stage, 2) they decide to act and move to Stage 4, or 3) they decide not to act and move to Stage 5 (Weinstein et al, 2008).

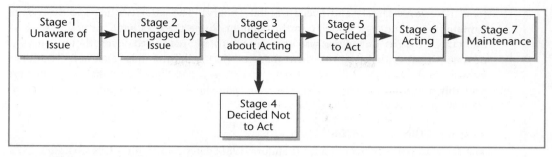

▲ **Figure 4.9** Stages of the Precaution Adoption Process Model (PAPM)

Source: From Weinstin, N. D., Sandman, P. M., & Blalock, S. J., "The Precaution Adoption Process Model" in *Health Behavior and Health Education: Theory, Research, and Practice,* 4th ed., K. Glanz, B. K. Rimer, and K. Viswanath, (Eds.), p. 127. Copyright © 2008 John Wiley & Sons, Inc. Reproduced with permission of John Wiley & Sons, Inc.

Once the people participate in the screening, they have initiated the behavior, and they are in Stage 6, Acting. Finally, if the people participate in the screening at the medically recommended intervals, they are in Stage 7, Maintenance. Note that this last stage of the PAPM is not applicable to some decision-making processes, for example, actions required only once in a lifetime, such as a vaccination that immunizes a person for life (Weinstein et al., 2008).

Interpersonal Theories

The category of interpersonal theories contains theories that "assume individuals exist within, and are influenced by, a social environment. The opinions, thoughts, behavior, advice, and support of the people surrounding an individual influence his or her feelings and behavior, and the individual has a reciprocal effect on those people" (Rimer & Glanz, 2005, p. 19). Research shows that social relationships can be a powerful influence on health and health behaviors (Heaney & Israel, 2008). As such, a number of theories have been created to explain concepts such as

- *Social norms*—"what are perceived to be true and acceptable" (Simons-Morton et al., 2012, p. 158)
- *Social learning*—learning that occurs in a social context
- *Social power*—ability to influence others or resist activities of others
- *Social integration*—structure and quality of relationships
- *Social networks*—"person-centered webs of social relationships" (Sharma & Romas, 2012, p. 283).
- *Social support*—"help obtained through social relationships and interpersonal exchanges" (Sharma & Romas, 2012, p. 284)
- *Social capital*—"the relationships and structures within a community, such as civic participation, networks, norms of reciprocity, and trust, that promote cooperation of mutual benefit" (Putnam, 1995, p. 66).
- *Interpersonal communication*

Because of space limitations, only three interpersonal theories are overviewed in this chapter, one that is well-established (Social Cognitive Theory) and two newer theories

(Social Network Theory and Social Capital Theory). The latter two may be theories in name only. As stated previously in this chapter, some theories have the term *model* in their title because that is the way they were initially identified. Even though there is now empirical evidence to call them theories, the model title has remained. The social network and social capital theories may have been called theories prematurely; they are probably more in the model stage. However, you should be aware of the main concepts in each one.

SOCIAL COGNITIVE THEORY (SCT)

The Social Cognitive Theory (SCT) (Bandura, 1986) dates back to the 1950s (Bandura, 1977; Rotter, 1954), when it was known as the Social Learning Theory (SLT). Some still refer to it as the SLT. In brief, the SCT asserts "that the social environment, the personal characteristics of the individual, and behavior interact and influence each other" (Crosby, Salazar, & DiClemente, 2013b, p. 164). Those who advocate the SCT believe that reinforcement contributes to learning. But the combination of reinforcement with an individual's expectations of the behavior's consequences is what determines the behavior. The SCT explains learning through its constructs. Unlike the other theories presented so far in this chapter, there is no diagram for the SCT nor is the interrelationship of its constructs specific in nature. Those constructs most often used in health education/promotion are presented in **Table 4.2**, along with an example of each.

SOCIAL NETWORK THEORY (SNT)

The term **social network** refers to the "person-centered web of social relationships" (Sharma & Romas, 2012, p. 283). Barnes, a sociologist who studied Norwegian villages (Barnes, 1954), created the term in the 1950s. He used it to describe villagers' social relationships and characteristics that were not traditional social units like families (Edberg, 2007; Heaney & Israel, 2008). Since that time, sociologists and professionals in various disciplines, including health education/promotion, have continued to study and use the social network concept.

Social epidemiological observational studies clearly document the beneficial effects of supportive networks on health status (Heaney & Israel, 2008). But some people question whether there is enough evidence to suggest a Social Network Theory (SNT). Heaney and Israel (2008) feel that the social network concept, and the closely related one of social support, are really not theories, but rather are concepts that describe social relationships. They feel that intervention studies are "needed to identify the most potent causal agents and critical time periods for social network enhancement" (p. 197). For example, it is not known how much social networking is needed to enhance health, or how much is too much. Also unknown are the characteristics of "good networks" that result in positive health behavior (i.e., regular exercise) versus characteristics of "bad networks" that lead to negative health behavior (i.e., smoking). We do know, however, that people who are part of social networks are healthier, as a whole, than those who are not involved in social networks.

Edberg (2007) described different types of social networks such as ego-centered networks and full relational networks (see **Figure 4.10**). He indicated that the key component to SNT is the relationships between and among individuals, including how those relationships influence beliefs and behaviors. He further stated that those using SNT need to consider the

TABLE 4.2 **Often-used constructs of the Social Cognitive Theory and examples of their application**

Construct	Definition	Example
Behavioral capability	Knowledge and skills necessary to perform a behavior	If people are going to exercise aerobically, they need to know what it is and how to do it.
Expectations	Beliefs about the likely outcomes of certain behaviors	If people enroll in a weight-loss program, they expect to lose weight.
Expectancies	Values people place on expected outcomes	How important is it to people that they become physically fit?
Locus of control	Perception of the center of control over reinforcement	Those who feel they have control over reinforcement are said to have internal locus of control. Those who perceive reinforcement under the control of an external force are said to have external locus of control.
Reciprocal determinism	"Environmental factors influence individuals and groups, but individuals and groups can also influence their environments and regulate their own behavior" (McAlister, Perry, & Parcel, 2008, p. 171)	Lack of use of vending machines could be a result of the choices within the machine. Notes about the selections from the nonusing consumers to the machine's owners could change the selections and change the behavior of the non-using consumers to that of users.
Observational learning	Learning by watching others	Provide the priority population with the opportunity to watch others modeling the desired behavior
Reinforcement (directly, vicariously, self-management)	Responses to behaviors that increase the chances of recurrence	Giving verbal encouragement to those who have acted in a healthy manner
Self-control, or **self-regulation**	Gaining control over own behavior through monitoring and adjusting it	If clients want to change their eating habits, have them monitor their current eating habits for seven days.
Self-efficacy	People's confidence in their ability to perform a certain desired task or function	If people are going to engage in a regular exercise program, they must feel they can do it.
Collective efficacy	Beliefs about the ability of the group to perform concerted actions that bring desired outcomes (McAlister et al., 2008, p. 171)	If a group of people is going to work to change a community's cultural toward healthy behavior, they must feel that they can do it.
Emotional-coping response	For people to learn, they must be able to deal with the sources of anxiety that surround a behavior.	Fear is an emotion that can be involved in learning, and people would have to deal with it before they could learn a behavior.

Source: From Created from Baranowski, T. Perry, C. L., & Parcel, G. S., (2002). "How Individuals, Environments, and Health Behavior Interact: Social Cognitive Theory," in K. Glanz, B.K. Riner & F.M. Lewis (Eds.), *Health behavior and health education: Theory, research, and practice,* 3rd ed., 165–184; McAlister, A.L., Perry, C.L. & Parcel, G.S. (2008). "How Individuals, Environments, and Health Behavior Interact: Social Cognitive Theory," in K. Glanz, B. K. Rimer, & K. Viswanath (Eds.), *Health behavior and health education: Theory, research, and practice,* 4th ed., 169–188; McKenzie, J. F., Neiger, B. L. & Thackery, R. (2013). *Planning, implementing, and evaluating health promotion programs: A primer,* 6th ed., Pearson, Boston, MA. Simons-Morton, B. G., McLeroy, K. R., & Wendel, M. L. (2012). *Behavior theory in health promotion practice and research.* Burlington, MA: Jones & Bartlett Learning.

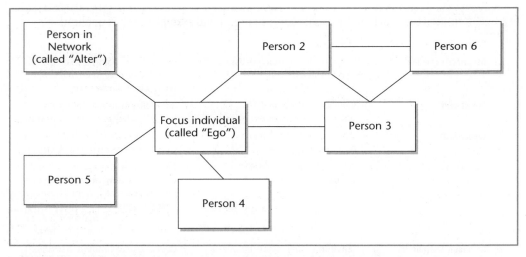

▲ **Figure 4.10** A simple sociogram, centered on a "focus individual" or ego

Source: From Edberg, M., *Essentials of Health Behavior: Social and Behavioral Theory in Public Health,* 1st ed., Fig. 5-1, p. 56. Copyright © 2007, Jones and Bartlett Publishers, Sudbury, MA. http://www. jblearning.com. Reprinted by permission.

following items when assessing a network's role on the health behavior of individuals who are part of the network (Edberg, 2007):

- Centrality versus marginality of individuals in the network: How involved is the person in the network?
- Reciprocity of relationships: Are relationships one-way or two-way?
- Complexity or intensity of relationships in the network: Do the relationships exist between two people, or are they multiplexed?
- Homogeneity or diversity of people in the network: Do all members of the network have similar characteristics, or are they different from one another?
- Subgroups, cliques, and linkages: Are there concentrations of interactions among some members? If so, do they interact with others, or are they isolated from others?
- Communication patterns in the network: How does information pass between the members in the network?

In summary, we know that social networks can impact health, but the specifics of who is most affected and how best to set up and use social networks are unknown. Even so, health education specialists who are planning interventions need to consider whether social networks should be a part of their strategy to bring about change. With the power of the Internet, the impact of social networks in the work of health education specialists will continue to grow.

SOCIAL CAPITAL THEORY

The term **social capital** got its start in political science and has been used in health education/promotion since the mid-1990s. An often-quoted definition is "the relationships and structures within a community, such as civic participation, networks, norms of reciprocity, and trust, that promote cooperation of mutual benefit" (Putnam, 1995, p. 66). "Social capital is a collective asset, a feature of communities rather than the property of individuals. As such, individuals both contribute to it and use it, but they cannot own it" (Warren, Thompson, & Saegert, 2001, p. 1).

"The influence of social capital is well documented" (Crosby et al., 2009). There are epidemiological studies that show that greater social capital is linked to several different positive outcomes (i.e., reduced mortality). There are also correlational studies that show a lack of social capital is related to poorer health outcomes (e.g., Kawachi, Kennedy, Lochner, & Prothrow, 1997). But as with social networks, a cause-effect relationship has not been established between social capital and better health. "Social capital does not provide theories of change, tools, or time lines for change; nor does it necessarily guarantee improved outcomes if social capital is improved" (Minkler & Wallerstein, 2005, p. 38). However, it does seem to have an impact on health.

Figure 4.11 provides a graphic representation of social capital. This particular figure includes the key concepts of Putman's (1995) definition of social capital and three different types of network resources: bonding, bridging, and linking social capital. These three types are differentiated based on the strength of the relationships between/among those people in the social network (Hayden, 2014). Originally, *bonding social capital*, sometimes referred to as exclusive social capital, was defined as "the type that brings closer together people who already know each other" (Gittell & Vidal, 1998, p.15). More recently, this concept was expanded to include people who are similar, or people who are members of the same group. Examples of bonding social capital include those who may be members in a service organization (e.g., Lions, Elks, American Legion) or religious community.

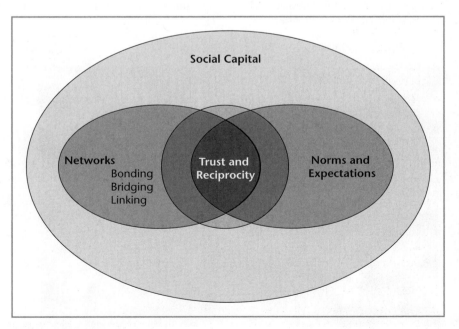

▲ **Figure 4.11** Social capital

Source: From Hayden, J., *Introduction to Health Behavior Theory*, 1st ed., Fig 9-3, p. 125. Copyright © 2009, Jones and Bartlett Publishers, Sudbury, MA. http://www.jblearning.com. Reprinted by permission.

Bridging social capital, sometimes referred to as inclusive social capital, was originally defined as "the type that brings together people or groups who previously did not know each other" (Gittell & Vidal, 1998, p. 15). Bridging social capital is now seen more as the resources people obtain from their interaction with others outside their group, who often are people with different demographic characteristics. An example is people from different parts of a community who come together to create a community park.

The most recently recognized and weakest (Hayden, 2014) network resource is *linking social capital*. This type of network resource comes from relationships between or among "individuals and groups in different social strata in a hierarchy where power, social status, and wealth are accessed by different groups" (U.K. Office of National Statistics, 2001, p. 11). An example may be where a boss and an employee are working together on a project.

As with social networks, it is important that health education specialists think about the concept of social capital when planning interventions. Although it is not an intervention in itself, it is a concept that needs to be considered and monitored.

Community Theories

This group of theories includes three categories of factors from the socio-ecological approach—organizational, community, and public policy. Organizational factors include rules, regulations, and policies of an organization that can impact health behavior. Community factors include social norms, whereas public policy includes legislation that can impact health behavior (see **Figure 4.12**). Theories associated with these three factors include theories of community organizing and community building (see Chapter 1), organizational change, the Diffusion Theory, and the Community Readiness Model (a stage model). The latter two are described in the following sections.

▲ **Figure 4.12** Public policy has become an important intervention strategy for health promotion.

DIFFUSION THEORY (DF)

The **Diffusion Theory (DF)** provides an explanation for the diffusion of innovations in populations. In health education/promotion, innovations come in the form of new ideas, techniques, behaviors, and programs. When people become "consumers" of an innovation, they are referred to as adopters. Rogers (2003) categorized adopters on the basis of when they adopt innovations. These categories include innovators, early adopters, early or late majority, and laggards. The rate at which people become adopters can be represented by the bell-shaped curve (see **Figure 4.13**).

Innovators are the first to adopt an innovation. They are venturesome, independent, risky, and daring. They want to be the first to do something. **Early adopters** are very interested in innovation, but they do not want to be the first involved. Early adopters are respected by others in the social system and looked at as opinion leaders.

Following the early adopters is the **early majority**. This group of people may be interested in the innovation but need some external motivation to get involved. These people, along with those in the late majority, make up the largest groups. The **late majority** comprises people who are skeptical. They will not adopt an innovation until most people in the social system have done so. The **laggards** are the last ones to get involved in an innovation, if they get involved at all.

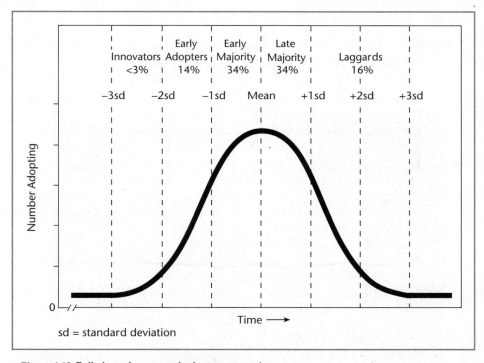

▲ **Figure 4.13** Bell-shaped curve and adopter categories

Following is an application of the Diffusion Theory. The health education staff at the Walkup Health Maintenance Organization (HMO) is beginning a new series of stress management classes for the HMO members. About 3 percent of the priority population (the innovators) will sign up and attend the classes as soon as they hear about the series. Shortly thereafter, another 14 percent (early adopters) will probably get involved, possibly after reading about the program's merits. At this point, the health education staff must work harder to attract others to the program. It will take constant reminders to get the early majority (~34 percent) involved. Buddy, peer, or mentoring programs might be needed to get the late majority (~34 percent) involved. The laggards (~16 percent) probably will not attend the series at all.

COMMUNITY READINESS MODEL (CRM)

The Community Readiness Model (CRM) is a stage theory for communities. Communities, like individuals, are in various stages of readiness for change. Yet, the stages of change for communities are not the same as for individuals. "The stages of readiness in a community have to deal with group processes and group organization, characteristics that are not relevant to personal readiness" (Edwards, Jumper-Thurman, Plested, Oetting, & Swanson, 2000, pp. 296–297). Although the CRM was developed initially to deal with alcohol and drug abuse, it also has been used in a variety of health and nutrition areas, environmental issues, and social programs (Edwards et al., 2000). The CRM has nine stages (Edwards et al., 2000):

1. *No Awareness.* The problem is not generally recognized by the community or leaders.

2. *Denial.* There is little or no recognition in the community that there is a problem. If recognition exists, there is a feeling that nothing can be done about the problem.

3. *Vague Awareness.* Some people in the community feel there is a problem and something should be done, but there is no motivation or leadership to do so.

4. *Preplanning.* There is a clear recognition by some that a problem exists and something should be done. There are leaders, but no focused or detailed planning.

5. *Preparation.* Planning is taking place but it is not based on collected data. There is leadership and modest support for efforts. Resources are being sought.

6. *Initiation.* Information is available to justify and begin efforts. Staff is either in training or has just completed training. Leaders are enthusiastic. There is usually little resistance and involvement from the community members.

7. *Stabilization.* The program is running, staffed, and supported by the community and decision makers. The program is perceived as stable with no need for change. This stage may include routine tracking, but no in-depth evaluation.

8. *Confirmation/Expansion.* Standard efforts are in place, which are supported by the community and decision makers. The program has been evaluated and modified, and efforts are in place to seek resources for new efforts. There is ongoing data collection to link risk factors and problems.

9. *Professionalism.* Much is known about prevalence, risk factors, and cause of problems. Highly trained staff members run effective programs aimed at the general population and appropriate subgroups. Programs have been evaluated and modified. The community is supportive but should hold programs accountable.

TABLE 4.3 **Community readiness stages and goals**

Stage	Goal
(1) *No Awareness*	Raise awareness of the issue.
(2) *Denial*	Raise awareness that the problem or issue exists in the community.
(3) *Vague Awareness*	Raise awareness that the community can do something.
(4) *Preplanning*	Raise awareness with the concrete ideas to combat condition.
(5) *Preparation*	Gather existing information to help plan strategies.
(6) *Initiation*	Provide community specific information.
(7) *Stabilization*	Stabilize efforts/programs.
(8) *Confirmation/Expansion*	Expand and enhance service.
(9) *Professionalism*	Maintain momentum and continue growth.

Source: Created from Edwards, R. W., Jumper-Thurman, P., Plested, B. A., Oetting, E. R., & Swanson, L. (2000). "Community Readiness: Research to Practice." *Journal of Community Psychology, 28* (3), 291–307.

A community's readiness can be assessed through interviews with key informants. As with other stage theories, once the stage of readiness is known, there are suggested processes for moving a community from one stage to the next. **Table 4.3** presents the nine stages and the goal for each stage.

▷ Planning Models

Good health education/promotion programs are not created by chance. "A systematic process is important in these endeavors" (Bartholomew, Parcel, Kok, Gottlieb, & Fernández, 2011). Well-thought-out and well-conceived models provide health education specialists with "frames" on which to build plans (see **Box 4.1**). Although many planning models have

BOX 4.1

Practitioner's Perspective

THEORIES AND PLANNING MODELS Trevor W. Newby

CURRENT POSITION/TITLE: Health Education Specialist, Senior

EMPLOYER: Idaho State Tobacco Prevention and Control Program (Project Filter)

MAJOR: Health Promotion

DEGREES: Master of Health Science in Health Promotion and Bachelor of Science in Health Promotion

INSTITUTION: Boise State University

How I obtained my job: During my graduate assistantship, I was fortunate to align myself with a number of individuals and professors that made me more marketable for employment upon graduation. Knowing I was ready to graduate, a professor forwarded me a job posting for a Senior Health Education Specialist position with the Idaho State Respiratory Health Program. While in this capacity, I've been able to work with a number of statewide programs and a variety of different organizations while taking part in a number of collaboration efforts related to Project Filter. My job has allowed me to work a great deal with marketing, evaluation, and reporting, and has provided me with countless networking and educational opportunities.

How I use theory in my job: At the state level, we are responsible for reporting

BOX

4.1

continued

progress in relation to tobacco prevention and control efforts to the Centers for Disease Control and Prevention (CDC). Because of this, we use a wide variety of theories, specifically those related to the stages of change, to assist us in achieving our work plan goals. This is very evident in the tobacco cessation services Project Filter offers to the general public through 1-800-QuitNow and Idaho.QuitNet.com. Both of these services utilize the behavior change model to help interested individuals to quit using tobacco.

Every model, strategy, or program that is implemented by Project Filter is evaluated to measure its effectiveness. Logic models are used as the marquee planning tool by CDC and other state programs to help strategize, plan, implement, and evaluate programs in most of the public health disciplines. In addition, Project Filter uses a variety of other methods to supplement the use of logic models in verifying programming effectiveness. These include use of work plans, quarterly and monthly reports from contracted agencies or groups, marketing analysis reports, event debriefing reports, and a variety of data collected from a host of different sources related to tobacco. This variety allows Project Filter to effectively plan, implement, and evaluate all facets of their programming efforts.

Recommendations for health education specialists: First, secure internship opportunities. Internship settings will not only provide valuable work experience that will put you ahead of other potential job seekers, but will also allow you to apply classroom learning while offering networking opportunities at the same time. The more internships you secure, the more diverse and enticing your portfolio will become for potential employers. Second, be proficient in grant writing. This is a valuable skill that is necessary in the public health profession. Third, take a number of marketing classes. Marketing plays an imperative role in public health. An agency could have the most dynamic program or resource available, but it won't provide any benefit unless it is effectively marketed to its intended audience. Lastly, don't be afraid to learn. Public health is a constantly evolving field with a wide variety of topics. In order to be a proficient educator, constant research and information gathering are critical.

Future of the health education/promotion profession: I consider the future of health education specialists in public health to be very positive. It has taken many years for businesses, lawmakers, and policy makers to realize the worth of proper prevention methods provided by public health professionals, but now the dynamic is changing. Prevention practices have already been proven to be effective with research surrounding tobacco. Prevention practices have saved millions of dollars in health care costs to tax payers in relation to tobacco use and have begun to change the social norm of tobacco use as a whole. I am certain prevention practices will play a vital role in the new health care reform as the government saves millions of dollars on secondary and tertiary clinical care by implementing effective prevention practices provided by public health professionals. This will provide many jobs to health education specialists in an increasingly changing and meaningful profession.

similar principles and common elements, those elements may have different labels. In fact, "there are important differences in sequence, emphasis, and the conceptualization of the major components that make certain models more appealing than others to individual practitioners" (Simons-Morton, Greene, & Gottlieb, 1995, pp. 126–127).

The following sections provide an overview of seven models used for planning health education/promotion programs. Although many more models exist, these seven have been

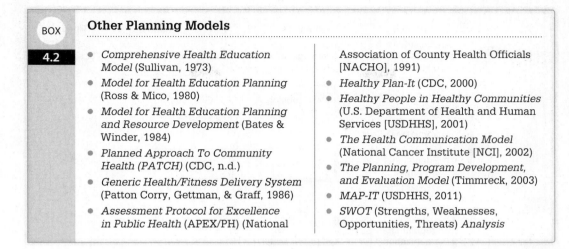

BOX 4.2

Other Planning Models

- *Comprehensive Health Education Model* (Sullivan, 1973)
- *Model for Health Education Planning* (Ross & Mico, 1980)
- *Model for Health Education Planning and Resource Development* (Bates & Winder, 1984)
- *Planned Approach To Community Health (PATCH)* (CDC, n.d.)
- *Generic Health/Fitness Delivery System* (Patton Corry, Gettman, & Graff, 1986)
- *Assessment Protocol for Excellence in Public Health* (APEX/PH) (National Association of County Health Officials [NACHO], 1991)
- *Healthy Plan-It* (CDC, 2000)
- *Healthy People in Healthy Communities* (U.S. Department of Health and Human Services [USDHHS], 2001)
- *The Health Communication Model* (National Cancer Institute [NCI], 2002)
- *The Planning, Program Development, and Evaluation Model* (Timmreck, 2003)
- *MAP-IT* (USDHHS, 2011)
- *SWOT* (Strengths, Weaknesses, Opportunities, Threats) *Analysis*

used successfully, and they represent a wide range of planning approaches. **Box 4.2** lists other planning models that may be just as good from a theoretical perspective, but currently they are not used as often. For more detailed explanations, see the original publications of the models.

PRECEDE-PROCEED

Currently, the best known planning model is **PRECEDE-PROCEED**. As its name implies, this model has two components. PRECEDE is an acronym that stands for *p*redisposing, *r*einforcing, and *e*nabling *c*onstructs in *e*ducational/*e*cological *d*iagnosis and *e*valuation. PROCEED stands for *p*olicy, *r*egulatory, and *o*rganizational *c*onstructs in *e*ducational and *e*nvironmental *d*evelopment (Green & Kreuter, 2005).

The PRECEDE-PROCEED model was developed over a period of 15 to 20 years. The PRECEDE framework was conceived in the early 1970s, whereas the PROCEED portion was developed in the early to mid-1980s. As shown in **Figure 4.14**, PRECEDE-PROCEED has eight phases. The first four phases, which make up the PRECEDE portion of the model, consist "of a series of planned assessments that generate information that will be used to guide subsequent decisions" (Green & Kreuter, 2005, p. 8). PROCEED also has four phases and "is marked by the strategic implementation of multiple actions based on what was learned from the assessments in the initial phase" (Green & Kreuter, 2005, p. 9).

At first glance, the PRECEDE-PROCEED model appears overly complicated. However, there is a logical sequence to the eight phases that outlines the health promotion planning process. The underlying approach of this model begins by identifying the desired outcome, then determines what causes it, and finally designs an intervention aimed at reaching the desired outcome. In other words, PRECEDE-PROCEED starts with the final consequences and works backward to the causes (McKenzie et al., 2013). **Table 4.4** provides an overview of the eight phases of this model.

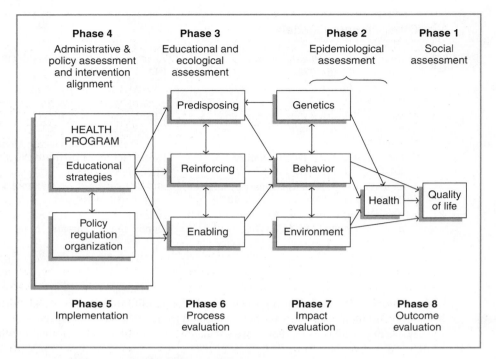

▲ **Figure 4.14** PRECEDE-PROCEED model for health program planning

Source: From Green, L. W., & Kreuter, M. W., *Health Program Planning: An Educational and Ecological Approach*, 4th ed., p. 17, Fig 1.5. Copyright © 2005 The McGraw-Hill Companies, Inc. Reprinted by permission.

TABLE 4.4 **The eight phases of the PRECEDE-PROCEED model**

Phase 1	**Social assessment** is "the assessment in both objective and subjective terms of high-priority problems or aspirations for the common good, defined for a population by economic and social indicators and by individuals in terms of their quality of life" (p. G-8), **situational analysis** is "the combination of social and epidemiological assessments of conditions, trends, and priorities with a preliminary scan of determinants, relevant policies, resources, organizational support, and regulations that might anticipate or permit action in advance of a more complete assessment of behavioral, environmental, educational, ecological, and administrative factors" (pp. G-7–8).
Phase 2	**Epidemiological assessment** is "the delineation of the extent, distribution, and causes of a health problem in a defined population" (p. G-3).
Phase 3	**Educational assessment** is "the delineation of factors that predispose, enable, and reinforce a specific behavior, or through behavior, environmental changes" (p. G-3), and **ecological assessment** is "a systematic assessment of factors in the social and physical environment that interact with behavior to produce health effects or quality-of-life outcomes" (p. G-3).
Phase 4a	**Intervention alignment** is matching appropriate strategies and interventions with projected changes and outcomes identified in earlier phases.
Phase 4b	**Administrative and policy assessment** is "an analysis of the policies, resources, and circumstances prevailing in an organizational situation to facilitate or hinder the development of the health program" (p. G-1).

continued

TABLE 4.4 *continued*

Phase 5	**Implementation** is "the act of converting program objectives into actions through policy changes, regulation, and organization" (p. G-5).
Phase 6	**Process evaluation** is "the assessment of policies, materials, personnel, performance, quality of practice or services, and other inputs and implementation experiences" (p. G-6).
Phase 7	**Impact evaluation** is "the assessment of program effects on intermediate objectives including changes in predisposing, enabling, and reinforcing factors, as well as behavioral and environmental changes, and possibly health and social outcomes" (p. G-5).
Phase 8	**Outcome evaluation** is an "assessment of the effects of a program on its ultimate objectives, including changes in health and social benefits or quality of life" (p. G-6).

Source: From Green, L. W., & Kreuter, M. W., *Health Program Planning: An Educational and Ecological Approach,* 4th ed. Copyright © 2005 The McGraw-Hill Companies, Inc. Reprinted by permission.

MATCH

MATCH is an acronym for Multilevel Approach To Community Health. This planning model (see **Figure 4.15**) was developed in the late 1980s (Simons-Morton, Simons-Morton, Parcel, & Bunker, 1988). Like the PRECEDE-PROCEED model, MATCH has also been used in a variety of settings. For example, several intervention handbooks created by the CDC used MATCH (Simons-Morton et al., 1995).

MATCH is a socio-ecological planning approach. It recognizes that intervention activities can and should be aimed at a variety of objectives and individuals. This approach is illustrated in Figure 4.15 by the various levels of influence.

The MATCH framework is recognized for emphasizing program implementation (Simons-Morton et al., 1995). "MATCH is designed to be applied when behavioral and environmental risk and protective factors for disease or injury are generally known and when general priorities for action have been determined, thus providing a convenient way to turn the corner from needs assessment and priority setting to the development of effective programs" (Simons-Morton et al., 1995, p. 155).

Intervention Mapping

Intervention Mapping is a relatively new model for planning health promotion programs (Bartholomew, Parcel, & Kok, 1998). It focuses on planning programs that are based on theory and evidence (Bartholomew et al., 2011). It also draws on multiple principles used in the PRECEDE-PROCEED and MATCH models.

Intervention mapping has six steps. The first step, *needs assessment*, includes two major components: (1) scientific, epidemiologic, behavioral, and social analysis of a priority population or community; and (2) an effort to get to know and understand the character of the priority population (Bartholomew et al., 2011).

Step 2, *matrices of change objectives*, specifies who and what will change as a result of the intervention (Bartholomew et al., 2011). Although the identification of goals and objectives is included in all planning models, intervention mapping makes a unique contribution in how this is carried out. In this step, planners create a matrix of change objectives for the intervention. By doing so, planners can more clearly see who and what will change as a result of the intervention.

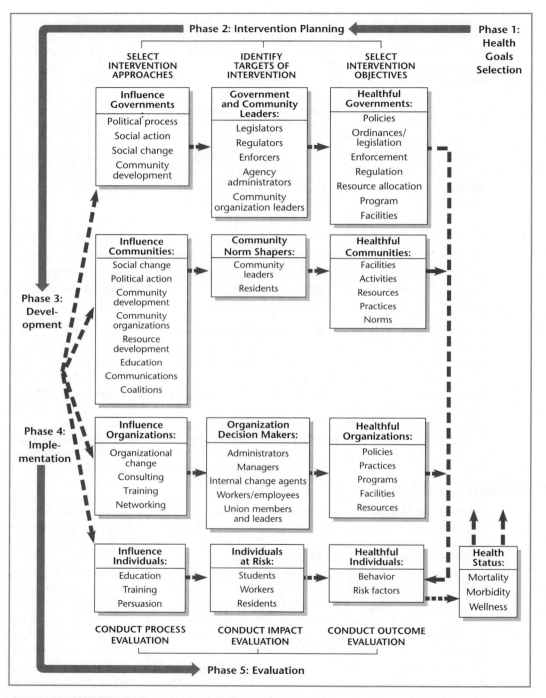

▲ **Figure 4.15** MATCH: Multilevel Approach To Community Health

In Step 3, *theory-based methods and practical applications*, planners work to identify theory-based methods and practical applications that hold the greatest promise to change the health behavior(s) of individuals in the priority population. Although planners seek theory-based methods, they also ensure that practical applications are selected and that final applications match the change objectives from the matrices.

In Step 4, *program production*, planners create the intervention details and materials and protocol needed for the program's implementation. This step is based on the methods and applications identified in Step 3.

Step 5, *adoption and implementation*, is like Step 2 in that it includes the development of matrices. However, these matrices focus on adoption and implementation performance objectives (Bartholomew et al., 2011). In other words, instead of concentrating on who and what will change within the priority population, the focus is on what will be done by whom among planners or program partners.

The sixth, and last, step of this model is *evaluation planning*. In this step, planners decide if determinants were well specified, if strategies were appropriately matched to methods, what proportion of the priority population was reached, and whether or not implementation was complete and executed as planned (Bartholomew et al., 2011).

CDCynergy

CDCynergy, or **Cynergy** for short, is a health communication planning model developed in 1997 by the Office of Communication at the CDC. It was first issued in 1998 (Parvanta & Freimuth, 2000). Cynergy was developed primarily for the CDC public health professionals who had responsibilities for health communication. However, because of widespread interest in the model, the CDC made it available to other health professionals in a variety of health education/promotion settings. Currently, CDCynergy is considered public domain, which means restrictions are not placed on copying or general use.

The basic edition of Cynergy presents a general methodology for health communication planning, a step-by-step guide, a reference library, and links to templates that allow tailored plans to be created (CDC, 2003). Cynergy uses six phases involving multiple steps to help planners: acquire a thorough understanding of a health problem and whom it affects; explore a wide range of possible intervention strategies for influencing the problem; systematically select the intervention strategies that show the most promise; understand the role communication can play in planning, implementing, and evaluating selected strategies; and develop a comprehensive communication plan (CDC, 2003). **Table 4.5** displays the six sequential, yet interrelated, phases, which are designed to build on the previous phases and prepare program planners for subsequent phases. Completion of these phases will lead to a strategic communication plan that is both science and audience based.

In addition to the basic edition of Cynergy, which is available in a Web version, CDC and its partners have produced content-specific editions of Cynergy to meet the particular needs of health education specialists addressing various health problems. There are content-specific editions for American Indian/Alaska Native Diabetes, Cardiovascular Disease, Diabetes, Emergency Risk Communication, Immunizations, Micronutrients, Social Marketing, STD Prevention, and Tobacco Prevention and Control (see Weblinks at the end of this chapter).

TABLE 4.5 *CDCynergy lite* (an abridged version of the CDCynergy health communication model)

Phase 1: Describe Problem

- Identify and define health problems that may be addressed by your program interventions.
- Examine and/or conduct necessary research to describe the problems.
- Assess factors and variables that can affect the project's direction, including strengths, weaknesses, opportunities, and threats (SWOT).

Phase 2: Analyze Problem

- List causes of each problem you plan to address.
- Develop goals for each problem.
- Consider strengths, weaknesses, opportunities, threats, and ethics of health (1) engineering, (2) communication/education, (3) policy/enforcement, and (4) community service intervention options.
- Select the types of intervention(s) that should be used to address the problem(s).

Phase 3: Plan Intervention

- Decide whether communication is needed as a dominant intervention or as support for other intervention(s).
  - If communication is used as a dominant intervention, list possible audiences.
  - If communication is to be used to support Community Services, Engineering, and/or Policy/ Enforcement interventions, list possible audiences to be reached in support of each selected intervention.
- Conduct necessary audience research to segment intended audiences.
- Select audience segment(s) and write communication objectives for each audience segment.
- Write a creative brief to provide guidance in selecting appropriate concepts or messages, settings, activities, and materials.

Phase 4: Develop Intervention

- Develop and test concepts, messages, settings, channel-specific activities, and materials with intended audiences.
- Finalize and briefly summarize a communication implementation plan. The plan should include:
  - Background and justification, including SWOT and ethics analyses
  - Audiences
  - Communication objectives
  - Messages
  - Settings and channels for conveying your messages
  - Activities (including tactics, materials, and other methods)
  - Available partners and resources
  - Tasks and timeline (including persons responsible for each task, date for completion of each task, resources required to deliver each task, and points at which progress will be checked)
  - Internal and external communication plan
  - Budget
- Produce materials for dissemination.

Phase 5: Plan Evaluation

- Determine stakeholder information needs.
  - Decide which types of evaluation (e.g., implementation, reach, effects) are needed to satisfy stakeholder information needs.
  - Identify sources of information and select data collection methods.
  - Formulate an evaluation design that illustrates how methods will be applied to gather credible information.
  - Develop a data analysis and reporting plan.

continued

TABLE 4.5 *continued*

Phase 5: Plan Evaluation

- Finalize and briefly summarize an evaluation implementation plan. The plan should include:
  - Stakeholder questions
  - Intervention standards
  - Evaluation methods and design
  - Data analysis and reporting
  - Tasks and timeline (including persons responsible for each task, date for completion of each task, resources required to deliver each task, and points at which progress will be checked)
  - Internal and external communication plan
  - Budget

Phase 6: Implement Plan

- Integrate, execute, and manage communication and evaluation plans.
- Document feedback and lessons learned.
- Modify program components based on feedback.
- Disseminate lessons learned and evaluation findings.

Source: Centers for Disease Control and Prevention (CDC), U.S. Department of Health and Human Services (USDHHS). 2003. *CDCynergy 3.0: Your Guide to Effective Health Communication (CD-ROM Version 3.0)*. Atlanta: Author.

SMART

Social marketing has been defined as "the application of commercial marketing technologies to the analysis, planning, execution, and evaluation of programs designed to influence the voluntary behavior of target audiences in order to improve their personal welfare and that of their society" (Andreasen, 1995, p. 7). This process offers benefits the audience wants, reduces barriers the audience faces, and uses persuasion to influence intentions to act favorably (Albrecht, 1997). The concept of social marketing is more than 30 years old, but its application to health education/promotion is much more recent (McDermott, 2000).

Even though the use of social marketing is relatively new in health education/promotion, several different authors (Andreasen, 1995; Bryant, 1998; Walsh, Rudd, Moeykens, & Moloney, 1993) have presented planning processes, models, or frameworks based on social marketing. The Social Marketing Assessment and Response Tool **(SMART)** is a social marketing planning framework developed by Neiger and Thackeray (1998) and influenced primarily by Walsh et al (1993). It is presented here because it provides a composite of other social marketing models, and because it has been used from start to finish on multiple occasions in several social marketing interventions (Neiger & Thackeray, 2002).

SMART is composed of seven phases (see **Table 4.6**). "Like other social marketing planning frameworks, the central focus of SMART is consumers. The heart of this model, composed of Phases 2 through 4, pertains to acquiring a broad understanding of the consumers who will be the recipients of a program and its interventions. These three phases seek to understand consumers before interventions are even developed or implemented. Though these phases (2–4) are displayed in linear fashion...they are typically performed simultaneously with members of the priority population" (McKenzie et al., 2013, p. 60).

TABLE 4.6 **The SMART model**

Phase 1: Preliminary Planning

- Identify a health problem and name it in terms of behavior.
- Develop general goals.
- Outline preliminary plans for evaluation.
- Project program costs.

Phase 2: Consumer Analysis

- Segment and identify the priority population.
- Identify formative research methods.
- Identify consumer wants, needs, and preferences.
- Develop preliminary ideas for preferred interventions.

Phase 3: Market Analysis

- Establish and define the market mix (4Ps).
- Assess the market to identify competitors (behaviors, messages, programs, etc.), allies (support systems, resources, etc.), and partners.

Phase 4: Channel Analysis

- Identify appropriate communication messages, strategies, and channels.
- Assess options for program distribution. Determine how channels should be used.
- Assess options for program distribution.
- Identify communication roles for program partners.

Phase 5: Develop Interventions, Materials, and Pretest

- Develop program interventions and materials using information collected in consumer, market, and channel analyses.
- Interpret the marketing mix into a strategy that represents exchange and societal good.
- Pretest and refine the program.

Phase 6: Implementation

- Communicate with partners and clarify involvement.
- Activate communication and distribution strategies.
- Document procedures and compare progress to timelines.
- Refine the program.

Phase 7: Evaluation

- Assess the degree to which the priority population is receiving the program.
- Assess the immediate impact on the priority population and refine the program as necessary.
- Ensure that program delivery is consistent with established protocol.
- Analyze changes in the priority population.

Source: Adapted from Walsh, R. E., et al. (1993). "Social Marketing for Public Health," *Health Affairs 12*(2), 104–119; and adapted from Neiger, B. L., & Thackeray, R. (1998). "Social Marketing: Making Public Health Sense." Paper presented at the annual meeting of the Utah Public Health Association, Provo, UT.

MAPP

MAPP is an acronym for Mobilizing for Action through Planning and Partnerships. It is a relatively new planning model created by the National Association of County and City Health Officials (NACCHO) to assist local health departments (LHDs) at the city or county level with planning. This model blends many of the strengths of the five planning models

▶ **Figure 4.16** Mobilizing for Action through Planning and Partnerships (MAPP) model

Source: National Association of County and City Health Officials, "Mobilizing for Action through Planning and Partnerships (MAPP) Model" from http://www.naccho.org/topics/infrastructure/mapp/upload/MAPP_Handbook_fnl.pdf. Reprinted by permission.

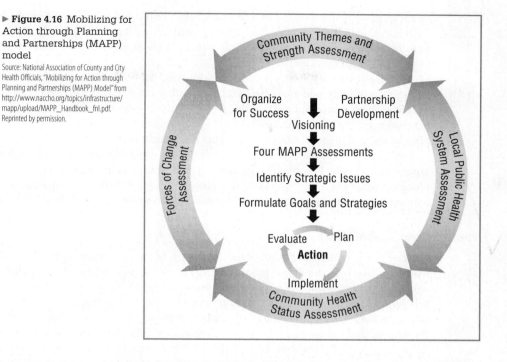

already presented in this chapter. The MAPP approach is designed to improve health and quality of life by mobilizing partnerships and taking strategic action (NACCHO, 2001).

MAPP is composed of multiple steps within six phases (see **Figure 4.16**). In the first phase of MAPP, Organizing for Success and Partnership Development, planners assess whether or not the MAPP process is timely, appropriate, and even possible. This involves assessing resources, including funding, personnel, and general interest of community members. If resources are not in place, the process is delayed. If resources are sufficient, the following work groups are created: (1) a core support team, which prepares most, if not all, of the material needed for the process; (2) the MAPP Committee, composed of key sponsors from the community who provide legitimacy and resources, and stakeholders who guide and oversee the process; and (3) the community itself, which provides input, representation, and decision making.

In Phase 2, Visioning, the community is guided through a process that results in a shared vision—what the ideal future looks like—and common values—principles and beliefs that will guide the remainder of the planning process (NACCHO, 2001). This phase is usually handled by a facilitator and involves anywhere from 50–100 participants, including the advisory committee, the MAPP committee, and key community leaders.

The strength and defining characteristic of MAPP are found in Phase 3, the Four MAPP Assessments. The four assessments include (1) the community themes and strengths assessment (community or consumer opinion); (2) the local public health system assessment (general capacity of the local public health system); (3) the community health status assessment (measurement of the health of the community by use of epidemiological data); and (4) the forces of change assessment (forces such as legislation, technology, and other environmental or social phenomena that do or will impact the community) (McKenzie et al., 2013). The four assessments help identify the gaps that exist between current status in the community and the vision identified in Phase 2, as well as strategic direction for goals and strategies (NACCHO, 2001).

In Phase 4, Identify Strategic Issues, a prioritized list of the issues facing the health of the community is developed. Only issues that jeopardize the vision and values of the community are considered. Important tasks in this phase include considering what would happen if certain issues are not addressed, understanding why an issue is strategic, consolidating overlapping issues, and identifying a prioritized list (McKenzie et al., 2013).

In Phase 5, Formulate Goals and Strategies, the goals and strategies to reach the vision are created. Finally, Phase 6, The Action Cycle, is similar to implementation and evaluation phases in other planning models. In this phase, implementation details are considered, evaluation plans are developed, and plans for disseminating results are made (NACCHO, 2001).

Generalized Model (GM)

As seen in the planning models presented so far, there are various approaches and frameworks on which to develop a program. Each model seems to have its own characteristics, whether it is the terminology used (e.g., predisposing, enabling, and reinforcing or analyze problem or consumer analysis), the number of components (e.g., eight phases versus six steps), or the progression through the phases or steps (e.g., circular, linear, or starting with the desired end and working backward). In other words, there are many ways to get from point A to point B. However, each of the models previously presented revolves around the five primary tasks incorporated in the **Generalized Model** (McKenzie et al., 2013). These five tasks are:

1. Assessing needs
2. Setting goals and objectives
3. Developing interventions
4. Implementing interventions
5. Evaluating results (see **Figure 4.17**)

"In addition, pre-planning is a quasi-step in the model but is not included formally since it involves actions that occur before planning technically begins" (McKenzie et al., 2013, p. 44). These tasks plus the quasi-step of pre-planning define planning and evaluation at its core.

To better understand the planning process in health education/promotion and the various models presented, consider the following scenario. A health education specialist was hired to develop health education/promotion programs in a corporate setting. She began her work with the quasi-step of pre-planning by trying to find out as much as possible about the "community" of this corporate setting and get those in the priority population involved in the program planning process. She did this by reading all the material she could find about the company. She also spent time talking with various individuals and subgroups in the company (i.e., new employees, longtime employees, management, clerical staff, labor representatives, etc.) to find out what they wanted from a health education/promotion program. In addition, she reviewed old documents of the company (i.e., health insurance records, labor agreements, written history of the company, etc.). As part of this background work, she

▲ **Figure 4.17** Generalized Model
Source: From McKenzie, J. F., Neiger, B. L., & Thackery, R., *Planning, Implementing and Evaluating Health Promotion Programs: A Primer*, 6th ed., p. 45, Fig. 3.1. Copyright © 2013. Reproduced by permission of Pearson, Boston, MA.

formed a program planning committee with representation from the various subgroups of the work force.

With the help of the planning committee, the health education/promotion specialist was ready to assess the needs of the priority population. She did this by reviewing the relevant literature, examining company health insurance claims, conducting a survey of employees, and holding focus groups with selected employees. As a result of the needs assessment, she was able to identify a target health problem. In this company, the problem was a higher than expected number of breast cancer cases in the priority population. This was a result in part of (1) the limited knowledge of employees about breast cancer, (2) the limited number of employees conducting breast self-examination (BSE), and (3) the low number of employees having mammograms on a regular basis.

With an understanding of the needs of the priority population, the health education specialist created specific objectives to increase the (1) employees' knowledge of breast cancer from baseline to after program participation, (2) number of women receiving mammograms by 30 percent, and (3) number of women reporting monthly BSE by 50 percent. Using these objectives, she planned multiple intervention activities:

1. An information sheet on the importance of BSE and mammography, for distribution with employee paychecks

2. A mobile mammography van on site every other month

3. Plastic BSE reminder cards, suitable for hanging from a showerhead, for distribution to all female employees

4. An article in the company newsletter covering the company's high rate of breast cancer and the new program to help women reduce their risk

5. Posters and pamphlets from the American Cancer Society in the company's lunchroom

Next, all of the listed intervention activities were carried out. Last, the health education specialist completed an evaluation to determine if there was an increase in knowledge, mammograms, and monthly BSE. As can be seen from this scenario, health education/promotion involves careful, systematic planning to achieve successful programs.

Summary

Health education/promotion is a multidisciplinary profession that has evolved from the theory and practice of other biological, behavioral, sociological, and health science disciplines. Many of the theories and models used in health education/promotion also have evolved from these other disciplines. This chapter presented an overview of the theoretical foundations and planning models of health education/promotion. Readers were introduced to the definitions of *theory, concept, construct, variable*, and *model*. A rationale was also provided to explain why it is important that health education specialists use theory in their work. Readers were then introduced to 12 of the behavior change theories that health education specialists use in their work. These theories were presented within the socio-ecological approach, which incorporates the seven levels of influence. There was also a distinction made between continuum theories and stage theories. And finally, overviews of seven planning models were provided.

Review Questions

1. Define each of the following and explain how they relate to each other.
   - *Theory*
   - *Concept*
   - *Construct*
   - *Variable*
   - *Model*
2. Why is it important to use theory in the practice of health education/promotion?
3. What are behavior change theories?
4. What are the seven levels of influence within the socio-ecological approach? How do they relate to behavior change theories?
5. Identify the 12 theories presented in this chapter that focus on health behavior change. Briefly describe each of the theories and name their components.
6. What is the difference between continuum theories and stage theories?
7. Explain why it might be important that health education specialists have a good understanding of stage models.
8. Name the seven planning models presented in this chapter, and list one distinguishing characteristic of each.
9. Of the seven planning models presented in this chapter, which one best known? Name the phases of this model.
10. What five components seem to be common to the planning models presented in this chapter?

▷ Case Study

Mike graduated a year ago with a bachelor's degree in health education. He felt extremely lucky to "beat out" 15 interviewees for the health education specialist position at the Lancaster County Health Department. Though the health department has a good reputation throughout the state, Mike is the only person on the staff hired to do health education.

Mike's supervisor, Dan Santoro, is Coordinator of Chronic and Infectious Disease for the health department. Santoro has worked for the department for about 30 years. He also holds a bachelor's degree from the same university Mike graduated from. However, Santoro received his degree in health and physical education before the implementation of the current community/public health education major.

Throughout Mike's tenure with the health department, he and Santoro have had a good working relationship. However, while planning a weight-loss program for a group of teenagers in the county, Mike ran into a situation that caused him some concern. After conducting a needs assessment and writing the program goals and objectives, he could not decide which behavior change theory to use to plan his intervention. He decided to seek Santoro's advice. When he asked Santoro what theory or model he would recommend, Santoro responded, "Theory-shmeary, you don't need to use that stuff, just skip the theory part and plan the intervention. This program needs to be up and running by the end of the month."

Based on this short conversation with Santoro, Mike was not sure how to proceed. During his undergraduate preparation at the university, Mike was told to "never plan an intervention that was not based on theory." Mike does not want to upset his supervisor, but he also knows that his program should be grounded in theory. What do you see as Mike's options at this point? What do you think Mike should do next? How would you solve this dilemma?

▷ Critical Thinking Questions

1. This chapter presented a number of different theories focusing on health behavior change. If you were trying to help a friend stop smoking, at the friend's request, what behavior change theory would you use to develop the intervention to help your friend? Defend why you selected this theory and explain how you would apply each of the constructs.

2. You have been invited by the Garber Corporation to interview for a newly created position in the company as a health education specialist. The position has been described as one that will focus on helping employees change their health behavior. As a part of the interview, the director of human resources asks you this question: "Of all the theories related to health education/promotion you studied in your college courses, which one do you think will have the greatest application to your work here at the Garber Corporation?" Defend your response.

3. What would you say to a person who asked you, "Tell me how the socio-ecological approach applies to changing health behavior?"

Activities

1. Interview a practicing health education specialist, asking about the theories and models the person has used in planning and implementing health education/promotion programs. Ask why those theories and models were used. Also, find out if the health education specialist has run into any problems trying to use the theories and models. Summarize the interview in a one-page paper.

2. Choosing and selecting from the components found in the planning models, create your own model. Draw a diagram of your model and, in two paragraphs, explain why you have included the components you did.

3. Pick one of the behavior change theories. Then choose a health behavior. In a one-page paper, explain how the theory can be applied to the health behavior you chose.

Weblinks

1. **http://www.naccho.org**
   National Association of County and City Health Officials
   At this Web site, the MAPP model is comprehensively presented and explained (search for "MAPP" on the homepage). To get access to the specifics you have to register. There is no cost to do so.

2. **http://www.healthypeople.gov/2020/implementing/default.aspx**
   Healthy People
   Choose the "Implement" tab on the HealthyPeople.gov Web site. It links to tools and strategies to help communities reach their health objectives.

3. **http://www.cdc.gov**
   CDCynergy
   Search the CDC homepage for "CDCynergy Health Communication" for an overview of *CDCynergy*, news and updates, information on all editions, current campaigns, practice areas, and resources. It also provides a link to the Web version of the original edition.

4. **http://www.uri.edu**
   Cancer Prevention Research Center (CPRC), University of Rhode Island
   Search the university's homepage for the Cancer Prevention Research Center, which is the home of the Transtheoretical Model of Change. Information about the model as well as measures that can be used to "stage" a person can be found at this site.

5. **http://people.umass.edu/aizen/tpb.html**
   Theory of Planned Behavior
   This is a Web page of Icek Ajzen, creator of the Theory of Planned Behavior. Information about the theory as well as example measures that can be used to measure the constructs of the theory can be found at this site.

6. **http://www.cancer.gov**
   National Cancer Institute (NCI)
   The National Cancer Institute presents the primer *Theory at a Glance: A Guide for Health Promotion Practice*. This volume explains why theories and models are important. It also

describes how to use theory. Explanations of several behavior change theories, as well as a couple of program planning models, are included. (Find it by searching at the NCI's homepage.)

7. http://www.cancer.gov/cancertopics/cancerlibrary/pinkbook

National Cancer Institute

This is the site where the entire 2002 edition of the Making Health Communication Programs Work, also called the Pink Book, can be downloaded.

 # References

Ajzen, I. (2006). *Theory of planned behavior diagram*. Retrieved May 19, 2013, from http://www.people.umass.edu/aizen/index.html.

Albrecht, T. L. (1997). Defining social marketing: Twenty five years later. *Social Marketing Quarterly, 3,* 21–23.

Andreasen, A. (1995). *Marketing sound change: Changing behavior to promote health, social development, and the environment.* San Francisco: Jossey-Bass.

Bandura, A. (1977). *Social learning theory.* Englewood Cliffs, NJ: Prentice-Hall.

Bandura, A. (1986). *Social foundations of thought and action.* Englewood Cliffs, NJ: Prentice-Hall.

Barnes, J. A. (1954). Class and committees in a Norwegian island parish. *Human Relations, 7,* 39–58.

Bartholomew, L. K., Parcel, G. S., & Kok, G. (1998). Intervention mapping: A process for developing theory- and evidence-based health education programs. *Health Education & Behavior, 25* (5), 545–563.

Bartholomew, L. K., Parcel, G. S., Kok, G., Gottlieb, N. H., & Fernández, M. E. (2011). *Planning health promotion programs: An intervention mapping approach* (3rd ed.). San Francisco: Jossey-Bass.

Bates, I. J., & Winder, A. E. (1984). *Introduction to health education.* Palo Alto, CA: Mayfield.

Bronfenbrenner, U. (1974). Developmental research, public policy, and the ecology of childhood (1974). *Child Development, 45* (1), 1–5.

Bronfenbrenner, U. (1979). *The ecology of human development: Experiments by nature and design.* Cambridge, MA: Harvard University Press.

Bryant, C. (1998). *Social marketing: A tool for excellence.* Eighth annual conference on social marketing in public health. Clearwater Beach, FL.

Centers for Disease Control and Prevention (CDC), U.S. Department of Health and Human Services (USDHHS). (2003). *CDCynergy 3.0: Your Guide to Effective Health Communication* (CD-ROM Version 3.0). Atlanta, GA: Author.

Centers for Disease Control and Prevention. (2000). *Healthy plan-it: A tool for planning and managing public health programs. Sustainable Management Development Program.* Atlanta, GA: Author.

Centers for Disease Control and Prevention (CDC), U.S. Department of Health and Human Services (USDHHS). (n.d.). *Planned approach to community health: Guide for local coordinators.* Atlanta, GA: Author.

Chaplin, J. P., & Krawiec, T. S. (1979). *Systems and theories of psychology* (4th ed.). New York: Holt, Rinehart & Winston.

Champion, V. L., & Skinner, C. S. (2008). The health belief model. In K. Glanz, B. K. Rimer, & K. Viswanath (Eds.), *Health behavior and health education: Theory, research, and practice* (4th ed., pp. 45–65). San Francisco: Jossey-Bass.

Crosby, R. A., Kegler, M. C., & DiClemente, R. J. (2009). Theory in health promotion practice and research. In R. J. DiClemente, R. A. Crosby, & M. C. Kegler (Eds.), *Emerging theories in health promotion practice and research* (2nd ed., pp. 4–17). San Francisco: Jossey-Bass.

Crosby, R. A., Salazar, L. F., & DiClemente, R. J. (2013a). How theory informs health promotion and public health practice. In R. J. DiClemente, L. F. Salazar, & R. A. Crosby. *Health behavior theory for public health: Principles, foundations, and application.* (pp. 27–44). Burlington, MA: Jones & Bartlett Learning.

Crosby, R. A., Salazar, L. F., & DiClemente, R. J. (2013b). Social cognitive theory applied to health behavior. In R. J. DiClemente, L. F. Salazar, & R. A. Crosby. *Health behavior theory for public health: Principles, foundations, and application.* (pp. 163–185). Burlington, MA: Jones & Bartlett Learning.

DiClemente, R. J., Crosby, R. A., & Kegler, M. (2009). *Emerging theories in health promotion practice and research* (2nd ed.). San Francisco: Jossey-Bass.

DiClemente, R. J., Redding, C. A., Crosby, R. A., & Salazar, L. F. (2013). Stage models for health promotion. In R. J. DiClemente, L. F. Salazar, & R. A. Crosby. *Health behavior theory for public health: Principles, foundations, and application.* (pp. 105–129). Burlington, MA: Jones & Bartlett Learning.

DiClemente, R. J., Salazar, L. F., & Crosby, R. A. (2013). *Health behavior theory for public health: Principles, foundations, and applications.* Burlington, MA: Jones & Bartlett Learning.

Edberg, M. (2007). *Essentials of health behavior: Social and behavioral theory in public health.* Sudbury, MA: Jones & Bartlett.

Edberg, M. (2015). *Essentials of health behavior: Social and behavioral theory in public health.* (2nd ed.) Burlington, MA: Jones & Bartlett Learning.

Edwards, R. W., Jumper-Thurman, P., Plested, B. A., Oetting, E. R., & Swanson, L. (2000). Community readiness: Research to practice. *Journal of Community Psychology, 28* (3), 291–307.

Fishbein, M., & Ajzen, I. (1975). *Belief, attitude, intention and behavior: An introduction to theory and research.* Reading, MA: Addison-Wesley.

Fisher, J. D., & Fisher, W. A. (1992). Changing AIDS risk behavior. *Psychological Bulletin, 111,* 455–474.

Fisher, J. D., Fisher, W. A., & Shuper, P. A. (2009). The informational-motivation-behavioral skills model of HIV preventive behavior. In R. J. DiClemente, R. A. Crosby, & M. C. Kegler (Eds.). *Emerging theories in health promotion practice and research* (2nd ed., pp. 21–63). San Francisco: Jossey-Bass.

Floyd, D. L., Prentice-Dunn, S., & Rogers, R. W. (2000). A meta-analysis of research on protection motivation theory. *Journal of Applied Social Psychology, 30,* 407–429.

Gittell, R., & Vidal, A. (1998). *Community organizing: Building social capital as a development strategy.* Thousand Oaks, CA: Sage.

Glanz, K., & Rimer, B. K. (1995). *Theory at a glance: A guide for health promotion practice* (NIH publication no. 95–3896). Bethesda, MD: National Institutes of Health, National Cancer Institute.

Glanz, K., Rimer, B. K., & Viswanath, K. (Eds.). (2008a). *Health behavior and health education: Theory, research, and practice* (4th ed.). San Francisco: Jossey-Bass.

Glanz, K., Rimer, B. K., & Viswanath, K. (2008b). Theory, research, and practice in health behavior and health education. In K. Glanz, B. K. Rimer, & K. Viswanath (Eds.), *Health behavior and health education: Theory, research, and practice* (4th ed., pp. 23–40). San Francisco: Jossey-Bass.

Goodson, P. (2010). *Theory in health promotion research and practice: Thinking outside the box.* Sudbury, MA: Jones & Bartlett.

Green, L. W., Glanz, K., Hochbaum, G. M., Kok, G., Kreuter, M. W., et al. (1994). Can we build on, or must we replace, the theories and models in health education? *Health Education Research, 9* (3), 397–404.

Green, L. W., & Kreuter, M. W. (2005). *Health program planning: An educational and ecological approach.* (4th ed.) Boston, MA: McGraw-Hill.

Hayden, J. (2009). *Introduction to health behavior theory.* Sudbury, MA: Jones & Bartlett.

Hayden, J. (2014). *Introduction to health behavior theory.* (2nd ed.). Burlington, MA: Jones & Bartlett Learning.

Heaney, C. A., & Israel, B. A. (2008). Social networks and social support. In K. Glanz, B. K. Rimer, & K. Viswanath (Eds.), *Health behavior and health education: Theory, research, and practice* (4th ed., pp. 189–210). San Francisco: Jossey-Bass.

Institute of Medicine (IOM). (2001). *Health and behavior: The interplay of biological, behavioral, and societal influences.* Washington, DC: National Academy of Sciences.

Kawachi, I., Kennedy, B. P., Lochner, K., & Prothrow-Stith, D. (1997). Social capital, income, equality, and mortality. *American Journal of Public Health, 87* (9), 1491–1497.

Kerlinger, F. N. (1986). *Foundations of behavioral research* (3rd ed.). Austin: Holt, Rinehart & Winston.

Luszczynska, A., & Sutton, S. (2005). Attitudes and expectations. In J. Kerr, R. Weikunat, & M. Moretti (Eds.), *ABC of behavior change: A guide to successful disease prevention and health promotion* (pp. 71-84). Edinburgh: Elsevier.

McAlister, A. L., Perry, C. L., & Parcel, G. S. (2008). How individual, environments, and health behaviors interact: Social cognitive theory. In K. Glanz, B. K. Rimer, & K. Viswanath (Eds.), *Health behavior and health education: Theory, research, and practice* (4th ed., pp. 169–188). San Francisco: Jossey-Bass.

McClendon, B. T., & Prentice-Dunn, S. (2001). Reducing skin cancer risk: An intervention based upon protection motivation theory. *Journal of Health Psychology, 6* (3), 321–328.

McDermott, R. J. (2000). Social marketing: A tool for health education. *American Journal of Health Behavior, 24* (1), 6–10.

McKenzie, J. F., Neiger, B. L., & Thackeray, R. (2013). *Planning, implementing, and evaluating health promotion programs: A primer* (6th ed.). Boston: Pearson.

McLeroy, K. R., Bibeau, D., Steckler, A., & Glanz, K. (1988). An ecological perspective for health promotion programs. *Health Education Quarterly, 15* (4), 351–378.

Minkler, M., & Wallerstein, N. (2005). Improving health through community organization and community building: A health education perspective. In M. Minkler (Ed.), *Community organizing and community building for health* (2nd ed., pp. 26–50). New Brunswick, NJ: Rutgers University Press.

Minkler, M., Wallerstein, N., & Wilson, N. (2008). Improving health through community organization and community building. In K. Glanz, B. K. Rimer, & K. Viswanath (Eds.), *Health behavior and health education: Theory, research, and practice* (4th ed., pp. 287–312). San Francisco: Jossey-Bass.

National Association of County and City Health Officials (NACCHO). (2001). *Mobilizing for action through planning and partnerships (MAPP)*. Washington, DC: Author.

National Association of County Health Officials (NACHO). (1991). *APEX/PH, Assessment protocol for excellence in public health*. Washington, DC: Author.

National Cancer Institute (NCI). (2002). *Making health communication programs work* (NIH Publication No. 02-5145). Washington, DC: U.S. Department of Health and Human Services (USDHHS).

Neiger, B. L., & Thackeray R. (1998). *Social marketing: Making public health sense*. Paper presented at the annual meeting of the Utah Public Health Association. Provo, UT.

Neiger, B. L., & Thackeray, R. (2002). Application of the SMART model in two successful social marketing campaigns. *American Journal of Health Education, 33,* 291–293.

Parvanta, C. F., & Freimuth, V. (2000). Health communication at the Centers for Disease Control and Prevention. *American Journal of Health Behavior, 24* (1), 18–25.

Patton, R. P., Corry, J. M., Gettman, L. R., & Graff, J. S. (1986). *Implementing health/ fitness programs*. Champaign, IL: Human Kinetics.

Petty, R. E., Barden, J., & Wheeler, S. C. (2009). The elaboration likelihood model of persuasion: Developing health promotions for sustained behavioral change. In R. J. DiClemente, R. A. Crosby, & M. C. Kegler (Eds.). *Emerging theories in health promotion practice and research* (2nd ed., pp. 185–214). San Francisco: Jossey-Bass.

Petty, R. E., & Cacioppo, J. T. (1986). The elaboration likelihood model of persuasion. In L. Berkowitz (Ed.). *Advances in experimental social psychology* (Vol. 19, pp. 123–205). New York: Academic Press.

Prentice-Dunn, S., & Rogers, R. W. (1986). Protection motivation theory and preventive health: Beyond the health belief model. *Health Education Research: Theory and Practice, 1* (3), 153–161.

Prochaska, J. (2005). Stages of change, readiness, and motivation. In J. Kerr, R. Weitkunat, & M. Moretti (Eds.), *ABC of behavior change: A guide to successful disease prevention and health promotion* (pp. 111–123). Edinburgh: Elsevier.

Prochaska, J. O. (1979). *Systems of psychotherapy: A transtheoretical analysis*. Homewood, IL: Dorsey Press.

Prochaska, J. O., & DiClemente, C. C. (1983). Stages and processes of self-change of smoking: Toward an integrative model of change. *Journal of Consulting and Clinical Psychology, 51* (3), 390–395.

Prochaska, J. O., Johnson, S., & Lee, P. (1998). The transtheoretical model of behavior change. In S. A. Shumaker, E. B. Schron, J. K. Ockene, & W. L. McBee (Eds.), *The handbook of health behavior change* (2nd ed., pp. 59–84). New York: Springer Publishing Company.

Prochaska, J. O, Redding, C. A., & Evers, K. E. (2008). The transtheoretical model and stages of change. In K. Glanz, B. K. Rimer, & K. Viswanath (Eds.), *Health behavior and health education: Theory, research, and practice* (4th ed., pp. 97–121). San Francisco: Jossey-Bass.

Prochaska, J. O., Redding, C. A., Harlow, L. L., Rossi, J. S., & Velicer, W. F. (1994). The transtheoretical model of change and HIV prevention: A review. *Health Education Quarterly, 24* (4), 471–486.

Putman, R. D. (1995). Bowling alone: America's declining social capital. *Journal of Democracy, 6* (1), 65–78.

Redding, C. A., Rossi, J. S., Rossi, S. R., Velicer, W. F., & Prochaska, J. O. (1999). Health behavior models. In G. C. Hyner, K. W. Peterson, J. W. Travis, J. E. Dewey, J. J. Foerster, & E. M. Framer (Eds.), *SPM handbook of health assessment tools* (pp. 83–93). Pittsburgh: The Society of Prospective Medicine.

Rimer, B. K., & Glanz, K. (2005). *Theory at a glance: A guide for health promotion practice* (2nd ed.). [NIH Pub. No. 05-3896]. Washington, DC: National Cancer Institute.

Rogers, E. M. (2003). *Diffusion of innovations* (5th ed.). New York: Free Press.

Rogers, R. W. (1975). A protection motivation theory of fear appeals and attitude change. *Journal of Psychology, 91,* 93–114.

Rogers, R. W. (1983). Cognitive and physiological processes in fear-based attitude change: A revised theory of protection motivation. In J. Caccioppo & R. Petty (Eds.), *Social psychophysiology: A sourcebook* (pp. 153–176). New York: Guilford.

Rosenstock, I. M. (1966). Why people use health services. *Milbank Memorial Fund Quarterly, 44,* 94–124.

Rosenstock, I. M., Strecher, V. J., & Becker, M. H. (1988). Social learning theory and the health belief model. *Health Education Quarterly, 15* (2), 175–183.

Ross, H. S., & Mico, P. R. (1980). *Theory and practice in health education.* San Francisco: Mayfield.

Rotter, J. B. (1954). *Social learning and clinical psychology.* New York: Prentice-Hall.

Salazar, L. F., Crosby, R. A., & DiClemente, R. J. (2013). Health behavior in context of the "new" public health. In R. J. DiClemente, L. F. Salazar, & R. A. Crosby. *Health behavior theory for public health: Principles, foundations, and applications.* (pp. 3–26). Burlington, MA: Jones & Bartlett Learning.

Sharma, M., & Romas, J. A. (2012). *Theoretical foundations of health education and health promotion* (2nd ed.). Sudbury, MA: Jones & Bartlett.

Simons-Morton, B. G., Greene, W. H., & Gottlieb, N. H. (1995). *Introduction to health education and health promotion* (2nd ed.). Prospect Hts., IL: Waveland Press, Inc.

Simons-Morton, B. G., McLeroy, K. R., & Wendel, M. L. (2012). *Behavior theory in health promotion practice and research.* Burlington, MA: Jones & Bartlett Learning.

Simons-Morton, D. G., Simons-Morton, B. G., Parcel, G. S., & Bunker, J. F. (1988). Influencing personal and environmental conditions for community health: A multilevel intervention model. *Family and Community Health, 1* (2), 25–35.

Spencer, L., Adams, T. B., Malone, S., Roy, L., & Yost, E. (2006). Applying the transtheoretical model to exercise: A systematic and comprehensive review of the literature. *Health Promotion Practice, 7* (4), 428–443.

Sullivan, D. (1973). Model for comprehensive, systematic program development in health education. *Health Education Report, 1* (1), (November/December), 4–5.

Timmreck, T. C. (2003). *Planning, program development, and evaluation* (2nd ed.). Boston: Jones & Bartlett.

Timmreck, T. C., Cole, G. E., James, G., & Butterworth, D. D. (2010). Health education and health promotion: A look at the jungle of supportive fields. Philosophies, and theoretical foundations. In J. M. Black, S. Furney, H. M. Graf, & A. E. Nolt (Eds.), *Philosophical foundations of health education* (pp. 67–78). San Francisco: Jossey-Bass.

U.K. Office of National Statistics, Social Analysis and Reporting Division. (2001). Social capital: A review of the literature. Newport, South Wales: Author.

U.S. Department of Health and Human Services (USDHHS). (2001). *Healthy people in health communities: A community planning guide using Healthy People 2010.* Washington, DC: Author.

U.S. Department of Health and Human Services (USDHHS). (2011). *MAP-IT: A guide to using Healthy People in your community.* Retrieved May 23, 2013, from http://www.healthypeople.gov/2020/implementing/default.aspx.

Walsh, D. C., Rudd, R. E., Moeykens, B. A., & Moloney, T. W. (1993). Social marketing for public health. *Health Affairs, 12,* 104–119.

Warren, M. R., Thompson, J. P., & Saegert, S. (2001). The role of social capital in combating poverty. In S. Saegert, J. P. Thompson, & M. R. Warren (Eds.). *Social capital and poor communities* (pp. 1–28). New York: Sage Foundation.

Weinstein, N. D. (1988). The precaution adoption process. *Health Psychology, 7,* 355–386.

Weinstein, N. D., Rothman, A. J., & Sutton, S. R. (1998). Stage theories of health behavior: Conceptual and methodological issues. *Health Psychology, 17,* 290–299.

Weinstein, N. D., & Sandman, P. M. (2002). The precaution adoption process model and its application. In R. J. DiClemente, R. A. Crosby, & M. C. Kegler (Eds.), *Emerging theories in health promotion practice and research: Strategies for improving public health* (pp. 16–39). San Francisco: Jossey-Bass.

Weinstein, N. D., Sandman, P. M., & Blalock, S. J. (2008). The precaution adoption process model. In K. Glanz, B. K. Rimer, & K. Viswanath (Eds.), *Health behavior and health education: Theory, research, and practice* (4th ed., pp. 123–147). San Francisco: Jossey-Bass.

Ethics and Health Education/Promotion

Chapter Objectives

After reading this chapter and answering the questions at the end, you should be able to:

- Identify and define the three major areas of philosophy.
- Define *ethics*.
- Explain the difference between ethics and morality.
- Explain why it is important to act ethically.
- Define *professional ethics*.
- Explain and briefly describe the two major categories of ethical theories.
- Identify principles that create a common ground for all ethical theories.
- Outline a guide for making ethical decisions.
- Identify ethical issues associated with the profession of health education/promotion.
- Explain how a profession can ensure that its professionals will act ethically.
- Define *code of ethics* and identify the source of the code available for health education specialists.

In recent years, there has been an increasing interest in ethical questions in all walks of life. The interest has become so great that it is difficult to avoid the topic of ethics in everyday living. Newspapers and television networks are constantly covering stories that involve ethical issues, many of which are related to health. Examples include genetic engineering, abortion, the right to die, nuclear waste storage, the marketing of harmful products such as tobacco in developing countries, the reduction of welfare benefits, health research, appropriate sexual behavior, and professional behavior, to name a few.

How is it that we determine what is ethical or unethical? By whose standards do we make such judgments? To answer these questions requires some background and perspective. In this chapter, we will provide the background and perspective to understand how ethics relates to the profession of health education/promotion. First, we will present key terms that relate to the study of ethics and examine the origin of ethics. Next we look at reasons why people should work from an ethical base. We will then briefly look at the theories used to create ethical "yardsticks" and how these theories can be used to make ethical decisions. Within this context, a sampling of ethical issues facing health education specialists today will be presented. Finally, we conclude with a discussion on how a profession can ensure that its professionals will act ethically.

▷ Key Terms and Origin

Ethics, the study of morality (Morrison, 2006), is one of the three major areas of philosophy. The other two are **epistemology**, the study of knowledge, and **metaphysics**, the study of the nature of reality (Thiroux, 1995). Ethics, or **moral philosophy** as it is often stated, dates back two thousand plus years to the Greek philosopher Socrates (470–399 B.C.), "who spent his days in the Athenian marketplace challenging people to think about how they lived" (White, 1988, p. 7). Though philosophers do not sit in the marketplace (or malls) today to challenge people, the behavior, actions, and values of people are constantly being examined for their appropriateness.

You will note that the word *ethics* was described using the words *moral* and *morality*. The reason for this is that both words, *ethics* and *morals*, have ancient Greek and Latin roots in the words *ethos* and *mores* and both mean *character*. Thus, most associate *good character* with we related ethical behavior (White, 1988). Sperry (2007) has made a distinction between morality and ethics saying that morality "is the activity of making choices and of deciding, judging, justifying, and defending those actions or behaviors called moral," whereas ethics is "the science of how choices are made or should be made" (p. 38). Pigg (2010) has stated that "*ethics* defines acceptable and unacceptable behavior within the norms of a particular group" (pp. 11–12), whereas "*morality* sets standards for right and wrong in human behavior" (p. 12). Nevertheless, to avoid confusion throughout the rest of this chapter, we will use **ethical** and **moral** to mean the same thing. "The important thing to remember here is that moral, ethical, immoral, and unethical, essentially mean, good, right, bad, and wrong, often depending on whether one is referring to people themselves or to their actions" (Thiroux, 1995, p. 3).

White (1988) refers to the words *good, right, bad*, and *wrong* as the labels people use when making ethical judgments about human actions. Some authors have used these words to define ethics. Feeney and Freeman (1999) state, "Ethics is the study of right and wrong, duty and obligation" (p. 5). In the end, factual knowledge is not the concern of ethics but rather the virtues and values that drive human conduct (Pozgar, 2013).

▷ Why Should People Act Ethically?

Because ethics is one of the three major areas of philosophy, a philosophical answer to the question of why people should act ethically is that to act ethically brings meaning or purpose to the life of an individual (McGrath, 1994). It provides a standard by which to live. Ethical living, in turn, provides for a better society for all. It is the right thing to do for society and self.

From a more personal viewpoint, observation has shown "that those who are ethical tend to lead healthier (both physically and psychologically), more emotionally satisfying lives" (McGrath, 1994, p. 131). "In fact, the ethical life promises rewards for everyone involved. Your friends and associates will obviously feel better about life and about you if you treat them decently. And they'll probably reciprocate, treating you the same way, which will make your life better" (White, 1988, pp. 84–85). In short, the ethical person is more mature, stronger, healthier, and more advanced and has a more fully developed personality than those who are not ethical (White, 1988).

From a professional viewpoint, those who implement community interventions (including health education specialists) have much to gain from ethical behavior. Rabinowitz (2013) has noted that it makes their programs more effective; it cements their standing in the community; it allows them to occupy the moral high ground when arguing the merits of their programs, and to exercise moral leadership in the community; and it assures that they remain in good standing legally and professionally. In short, ethics help guide our decision making and assist us in making better choices.

Professional Ethics

Whereas personal values and morality may guide us in our everyday living, it is important to note that they may not be sufficient to guide our professional behavior. People come to their work with different personal experiences. Because of these different experiences, they do not hold the same values nor have they learned the same moral lessons. Even those who hold the same beliefs may not apply them in the same way in a professional setting (Feeney & Freeman, 1999). Thus, in a work setting, individuals are guided by professional ethics. **Professional ethics** focuses on the "actions that are right and wrong in the workplace and are of public matter. Professional moral principles are not statements of taste or preference; they tell practitioners what they ought to do and what they ought not do" (Feeney & Freeman, 1999, p. 6). Coming to an understanding of what behaviors are appropriate in a professional role is referred to as *professional socialization* (Morrison & Furlong, 2014).

Ethical behavior is expected from professionals. "'Ethics' delineates what we consider acceptable and unacceptable conduct regarding professional practice in Health Science education. Ethical conduct is particularly important to professional health educators, since we belong to a profession with a mission to serve the individual" (Pigg, 1994, p. iii). Health education/promotion is a profession with much human interaction. Dorman (1994) adds, "As writers, reviewers, and scientists we must insist on the highest of ethical practices in publication and research. As practitioners, we must seek to actively practice ethical behavior in our service and teaching. Individually, we must aspire for a reputation which reflects a life of personal integrity. The wisdom of King Solomon probably puts it best: '*A good name is more desirable than great riches; to be esteemed is better than silver or gold*'" (p. 4). Or, as Pigg (2006) stated when he summarized the lesson on integrity he learned from observing his father throughout life, "When fame and fortune fade, only our reputations remain as important but fragile reflections of our true nature" (p. 41).

Within the larger realm of *professional ethics* there may be some subsets of ethical behavior that are specific to certain tasks of the professional. For example, among the seven responsibilities of health education specialists is Responsibility IV "Conduct Evaluation and Research Related to Health Education" (National Commission for Health Education Credentialing [NCHEC], 2010) (see the discussion of the responsibilities in Chapter 6). To conduct evaluation and research, health education specialists need to be aware not only of appropriate general professional ethics but also of ethical behavior as it relates to the evaluation and research processes. Such behavior falls under the area of *research ethics*. **Research ethics** "comprises principles and standards that, along with underlying values, guide appropriate conduct relevant to research decisions" (Kimmel, 2007, p. 6). An ethical principle associated with the research

Examples of Ethical Issues Related to Research

The research process includes a number of steps that could have ethical ramifications. Examples of such issues are presented based on whether it is a consideration before the research begins, during the research process, or after the research is complete.

Before the research begins

- Selecting a research topic; must weigh risk (harm) to benefit (positive value)
- Recruiting participants: equitable opportunity to participate; voluntary participation; concern for vulnerable groups
- Institutional Review Board approval of research protocol
- During the research process
  - Obtaining participant consent and/or assent
  - Using deception (active or passive) as part of the intervention

- Participant privacy: anonymity or confidentiality
- Using an untreated comparison or control group
- Data analysis: careless use of data; manipulation of data; selective use or elimination of data; over-analysis of data

After the research is complete

- Reporting results: what to report; protecting confidentiality; declaring conflict of interest; disclosing sponsorship
- Sharing results with participants; debriefing experimental, control, and comparison groups
- Publication/presentation of results: determining authorship and order of authors; avoiding duplication of published works, fragmentation into several publications, and plagiarism

process is the concept of voluntary participation. That is, potential research participants should not be forced or coerced into participating in a research study, but rather should do so on a voluntary basis (see **Box 5.1** for other issues related to research process).

▷ Ethical Theories

Philosophers do not speak with a common voice about the standards of morality. Depending on the ethical theory espoused, one philosopher may see a certain behavior as moral or ethical, whereas another may see the same behavior as immoral or unethical. For example, one philosopher may see corporal punishment as a moral action to punish a person for murder, and the other sees the taking of another life, for whatever reason, as immoral. The purpose of this section is not to present a detailed description of ethical theories—that has been done elsewhere—but to categorize and summarize the better-known theories (see **Table 5.1**) and to suggest ways by which their content can be applied to health education/promotion practice.

Ethical theories provide frameworks whereby health education specialists and others are able to evaluate whether human actions are acceptable (Shive & Marks, 2006). The primary means by which ethical theories have been categorized has been to place them in the category of deontology (**formalism**, or **nonconsequentialism**, as some refer to it) or teleology (or **consequentialism** as some refer to it) theories. **Deontological theories** (from Greek *deontos*, "of the obligatory" or *deon* meaning duty) "are those that claim that certain actions are inherently right or wrong, or good or bad, without regard for their consequences"

TABLE 5.1 **Summary of ethical theories**

Category	Primary Reasoning	Examples of Such Theories
Deontology (also known as formalism or nonconsequentialism)	The end does not justify the means.	Natural law morality, deontological ethics, existentialism
Teleology (also known as consequentialism)	The end does justify the means.	Contractarian ethics, utilitarianism, pragmatism

(Reamer, 2006, p. 65). For example, a deontologist would argue that lying to a client or patient is wrong even if it is done to help that person. According to this theory, the mere act of lying is wrong, regardless of the benefits it may bring. Deontology theories involve making decisions based on a moral code or rules (Pozgar, 2013)—that is to say, the end (the consequences) *does not* justify the means (the act).

Teleological theories (from Greek *teleios*, "brought to its end purpose"), on the other hand, evaluate the moral status of an act by the goodness of the consequences (Reamer, 2006). If the act produces good or happiness, it is morally okay; if it does not, it is immoral. Using the same example of lying to a patient or client, if the consequences turned out okay, the consequentialist would see this act as morally okay. In short, this category of ethical theories states that the end *does* justify the means.

As can be seen from these descriptions of formalism and consequentialism, the primary point of contention is whether or not the means justify the end. "Is there a way to reconcile these two approaches to ethics, or must we simply make a choice between them?" (Mellert, 1995, p. 133). Most people would say that neither category of ethical theory can answer all moral questions in their lives. In fact, Summers (2014) has stated, "humans have yet to develop an ethical theory that will satisfactorily handle all issues" (p. 62). There are times when deontology provides guidance for the ethical way to act, whereas teleology is best in other situations. What this means is that each person must carefully study the ethical theory options, combine what is compatible and resolve what is inconsistent in those options, and attempt to work out a moral consensus for herself and society (Mellert, 1995). This is not an easy process. Many times, philosophical questions and problems are abstract or conceptual in nature. For example, is there ever a time when it is okay for a health education specialist to lie to his supervisor? Such questions are answered through philosophical thought, using reason, logic, and argument. Thus, the most important tool people can use to find these answers is the mind.

When analyzing an ethical problem, people need to depend more on thinking than feeling—using their minds and not their hearts (White, 1988). For example, if a person says, "I feel that abortion, no matter when it occurs, is morally wrong," that person is really saying there is something about abortion that makes her uneasy, unhappy, or distressed. This person is expressing a feeling, not a moral position. This person's feelings would be better stated if she were to say, "Abortion makes me feel upset." However, if a person states that abortion is immoral, then she should be prepared to provide specific reasons for holding this belief (White, 1988). For example, she may hold the belief that life begins at conception and having an abortion is ending the life of another human being. It is for these reasons that answering ethical questions is a thinking, not a feeling, process. Or, as Penland and Beyrer (1981) have stated, "If ethics is to have personal meaning it demands thoughtful examination.

The answers to ethical questions are found by looking within, examining our personal belief systems and values, and using our intelligence to integrate what we have learned and what we have experienced with what we believe and value" (p. 6).

▷ Basic Principles for Common Moral Ground

As was shown in the previous section, deontoloists and teleologists are not in agreement when it comes to the rationale to be used in making moral decisions. No single ethical theory can answer every ethical question to the satisfaction of all, yet, to live in a moral society, all must be able to work from a common moral ground. "We must search for a larger meeting ground in which the best of all these theories and systems can operate meaningfully with a minimum of conflict and opposition" (Thiroux, 1995, p. 172).

To help us with this common ground, Thiroux (1995) has identified five basic principles that can apply to human morality, regardless of the embraced theory. The principles do not provide the answers to how one should behave, but rather help to provide a foundation for making ethical decisions. The first is the **value of life** principle. This is the most basic of principles. Without living human beings, there can be no ethics. Thiroux (1995) has specifically stated this principle as "human beings should revere life and accept death" (p. 180). This means that no life should be ended without strong justification. This, for example, is why topics such as abortion, suicide, euthanasia, and capital punishment raise a number of ethical questions.

The second is the principle of **goodness (rightness)**. "Good" and "right" are at the core of every ethical theory. Theorists may disagree on what is good and bad and right and wrong, but they all strive for goodness and rightness. "'Good' should not only be in abstract, but it should be seen in relation to (other) human beings. As an example, a person who is suicidal may no longer value his or her life as 'good,' but that person's mother may have a very different concept of the value of her child's life" (Tschudin, 2003, p. 56).

The principle of goodness includes two parallel principles of ethics: (1) the principle of **nonmaleficence** and (2) the principle of **beneficence**, or **benevolence**. "Briefly, nonmaleficence refers to the non-infliction of harm to others" (Balog et al., 1985, p. 91). Further, nonmaleficence can "be broken into three components: not inflicting harm, preventing harm, and removing harm when it is present" (Greenberg, 2001, p. 3). Though the concepts presented in this explanation of nonmaleficence are seemingly straightforward, the application of the concepts can be difficult. For example, what is meant by harm? Are there degrees of harm like "a little harm" and "a lot of harm"? Must an action produce no harm to be acceptable from an ethical point of view? These are difficult questions to answer and make some situations difficult to respond to in an ethical way.

"Beneficence implies more than just avoiding doing harm" (Summers, 2014, p. 49). It "describes the principle of doing good, demonstrating kindness, showing compassion, and helping others" (Pozgar, 2013, p. 9). In the bioethical realm, nonmaleficence and beneficence make up the "benefit-harm ratio" in which, ideally, benefits outweigh costs and in which the "minimization of harm" rather than the "maximation of good" is more strongly emphasized (Fox & Swazey, 1997).

Thiroux's third principle is the principle of **justice (fairness)**. This principle deals with people treating other people fairly and justly in distributing goodness (benefits) and badness (burdens) (Summers 2014; Thiroux, 1995). Justice can be examined in two ways—(1) *procedural* and (2) *distributive* (Summers, 2014). **Procedural justice** deals with whether or not fair procedures were in place and whether those procedures were followed, while **distributive justice** deals with the allocation of resources (Summers, 2014). Does this mean that all people will always get their fair share of goodness and badness? No, but it does mean everyone will have an equal chance at obtaining the good (Thiroux, 1995). "The bottom line is that one has indeed acted justly toward a person when that person has been given what she or he is due or owed" (Balog et al., 1985, p. 90). For example, should only those who are able to pay for them receive health education/promotion services, or should only the poor shoulder all of the burden?

The fourth principle of this common moral ground is that of **truth telling (honesty)**. At the heart of any moral relationship is communication. A necessary component of any meaningful communication is telling the truth, being honest. This may be the most difficult principle to live by. This is not to say that people will never lie or that lying might be justified, but there is a need for a strong attempt to be truthful. In the end, morality depends on what people say and do (Thiroux, 1995). Health education specialists working in a clinical setting may be faced with this principle when caught in a situation in which an ill child (and a minor by law) asks about his or her health problem, but the child's parent or guardian has strictly forbidden such communication.

The fifth principle is that of **individual freedom (equality principle or principle of autonomy)**. (See **Figure 5.1**.) "The word *autonomy* comes from the Greek words *autos* ("self") and *nomos* ("rule," "governance," or "law") and originally referred to as self-governance in Greek city-states" (Greenberg, 2001, p. 3). "This principle means that people, being individuals with individual differences, must have the freedom to choose their own ways and means of being moral within the framework of the first four basic principles" (Thiroux, 1995, p. 187). This is to say that individual freedom is limited by the other four principles. Underlying the principle "of autonomy is the idea that we are to respect others for who they are" (Summers, 2014, p. 50). This is a principle that health education specialists deal with on a regular basis, specifically as

▲ **Figure 5.1** Individual freedom is an important principle of human morality.

it relates to helping others engage in enhancing health behavior. Health education specialists need to respect the rights of others to deliberate, choose, and act (Balog et al., 1985).

With the grounding of the ethical theories and the establishment of these basic principles, let us examine the process of making ethical decisions.

▷ Making Ethical Decisions

"Ethical decision making in health education, as in other areas, involves determining right and wrong within situations where clear demarcations do not exist or are not clearly apparent to the decision maker.... To be considered a professional health educator, one must possess requisite skill and knowledge in making individual decisions. And, in making decisions it is imperative that one has analyzed his or her decisions in terms of standards of right and wrong, good and bad" (Balog et al., 1985, p. 88). To decide and, in turn, act in an ethical manner, people must rely on their values, principles, and ethical thinking. To assist in this process, a number of authors (e.g., Balog et al., 1985; Fisher, 2003; Mellert, 1995; Melnick, 2015; Nelson, 2005; Reamer, 2006; Remley & Herlihy, 2007; Svara, 2007; Thompson, Melia, & Boyd, 2000) have presented guides for applying the concepts presented previously in this chapter to everyday ethical decision making. Though the number of steps and labels used to identify the steps are different from guide to guide, they are similar in that they provide a framework for making an ethical decision. Because of the limitation of space, we are presenting a single approach (see **Figure 5.2**) to ethical decision making that blends the ideas and is representative of these guides.

The ethical decision-making process should begin long before any ethical problems surface. The process begins when a person develops and sustains a professional commitment to doing

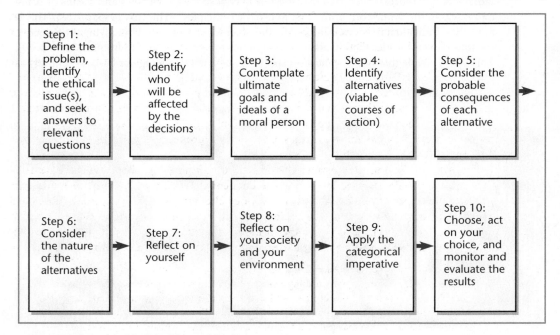

▲ **Figure 5.2** Steps in ethical decision making
Sources: Adapted from: Balog et al., (1985); Mellert (1995); Nelson (2005); Reamer (2006); Remley & Herlihy (2007); Svara, (2007).

what is right (Fisher, 2003). Such a commitment will go a long way toward creating a work environment that can prevent many ethical problems. This is not to say that all ethical problems will be avoided. Ethical problems can arise in situations in which two or more ethical principles appear to be in conflict, in unforeseen reactions from those with whom health education special-ist may work, or in unexpected events (Fisher, 2003). However, having a commitment to doing what is right becomes a form of "primary prevention" for many ethical problems.

Closely aligned with a commitment to doing what is right, is familiarity with what the health education/promotion profession expects of practicing professionals. Stated differ-ently, what are the expected norms for those who practice health education/promotion? Such expectations can be found in the profession's code of ethics. With a commitment to doing what is right and knowing what is expected of a practicing health education specialists are enhancing their *moral sensitivity*. Rest and colleagues (1999) have explained **moral sen-sitivity** as being aware that an ethical problem exists and having an understanding of what impact different courses of action may have on the people involved.

The first step to take when confronted with an ethical decision is to define the problem/concern, identify the ethical issue(s), clarify the facts, and seek answers to relevant questions (Mellert, 1995; Melnick, 2015; Nelson, 2005; Reamer, 2006; Remley & Herlihy, 2007; Svara, 2007). This first step is one of clarification and gathering relevant information. Several ques-tions need to be answered. What is the problem/concern that makes you believe there is an ethical decision to be made? Is there a legal question that needs to be answered? What do you know? What do you need to find out? Does a decision have to be made? If so, by when, and in what context? Are these decisions within the realm of your authority, or does someone else with other responsibilities/authority/resources determine them?

Second, identify the individuals, groups, and organizations that are likely to be affected by this ethical decision (Nelson, 2005; Reamer, 2006) and what stakes they have in the outcome (Svara, 2007). When making an ethical decision, it is important to understand all who will be impacted because one solution may create additional ethical problems for others.

Third, "contemplate the ultimate goals and ideals for which you as a moral person are striving. What are the most noble human aspirations that pertain to this concrete situation?" (Mellert, 1995, p. 156). How should you as an ethical person want to act in this situation? Consider the ethical theory you embrace and the principles for common ethical ground. How do these goals and ideals apply to this decision? Ultimate goals and ideals do not always apply to every decision and sometimes may not be appropriate, but, to the extent that they do apply, let them help with the decision.

Fourth, identify all the possible alternatives to solving the problem (viable courses of action), the people involved in each, and the potential benefits and risks of each (Reamer, 2006). It is important to brainstorm the various alternatives to help organize subsequent analysis (Reamer, 2006). Consider ethical and health theories, a code of ethics (Melnick, 2015), and consult with colleagues and, if necessary, experts. Be aware that there may not be a "best alternative, you may have to deal with an ethical dilemma. An **ethical dilemma** is

a situation that forces a decision that involves breaking some ethical norm or contradicting some ethical value. It involves making a decision between two or more possible actions in which any one of the actions can be justified as being right decision, but whatever action is taken, there always remains some doubt as to whether the correct course of action was chosen. The effect of an action may put others at risk, harm others, or violate the rights of others (Pozgar, 2013, pp. 534–535).

Fifth, "consider the probable consequences of each alternative" (Mellert, 1995, p. 157). Look at both the short- and long-term consequences of each alternative. How will these consequences affect you, others, and the environment? In other words, weigh the strengths and weaknesses of the alternatives based on the consequences (Balog et al., 1985). Maybe the consequences are different, or maybe they are not and thus, may not be important in the final decision.

Sixth, "consider the nature of the alternatives" (Mellert, 1995, p. 157). Consider the deontologist approach to the decision-making process in selecting an alternative. Does the alternative lead to an act or a behavior that is wrong, according to the natural law hypothesis? Would you be violating anyone's basic rights? Does it go against basic human ideals and intrinsic moral values? If you answer *yes* to any of these questions, you do not need to eliminate the alternative from further consideration but should give greater consideration to alternatives that do not violate this portion of your reflection.

Seventh, "reflect on yourself" (Mellert, 1995, p. 157). What impact will a proposed course of action have on you as a moral person? Will it enhance or detract from your moral stature? If it detracts, then maybe other alternatives should be considered. If you cannot accept a course of action "as part of your inner self and as data for your own moral growth, then there must be something morally questionable about it" (Mellert, 1995, pp. 157–158). Although you may be striving to be objective as you work toward a decision, be aware that your emotions will also play a part. Your emotions will influence your judgment and may help guide you in your decision-making (Remley & Herlihy, 2007).

Eighth, "reflect on your society and your environment" (Mellert, 1995, p. 158). Will your action mesh with that of society and the environment? Moral acts are unselfish acts in that they do not prefer one's own interests at the expense of the interests of others (Mellert, 1995). Will society in general see your action as morally correct? (See **Figure 5.3**.)

▶ **Figure 5.3** An anti-abortion rally

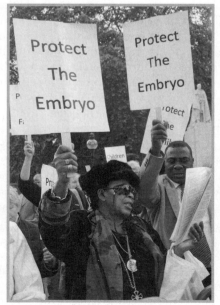

Ninth, "apply the categorical imperative" (Mellert, 1995, p. 158). Would you want your course of action to be a role model for others? If others were faced with the same decision, is this how you would want them to act?

Tenth, choose the best alternative, provide a reasoned justification for the choice (Svara, 2007), "act courageously and decisively" (Mellert, 1995, p. 158), monitor and evaluate the results, and if necessary make adjustments (Svara, 2007). "Choosing among conflicting options is difficult, but at least one can feel confident that the choice did not ignore an important alternative" (Svara, 2007, p. 109). Having said this, you still may not feel comfortable after the choice has been made.

Context of Ethical Decision Making

In considering the components in this decision-making process, it is important to note that moral decision-making does not occur in a vacuum (Mellert, 1995). If it did, every decision would be resolved with the "right" alternative for all. Each decision is surrounded by the context in which it must be made. Mellert feels that, when working through the process, a person must consider and be aware of the context. When making ethical decisions, people must have a sense of the following:

1. **Place.** Be aware of the appropriateness of an action in a particular environment. One action may be appropriate in one setting but not in another.

2. **Time.** Be aware of the history leading up to the decision and other similar decisions. Learn from past decisions.

3. **Identity.** Who am I? How does this moral decision relate to me?

4. **Social relationships.** Be aware that making moral decisions will impact social relationships. There is a good chance that not everyone will agree with your decision and action.

5. **The ideal.** When making a moral decision, aim for the most noble ideals of humanity.

6. **The concrete.** Never lose sight of the fact that choices arise from concrete events.

7. **Seriousness.** When making a moral decision, do so with an attitude that is appropriate to the situation.

▷ Applying the Ethical Decision-Making Process

Now let us see if we can apply this decision-making process to the profession of health education/promotion. A health education specialist, let's call her Anne, is employed by an organization and is in charge of the organization's employee health promotion program. Based on the results of the health risk assessments (HRA) taken by employees, Anne is aware that one employee, "high up in the organization" (e.g., school principal, department manager), is a consistent abuser of alcohol. The person's supervisor is aware of the situation but has ignored it. The employee in question is well liked within the organization and is a good employee. To the best of Anne's knowledge, alcohol has not impacted this person's work performance, but she feels it has the potential to do so. Anne is not sure if the alcohol has impacted the employee's personal life. What should Anne do with this information? Let's look at how we might analyze this situation using the 10-step process presented on the previous pages.

Step 1. Define the problem, identify the ethical issue, and gather relevant information.

The problem is that the employee is abusing a substance and the health education specialist knows it, as does the employee's supervisor. Is it an ethical problem? Anne knows that an alcohol-impaired person can harm himself or herself and others, either intentionally or unintentionally, and thus has an obligation to protect their health (see Article I, Section 4, of Appendix A). Anne also knows she has an obligation to protect the privacy of the employees (see Article I, Section 6, of Appendix A). This appears to be an ethical situation to Anne because of the two competing issues. Anne has decided to get more information before acting. She decides to look at the employee handbook to see if anything like this appears there. She also decides to ask her own supervisor for guidance and check with the Human Resources (HR) Department for information. And, last, she looks to see when the employee is scheduled for his or her HRA feedback appointment.

Step 2. Identify who will be affected.

Anne is aware that, depending on what actions are taken, the parties impacted by those actions are the employee, his or her supervisor, the organization and its reputation, family members of the employee, and even Anne herself and her supervisor.

Step 3. Contemplate the ultimate goals and ideals.

Anne wants to do what is ethically right. From a theoretical point of view, Anne embraces the deontological viewpoint of dealing with ethical situations. In other words, she believes that the ends do not justify the means. She is trying to make sense of how that applies to this situation.

Step 4. Identify the alternatives (viable courses of action).

Anne sees the following as viable courses of action: (1) Approach the employee's supervisor and ask him or her to handle it; (2) Talk to the employee about it at his or her scheduled HRA feedback appointment; (3) Turn the information over to the HR Department to let someone there deal with the problem; (4) Turn the information over to the her supervisor so that it can be dealt with at the managers' level; (5) Do nothing until something happens because of the employee's alcohol use; or (6) Do nothing at all.

Step 5. Consider the consequences of the alternatives.

Here are the consequences Anne sees with each of the alternatives she identified in Step 4: Alternative 1—The supervisor may do nothing or may now be forced to act because someone else is aware of the situation. This may lead to the employee's dismissal, or the employee may get the help he or she needs, or the supervisor may decide not to act on the information. Alternative 2—This alternative would protect the employee's privacy, bring the problem to the attention of the employee, and let the employee act without others knowing about it. Anne also knows that the employee may not take the feedback session well and "blow up" at Anne. Alternative 3—This alternative places the situation in the hands of those trained to deal with them effectively. Depending on the organization's policy, it may also lead to the employee's dismissal, or the employee may get the help he or she needs. Alternative 4—Similar to Alternatives 2 and 4, it places the problem in someone else's hands and would probably have much the same consequences as those two alternatives. Alternative 5—Nothing may ever come of the employee's alcohol abuse, or some serious harm may come to the employee or someone around him or her. Or Alternative 6—Doing nothing at all, which would change nothing. The employee possibly will continue as a good employee with no problem for himself or herself or others, or harm could come to the employee, his or her coworkers, or members of the employee's family.

Step 6. Consider the nature of the alternatives.

Anne does not feel that by acting she would be violating any human ideals or intrinsic moral rules or values. She does feel, however, that she cannot do "nothing." She does not like the alternatives, but she feels an ethical obligation to act. Anne may be facing an ethical dilemma.

Step 7. Reflect on yourself.

Anne knows that if she does nothing, she will not be able to live with herself because she sees herself as a moral person. But she is concerned about being seen as the "goody-goody" employee or even a "tattle tale" or an employee that cannot be trusted with confidential information.

Step 8. Reflect on society and the environment.

Anne had a hard time reasoning through this step of the process. Because a large percentage of U.S. adults consume alcohol, she feels that society in general may see the employee's situation as "none of her business." But she still sees a need to act.

Step 9. Apply the categorical imperative.

Anne feels she needs to act because it is her duty. She wonders what kind of health education specialist she would be if she were not concerned about the health of a coworker and the possible harm that coworker could bring to self or others. She feels that she needs to be a role model for others.

Step 10. Choose an alternative, provide a rationale, act, and monitor the results.

Anne decided to act by talking to the employee about the alcohol abuse at his or her scheduled HRA feedback appointment. She chose this approach not only because it does not violate the employee's privacy, but it also tries to protect both the employee's health and that of those around him or her. If this approach does not induce the employee to change, Anne feels that she may need to take further action.

As you can see, moral decisions are not easy to make. They are not to be taken lightly, and responsible action is important. Remember, this decision will not occur in a vacuum; the "ideal" decision may not be the best decision. What do you think about Anne's actions?

▷ Ethical Issues and Health Education/Promotion

As noted at the beginning of this chapter, ethical concerns interface with all aspects of our lives. That includes our professional lives too. "Ethical issues permeate almost every decision and action undertaken in health education" (Goldsmith, 2006, p. 33). Although some of the ethical issues faced by health education specialists are specific to the profession, such as the ethical issues surrounding getting clients to begin a health-enhancing behavior, using interventions to protect and promote at the population level, and dealing with the potential pervasiveness of most things in life impacting peoples health (Dawson & Verweij, 2007), the majority of concerns affecting most professions are similar (Hiller, 1987). Here are some situations that are specific to preventive care and public health programs.

Bayles (1989) has organized the substantive obligations of professions and professionals, regardless of the profession, from which most professional ethical situations arise. The following is a list of these obligations, with several questions that relate the obligations to the practice of health education/promotion. [Note: These obligations closely align with the *Code of Ethics for the Health Education Profession* (Coalition of National Health Education Organizations [CNHEO], 2011).]

1. **Obligations and availability of services.** The primary issue related to this obligation is the equality of opportunity for making professional services available to all citizens. Examples of ethical issues associated with this obligation include the right to legal counsel, access to health care, and refusal to accept clients for lack of ability to pay. (Who should receive health education/promotion? What about clients who are hard to reach? In what settings should it be offered? Should clients have to pay for health education/ promotion, or should health education/promotion be denied if a person cannot pay? Should health education specialists ever terminate an intervention before it is complete? Is there ever a time when a health education specialist should use an intervention in which the possible outcomes are questionable?)

2. **Obligations between professionals and clients.** Once the services of a professional have been secured, a number of ethical issues can arise from the professional–client relationship. (See **Figure 5.4**.) "The fiduciary model presents the best ethical ideal for the professional-client relationship" (Bayles, 1989, p. 100). In such a model, the professional is honest, candid, competent, loyal, fair, and discrete. At the same time, the client keeps commitments to the professional, is truthful to the professional, and does not request unethical acts from the professional. (Is there ever a time when health education specialists should not be candid or honest with their clients? How should health education specialists respond when their clients ask them about their personal behavior?

▶ **Figure 5.4** The professional–client relationship is an obligation that is often encountered by health education specialists.

BOX

5.2

Informed Consent: An Ethical Obligation

The term "**informed consent**" is often associated with medical procedures or research projects, but it is also important in health education/promotion. The concept behind informed consent is that people—whether patients, research participants, or participants in a health education/promotion program—should be given sufficient information from which to make informed choices about whether or not they want a certain medical procedure, or to participate in a research project or health education/promotion program. From an ethical standpoint, it is based on the common ground principle of individual freedom. That is, freedom to choose after being well informed on the consequences of participation.

Though receiving a medical procedure or participating in a clinical trial often carries more risks than participating in a health education/promotion program, individuals should not be allowed to participate in any health education/promotion program without giving their informed consent (McKenzie, Neiger, & Thackeray, 2013). In practice, the informed consent process should include: (1) the health education specialist discussing the details of the program (i.e., purpose of the program, description of the intervention, risks and benefits associated with participation, alternative programs that will accomplish the same thing, and the freedom to discontinue participation at any time) with the prospective participant; (2) the participant having an opportunity to ask questions about the program; (3) the participant understanding what he or she has been told; and (4) the participant signing a written informed consent document (Cottrell & McKenzie, 2011).

Is there ever a time when health education specialists should not obtain informed consent before proceeding with an intervention?) (See **Box 5.2**.)

3. **Obligations to third parties.** This obligation revolves around what others need to know about the professional–client relationship. Often professionals are confronted with the issue of whether or not to share client information with family members of the client, people in a supervisory capacity (e.g., teachers, employers), legal authorities (e.g., police, lawyers), or peers (e.g., professional colleagues). (What duty does a health education specialist have to share information with a student's parents when the student has shared the information with the health education specialist in confidence? Is there ever a time when a health education specialist can share confidential information? How about with the insurance company of a client? With the client's employer?) (See **Box 5.3**.)

4. **Obligations between professionals and employers.** Employed professionals have obligations to employers that are similar to the obligation they have to their clients (see #2). "However, the obligation to obey employers is stronger than an obligation to clients. It includes acting as, and only as, authorized" (Bayles, 1989, p. 158). On the other hand, "employers' obligations to professional employees are universal, role related, and contractual" (Bayles, 1989, p. 159). Ethical issues related to this obligation often involve due process, confidentiality, and professional support. (Should health education specialists always implement "company" policy when they know it is wrong or could bring harm to a client? What if a health education specialist has a conflict of interest between his personal life and what his employer says he must do? Is there ever a time when health education specialists should publicly speak against their employers?)

5. **Obligations to the profession.** "These obligations rest on the responsibilities of a profession as a whole to further social values" (Bayles, 1989, p. 179). Issues associated

---

Privacy, HIPAA, and GINA

One of the most basic concepts associated with providing a service (e.g., health education) to other people is that of privacy. **Privacy** has been defined as "the claim of individuals, groups, or institutions to determine for themselves when, how, and to what extent information about them is communicated to others" (Westin, 1968, p. 7). Thus, when people have agreed to participate in a health education/promotion program, it becomes the duty of the health education specialist to protect the information provided by participants.

The importance of privacy for health education specialists, and all others associated with health care, was further emphasized with the enactment of the Health Insurance Portability and Accountability Act of 1996 (officially known as Public Law 104-191 and referred to as HIPAA) and the Genetic Information Nondiscrimination Act of 2008 (officially known as Public Law 110-233 and referred to as GINA). The HIPAA and GINA regulations apply to protected health information (PHI), whether transmitted orally, in writing, or electronically, that is generated by an employer, a health plan, a health clearinghouse, or a healthcare provider, or in connection with financial or administrative activities related to health care (Fisher, 2003). Failure to implement the standards can lead to civil and criminal penalties (U.S. Department of Health and Human Services [USDHHS], n.d.). The two techniques that are used to protect the privacy of program participants are anonymity and confidentiality. **Anonymity** exists when no one, including those conducting the program, can relate a participant's identity to any information pertaining to the program. In applying this concept, health education specialists would need to ensure that collected information had no identifying marks attached to it such as the participant's name, social security number, or any other less common information. In practice, because of the nature (the need to know about the participants) of most health education/promotion programs, anonymity is not often used. Its most common application in health education/promotion is in conducting research projects.

On the other hand, the concept of confidentiality is common in health education/promotion programs. **Confidentiality** exists when only those responsible for conducting a program can link information about a participant with the individual and do not reveal such information to others. Thus, health education specialists need to take every precaution to protect participants' information. Often this means keeping the information "under lock and key" while the program is being conducted, then destroying (e.g., shredding) the information when it is no longer needed.

---

with this obligation include conducting research, reforming the profession, and maintaining respect for the profession. (Is there ever a reason why health education specialists should not behave in a professional manner? What duty does a health education specialist have to report the inappropriate behavior of a colleague? What obligations do health education specialists have to keep up-to-date on the content of their fields?)

Having identified problems that may cut across all professions, let us examine those that are more specific to health education/promotion. First, Penland and Beyrer (1981) state that ethical issues are defined by two criteria. "First they must be 'issues'; that is, there must be controversy related to the problem or topic. There must be 'two sides,' supported by people with two different viewpoints" (p. 6). Issues, by definition, are controversial. For example, the need for youth to know sexual information is not an issue; however, from whom and when such information should be provided may be an issue.

"The second criterion for an ethical issue in health education is that it must involve a question of right and wrong" (Penland & Beyrer, 1981, p. 6). "Can health education/promotion programs in the worksite change health behavior?" may be a controversial issue, but it does not deal with rightness and wrongness. Thus, it is not an ethical issue, but "does an employer have the right to make all employees attend the health education/promotion program?" is an ethical issue.

Now that we know what comprises an ethical issue, let us look at some of the ethical issues health education specialists are likely to face. The literature is abundant with examples of ethical issues in health education/promotion. Issues cited include abstinence-only and abstinence-plus sexuality education (Wiley, 2002), community organization and community participation (Minkler, Pies, & Hyde, 2012), ethics instruction (Modell & Citrin, 2002), health education research (Bastida, Tseng, McKeever, & Jack, 2010; Buchanan et al., 2002; Minkler et al., 2002; Minkler, Vasquez, Tajik, & Petersen, 2008), health disparities (Shaw-Ridley & Ridley, 2010), health literacy (Marks, 2009), health promotion evaluation (Thurston, Vollman, & Burgess, 2003), health risk appraisals (Society of Prospective Medicine [SPM], 1999), health screenings (Melnick, 2015), practice of health education/practice (Kahan, 2012; Shive & Marks, 2006), research/scientific inquiry/publishing (Margolis, 2000; McKenzie, Seabert, Hayden, & Cottrell, 2009; Pigg, 1994, 2006; Price & Dake 2002; Price, Dake, & Islam 2001), service by health education specialists (Price, Dake, & Telljohann, 2001; Young & Valois, 2010), social marketing (Rothschild, 2000; Siegel & Lotenberg, 2007), the teaching of health (Telljohann, Price, & Dake, 2001), topical areas (Eve, Marty, McDermott, Klasko, & Sanberg, 2008), and the teaching of ethics (Goldsmith, 2006). McLeroy, Bibeau, and McConnell (1993) have identified other areas of ethical concern, which reflect the inclusion of health education as a component of health promotion. The major categories of issues raised by McLeroy and colleagues (1993) include:

1. "Assigning individual responsibility to the victim for becoming ill due to personal failures" (p. 314)—for example, becoming ill because one does not exercise, or continues to use tobacco products.

2. "Attempting to change individuals and their subsequent behaviors rather than the social environment that supports and maintains unhealthy lifestyles" (p. 314)—for example, telling employees to manage their stress when it is environmental stressors causing the stress.

3. Using "system interventions to promote health behaviors" (p. 315)—for example, public policy strategies or coercive strategies to modify unhealthy actions.

4. Overemphasizing behavior change as a program outcome instead of focusing more on changes in the social and physical environment.

5. Overemphasizing the importance of health, forgetting that health is a means to an end, not an end in itself.

6. Educating the public on the concept of risk and how to properly use risk factor information.

7. Underemphasizing professional behavior, regardless of the health education/promotion setting—for example, keeping up-to-date, serving as a role model, and providing ethics education for the next generation of health education specialists.

As you can see, there are a number of ethical issues that can arise in the process of carrying out the work of a health education specialist. Rabinowitz (2010) has provided several issues that need to be considered when planning, implementing, and evaluating community interventions. They are presented in **Box 5.4.**

BOX

5.4

Ethical Issues that Need to Be Considered with Community Interventions

1. **Confidentiality.** Probably the most familiar of ethical issues—perhaps because it's the one most often violated—is the expectation that communications and information from participants in the course of a community intervention or program (including conversations, written or taped records, notes, test results, etc.) will be kept confidential.

2. **Consent.** There are really three faces of consent: program participants giving program staff consent to share their records or information with others for purposes of service provision; participants giving informed consent to submit to particular medical or other services, treatment, research, or program conditions; and community members consenting to the location or operation of an intervention in their neighborhood.

3. **Disclosure.** Like consent, disclosure in this context has more than one meaning: disclosure to participants of the conditions of the program they're in; disclosure of participant information to other individuals, agencies, etc.; and disclosure—by the program and by the affected individuals—of any conflict of interest that the program represents to any staff or board members.

4. **Competence.** By offering services of any kind, an organization is essentially making a contract with participants to do the job it says it will do. Implied in that contract is that those actually doing the work, and the organization as a whole, are competent to accomplish their goals under reasonable circumstances.

5. **Conflict of interest.** A conflict of interest is a situation in which someone's personal (financial, political, professional, social, sexual, family, etc.) interests could influence his judgment or actions in a financial or other decision, in carrying out his job, or in his relationships with participants. In community interventions, conflicts of interest may change—to the community's disadvantage—how a program is run or how its money is spent.

6. **Grossly unethical behavior.** This is behavior far beyond the bounds of the normally accepted ethical standards of society. In some cases, grossly unethical behavior may stem from taking advantage of a conflict of interest situation. In others, it may be a simple case of dishonesty or lack of moral scruples. Both individuals and organizations can be guilty of some instances of it, and in both cases it is often a result of someone managing to justify the unjustifiable. Community programs need to be clear about their own ethical standards, and to hold individuals to them and to any other standards their professions demand. In most cases, staff members guilty of grossly unethical behavior should be dismissed as quickly as possible, and prosecuted where that is appropriate.

7. **General ethical responsibilities.** Ethical behavior for a community intervention is more than simply following particular professional codes and keeping your nose clean. It means actively striving to do what is right for participants and for the community, and treating everyone—participants, staff members, funders, the community at large—in an ethical way.

Source: From Rabinowitz, P., edited by Berkowitz and Brownlee. (2010). "Ethical Issues in Community Interventions," *The Community Tool Box: Ethical Issues in Common Interventions.* Reproduced by permission of the Work Group for Community Health and Development, The Community Tool Box: http://ctb.ku.edu.

▷ Ensuring Ethical Behavior

The majority of this chapter has been used to examine ethical theory, identify and deal with ethical issues, and discuss why it is important to act ethically. What we have yet to discuss is the answer to the question "how the profession can ensure that professionals will behave ethically?" The answer is it cannot. Professionals who act unethically usually do so (1) for personal financial gain and reputation and (2) for the benefit of clients or employers without considering the effects on others (Bayles, 1989). However, a profession can put procedures into place to work toward ethical behavior by all.

Some procedures put in place by professions are limited, in some form, to those who are in professional preparation programs and those who have already been admitted to the profession. Traditional ways of doing this have been through (1) selective admissions into academic programs, (2) retention standards to remain in academic programs, (3) graduation from academic programs, (4) completion of internships, (5) the process of becoming credentialed (i.e., certified or licensed to practice), and (6) continual updating to retain the credential. While proceeding through these steps, individuals may have to provide evidence of good moral character.

Once in the profession, professionals are expected to behave according to a system of norms. As noted previously in this chapter, this system of norms (or professional moral consensus, as some refer to it) is often placed in writing and referred to as a code of ethics. More specifically, a **code of ethics** is a "document that maps the dimensions of the profession's collective social responsibility and acknowledges the obligations individual practitioners share in meeting the profession's responsibilities" (Feeney & Freeman, 1999, p. 6). Such a document is usually useful not only for the professional but also for those who use the services of the professional. An ethical code's principal function is to "organize in a systematic way basic ethical standards, rules, and principles of professional conduct" (Pritchard, 2006, p. 85). In other words, "codes serve to *constrain* and set limits by identifying behaviors that should be avoided. They *guide* or instruct by identifying obligations and desirable qualities" (Svara, 2007, p. 75). And, "they can *inspire* and set forth the board goals that the adherents are supposed to promote" (Svara, 2007, p. 76). They also provide the consumers of health education/promotion services with an understanding of what they should expect from the provider.

Svara (2007) has noted that most codes of ethics have four different types of statements in them. They include (1) "don't" statements (which cover prohibited activities or behaviors), (2) obligations and responsibilities (which set forth the things one must or should do), (3) virtues, personal qualities, and/or values (which state how one should be rather than what one should do), and (4) aspirations (which state desirable conditions that one seeks to promote as opposed to actions or personal qualities). **Box 5.5** lists these four different types of statements and references to where they may be found in the *Code of Ethics for the Health Education Profession* (CNHEO, 2011).

In addition to a code of ethics, a profession should also have a means by which to deal with (discipline) professionals who violate the code of ethics. "A wide range of enforcement mechanisms are possible" (Taub, Kreuter, Parcel, & Vitello, 1987, p. 82). Such mechanisms may range from self-monitoring (also referred to as self-regulating) to a more formal process in which a committee of peers reviews ethics cases. When self-monitoring is used, charges of the ethical violation "might be conveyed directly to the professional charged with the violation. That person would then be responsible for resolving the situation. This procedure

> **BOX 5.5**
>
> ## Types of Ethical Statements and Examples Found in the *Code of Ethics for the Health Education Profession*
>
> **"Don't" statements**
>
> Ex. There are no "Don't" statements in the *Code of Ethics for the Health Education Profession* (CNHEO, 2011), but they are assumed. All statements are made in the positive of what health education specialists will do, not what they shouldn't do. For example, instead of saying that health education specialists should never violate one's right to privacy, Article I, Section 6 states "Health Educators are ethically bound to respect, assure, and protect the privacy, confidentiality, and dignity of individuals" (CNHEO, 2011, p. 2).
>
> **Obligations and Responsibilities**
>
> Ex. Article IV, Section 6—"Health Educators communicate the potential outcomes of proposed services, strategies, and pending decisions to all individuals who will be affected" (CNHEO, 2011, p. 4).
>
> **Virtues, Personal Qualities, and/or Values**
>
> Ex. Article I, Section 8—"Health Educators respect and acknowledge the rights of others to hold diverse values, attitudes, and opinions" (CNHEO, 2011, p. 2).
>
> **Aspirations**
>
> Ex. Article VI, Section 2—"Health Educators strive to make the educational environment and culture conducive to the health of all involved, and free from all forms of discrimination and harassment" (CNHEO, 2011, p. 6).

works well when there is peer pressure for professionals to behave consistent with a clearly identifiable set of standards and rules of professional conduct" (Gold & Greenberg, 1992, p. 143). When ethical violations are reviewed by an ethics committee of the profession or as part of a professional organization, the "committees usually have the authority to recommend sanctions against members who are judged to behave unethically" (Gold & Greenberg, 1992, p. 143). First or minor violations of ethical behavior often carry disciplinary measures of "warnings." Repeated or major violations can lead to more serious penalties like limitations on the ability to practice and "even outright expulsion from the profession (that is, decertification or rescinding the member's license to practice)" (Gold & Greenberg, 1992, p. 145). In determining the sanctions, review committees may base their decision on a variety of factors including but not limited to (1) the type of violation (e.g., violation of privacy vs. sexual misconduct), (2) number of prior violations by the professional, (3) the willfulness of the violation, and (4) the level of responsibility of the professional (Svara, 2007).

Ensuring Ethical Behavior in the Health Education/Promotion Profession

In the previous section, we identified a number of steps that a profession can take to try to ensure ethical behavior from its professionals. Let's look at how the health education/promotion profession has dealt with this, starting with admission into a health education professional preparation program at a college or university.

Currently, the admission procedure into the profession of health education/promotion is not clear. Some colleges and universities preparing health education specialists have selective admission standards, but most have open admissions, meaning that students can enter the health education/promotion program if admitted to the institution. Once in the program, all academic institutions have retention standards and graduation requirements, however minimal they may be—minimum grades in certain courses or a grade point average of 2.0 on a 4-point scale. Other institutions may have a minimum overall grade point average or minimum grade point average in certain professional courses to be admitted into student teaching an or an internship. With regard to the amount of education required in the profession, a bachelor's degree is required to sit for the certified health education specialist (CHES) examination (see Chapter 6); however, there is no consensus in the profession that a bachelor's degree should be the standard. Many feel a master's degree is more appropriate. Regardless of whether a bachelor's or master's degree is required to take the credentialing examination, the earned credentials (CHES or MCHES) are not universally accepted, either in or out of the profession, as necessary to practice health education/promotion.

The profession of health education/promotion has had a code of ethics for a number of years. The first was created in 1976 by the Society for Public Health Education (SOPHE). That code was later revised in 1983 and abridged in 1993. Though that code was developed more than 35 years ago, it was not universally adopted by the profession. In 1984, SOPHE and the Association for the Advancement of Health Education (AAHE; last known as the American Association for Health Education) appointed a joint committee to develop a profession-wide code of ethics. That committee was not able to create a profession-wide code of ethics. Further, in April 1994, AAHE developed another code, the "Code of Ethics for Health Educators." However, in 1995, the National Commission for Health Education Credentialing, Inc. (NCHEC) (see Chapter 6 for more on NCHEC) and Coalition of National Health Education Organizations (CNHEO) (see Chapter 8 for more on CNHEO) cosponsored a conference, "The Health Education Profession in the Twenty-First Century: Setting the Stage," at which it was recommended that efforts be expanded to develop a profession-wide code of ethics. Soon after that conference the CNHEO began work on such a code. After several years of work, in 1999 the *Code of Ethics for the Health Education Profession* was created and approved by all members of CNHEO, thus replacing the earlier codes developed by SOPHE and AAHE. That code was updated in 2011 (see Appendix A for a copy of the code and more information on its development). However, like the codes before it, this code does not include a formal procedure for enforcement. So currently, the profession has informal enforcement via "the subtle influences colleagues exert on one another" (Iammarino et al., 1989, p. 104). "One of the true weaknesses of our present code of ethics is no accountability to its standards" (Goldsmith, 2006, p. 36).

As can be seen from this analysis, the health education/promotion profession is moving in the right direction but still has much opportunity to refine its ethical foundations.

Summary

Ethical questions impact all aspects of life. Individuals on both a personal and professional level are constantly being confronted with ethical situations. To deal with these situations, people must have a basic understanding of how to make an ethical decision. To prepare readers for this task, this chapter presented key terms, such as philosophy, ethics, and morals; the philosophical, practical, and professional viewpoints of why people and professionals should work from an ethical base; the two major categories of theories (deontology and teleology) used to create ethical "yardsticks" for making ethical decisions; a set of principles and a guide for ethical decision making; a sampling of the ethical issues facing health education specialists today; and a discussion about how a profession can ensure that its professionals will act ethically.

Review Questions

1. What are the three major areas of philosophy? What does each of them mean?
2. In your own words, how do you define *ethics?*
3. What do the definitions of *ethics* and *morals* share? How are they different?
4. Why is it important to act ethically?
5. What is meant by the term *professional ethics?* What is *research ethics?*
6. How would you summarize the difference between the two major categories of ethical theories (deontology and teleology)?
7. What are Thiroux's five principles that create a common ground for all ethical theories?
8. What should be included in a process for making ethical decisions?
9. What is meant by the term *moral sensitivity?*
10. Name five ethical issues currently facing the profession of health education/promotion.
11. What can a profession do to ensure that its professionals will act ethically?
12. Define *code of ethics.*

Case Study

Sue accepted a position as a patient educator with the Franklin County Hospital after graduating with her bachelor's degree last spring. She is one of five health education specialists employed by the patient education department. About three months after Sue was hired, she observed Tom, the most experienced patient educator in the department, engage in what she believed was unethical behavior. Sue observed Tom accepting a really nice windbreaker (worth about $80) from a pharmaceutical company representative. In return, the pharmaceutical rep asked Tom to recommend the pharmaceutical company's glucometer during the diabetes education sessions he ran. Tom said that "that would be no problem." Do you agree with Sue—do you think this is unethical behavior? On what ethical principles do you base your response? Is there something in the *Code of Ethics for the Health Education Profession* (Appendix A) that supports your position? Say you agree with Sue; what would be your course of action? Do you think Tom's supervisor should be involved? Why or why not? Do you think Tom should be sanctioned by the profession? If so, how could it be enforced?

Critical Thinking Questions

1. Do you think it is ethical to use disincentives to change people's health behavior? For example, charging smokers more for life insurance, or fining a person for not wearing a safety belt or motorcycle helmet. Provide a rationale for your response.

2. If you were asked by one of your professors to help design a professional ethics course for health education/promotion majors or minors at your college/university, what would you suggest be included in the course? Why?

3. Several professions (e.g., medicine and law) have procedures for dealing with members' unethical behavior. In fact, if the offense is extreme enough a lawyer can be disbarred and a physician could lose his or her license to practice medicine. Do you think the profession of health education/promotion should create a similar process to review unethical behavior and if necessary take away the certification of certified health education specialists (CHES or MCHES)? Defend your response.

4. Do you think that all health education/promotion majors/minors should be required to take an ethics course while in college? Why or why not? If you responded yes to the question, do you think that a general ethics course open to all university students would be sufficient, or do you think the course should be specific to the profession? Why?

▶ Activities

Directions for activities 1–4. You will find four scenarios that include an ethical issue. Using the 10-step decision-making process put forth in this chapter, write a response to one of the scenarios. Include in your response a paragraph for each of the 10 components. Your 10 paragraphs should state your course of action.

1. You have been hired to work for the city health department to complete a project that was begun by your predecessor and funded with money from a local foundation. The grant requires the health department to develop X number of programs on the topic of hepatitis and then to present these programs to X number of people representing specific priority groups in the community. After being hired, you discover that the administrator of the grant, your supervisor, has not adhered to the grant guidelines. Only half the number of programs have been developed as the grant required. Further, the number of presentations is less than required, and presentations have been given to people not in the identified priority groups. In addition, your supervisor has taken some of the travel funds allocated to pay for your travel to and from presentations and has diverted them into his personal travel fund to attend a national conference in Las Vegas. It is now time for you to develop your year-end report, which will be sent directly to the local foundation office. Your supervisor has provided you with a copy of the original grant proposal and says to make sure your figures agree with those in the proposal. In other words, he expects you to "fudge" the data. What will you do?

2. As the health and fitness director of a large corporate wellness program, you have been asked to provide data to your supervisor that supports the effectiveness of your program. The trend in the company has been to cut programs that do not "carry their weight." The "bottom line" is important. In your review of the data related to your program, it is obvious that the data are not strong. However, in fairness to you, the program has been in operation for only two years, and it is too early to see the type of results management is looking for. You are the only one who has access to the data, and no one will know if the data you submit are accurate. How will you handle this situation?

3. You are a high school health teacher. The board of education has just adopted a policy that prohibits the teaching or discussing of information related to contraceptives or abortion in the district. The only approach that can be mentioned in the classroom is abstinence. You have read research that indicates that the abstinence approach is not as

effective as some may think. After class one day, one of your students approaches you and informs you that she is pregnant. She requests your help and asks for the name and location of an abortion clinic. She also asks that you not tell anyone else about this. What will you do?

4. You are the health education specialist for a large city hospital. Your supervisor has asked you to develop a program on "safer sex" practices for the gay and lesbian population. The program is to be made available to lesbian and gay groups in the community. Because of your strong religious convictions, your personal values and beliefs are opposed to the gay/lesbian lifestyle and the "safer sex" approach. In addition, you feel uncomfortable dealing with homosexuals in general and especially with anyone who is HIV-positive. How will you handle this situation?

5. Read thoroughly the *Code of Ethics for the Health Education Profession* presented in Appendix A, then provide written answers to the following questions.
   - What is your overall opinion of the code? Does it include everything you thought it would? Were there any surprises?
   - Do you think it should include any "Don't" statements? (Refer back to Box 5.5) If yes, which ones? If no, why not?
   - Is there anything in the code you feel should not be there? If so, what and why?
   - If you could add something else to the code, what would it be?
   - Do you think the profession should incorporate a means of enforcement in the code? Why or why not?

6. Select one of the ethical theories presented in Table 5.1 to study further. Find and read from other sources explaining the theory. Then write a three-page paper on the theory's application to the practice of health education/promotion.

7. Make an appointment to meet with one of your professors or with a practicing health education specialist. Inform him or her that you would like to spend about 15 to 20 minutes discussing professional ethics. At the meeting ask him or her if he or she has ever observed a professional situation that involved an ethical situation. If so, ask him or her to describe the situation without revealing the parties who were involved. Then ask how the situation was resolved. After your meeting, summarize in writing the discussion and compare the steps taken in the situation to the components of the 10-step process presented in this chapter. Do you think the situation was handled properly? Why or why not?

 ## Weblinks

1. **http://www.cnheo.org**

   Coalition of National Health Education Organizations (CNHEO)

   This is the home page for the CNHEO. The coalition has as its primary mission the mobilization of the resources of the health education/promotion profession to expand and improve health education/promotion, regardless of the setting. At this site you can print out a copy of the *Code of Ethics for the Health Education Profession.*

2. **http://www.ethics.org/**

   Ethics Resource Center (ERC)

   The ERC is a nonprofit, nonpartisan educational organization dedicated to independent research that advances high ethical standards and practices in public and private institutions.

3. http://www.professionalethics.ca/

Professional Ethics

This is a Canadian Web site that provides a wide variety of resources on various topics related to professional ethics. One special feature of this Web site is the presentation of a number of up-to-date articles on professional ethics. It also has links to several other ethics-related Web sites.

4. http://www.hhs.gov

U.S. Department of Health and Human Services (USDHHS)

Search the USDHHS homepage for "Health Information Privacy"; this will bring you to a page where you can get more information about the National Standards to Protect the Privacy of Personal Health Information.

5. http://appe.indiana.edu/

Association for Practical and Professional Ethics (APPE)

The APPE is professional organization that works to advance scholarship, education, and practice in practical and professional ethics. It offers both individual and institution memberships.

References

Balog, J. E., Shirreffs, J. H., Gutierrez, R. D., & Balog, L. F. (1985). Ethics and the field of health education. *The Eta Sigma Gamma Monograph Series, 4* (1), 65–110.

Bastida, E. M., Tseng, T-S., McKeever, C., & Jack, Jr., J. (2010). Ethics and community-based participatory research: Perspectives from the field. *Health Promotion Practice, 11* (1), 16–20.

Bayles, M. D. (1989). *Professional ethics* (2nd ed.). Belmont, CA: Wadsworth.

Buchanan, D., Khoshnood, K., Stopka, T., Shaw, S., Santelices, C., & Singer, M. (2002). Ethical dilemmas created by the criminalization of status behaviors: Case examples from ethnographic field research with injection drug users. *Health Education & Behavior, 29* (1), 30–42.

Coalition of National Health Education Organizations (CNHEO). (1999). *Code of ethics for the health education profession.* Retrieved May 30, 2013, from http://cnheo.org/ethics.html.

Cottrell, R. R., & McKenzie, J. F. (2011). *Health promotion and education research methods: Using the five-chapter thesis/dissertation model* (2nd ed.). Sudbury, MA: Jones & Bartlett.

Dawson, A., & Verweij, M. (Eds.). (2007). *Ethics, prevention, and public health.* New York: Oxford University Press, Inc.

Dorman, S. M. (1994). The imperative for ethical conduct in scientific inquiry. In R. M. Pigg (Ed.), Ethical issues of scientific inquiry in health science education. *The Eta Sigma Gamma Monograph Series, 12* (2), 1–5.

Eve, D. J., Marty, P. J., McDermott, R. J., Klasko, S. K., & Sanberg, P. R. (2008). Stem cell research and health education. *American Journal of Health Education, 39* (3), 167–179.

Feeney, S., & Freeman, N. K., (1999). *Ethics and the early childhood educator.* Washington, DC: National Association for the Education of Young Children.

Fisher, C. B. (2003). *Decoding the ethics code: A practical guide for psychologists.* Thousand Oaks, CA: Sage Publications.

Fox, R. C., & Swazey, J. P. (1997). Medical morality is not bioethics: Medical ethics in China and the United States. In N. S. Jecker, A. R. Jonsen, & R. A. Pearlman (Eds.), *Bioethics: An introduction to history, methods and practice* (pp. 237–251). Sudbury, MA: Jones and Bartlett.

Gold, R. S., & Greenberg, J. S. (1992). *The health education ethics book.* Dubuque, IA: Wm. C. Brown Publishers.

Goldsmith, M. (2006). Ethics in health education: Issues, concerns, and future directions. *The Health Education Monograph Series: Foundations of Health Education, 23* (1), 33–37.

Greenberg, J. S. (2001). *The code of ethics for the health education profession: A case study book.* Boston: Jones & Bartlett Publishers.

Hiller, M. D. (1987). Ethics and health education: Issues in theory and practice. In P. M. Lazes, L. Kaplan, & G. A. Gordon (Eds.), *The handbook of health education* (pp. 87–108). Rockville, MD: Aspen.

Iammarino, N. K., O'Rourke, T. W., Pigg, R. M., & Weinberg, A. D. (1989). Ethical issues in research and publication. *Journal of School Health, 59* (3), 101–104.

Kahan, B. (2012). Using a comprehensive best practices approach to strengthen ethical health-related practice. *Health Promotion Practice, 13,* 431–437.

Kimmel, A. J. (2007). *Ethical issues in behavioral research: Basic and applied perspectives* (2nd ed.). Malden, MA: Blackwell Publishing.

Margolis, L. (2000). Commentary: Ethical principles for analyzing dilemmas in sex research. *Health Education & Behavior, 27* (1), 24–27.

Marks, R. (2009). Ethics and patient education: Health literacy and cultural dilemmas. *Health Promotion Practice, 10* (3), 328–332.

McGrath, E. Z. (1994). *The art of ethics: A psychology of ethical beliefs.* Chicago: Loyola University Press.

McKenzie, J. F., Neiger, B. L., & Thackeray, R. (2013). *Planning, implementing, and evaluating health promotion programs: A primer* (6th ed.). Boston: Pearson.

McKenzie, J. F., Seabert, D. M., Hayden, J., & Cottrell, R. R. (2009). Textbook writing: A form of professional development. *Health Promotion Practice, 10* (1), 10–14.

McLeroy, K. R., Bibeau, D. L., & McConnell, T. C. (1993). Ethical issues in health education and health promotion: Challenges for the profession. *Journal of Health Education, 24* (5), 313–318.

Mellert, R. B. (1995). *Seven ethical theories.* Dubuque, IA: Kendall/Hunt.

Melnick, A. L. (2015). Case finding: Screening, testing, and contact tracing. In R. Gaare Bernheim, J. F. Childress, R. J. Bonnie, and A. L. Melnick (Eds.). Essentials of public health ethics (pp. 119–143). Burlington, MA: Jones & Bartlett Learning.

Minkler, M., Fadem, P., Perry, M., Blum, K., Moore, L., & Rogers, J. (2002). Ethical dilemmas in participatory action research: A case study from the disability community. *Health Education & Behavior, 29* (1), 14–29.

Minkler, M., Pies, C., & Hyde, C. A. (2012). Ethical issues in community organizing and building. In M. Minkler (Ed.). *Community organizing and community building for health* (3rd ed., pp. 110–129). New Brunswick, NJ: Rutgers University Press.

Minkler, M., Vasquez, V. B., Tajik, M., & Petersen, D. (2008). Promoting environmental justice through community-based participatory research: The role of community and partnership capacity. *Health Education & Behavior, 35* (1), 119–137.

Modell, S. M., & Citrin, T. (2002). Ethics instruction in an issues-oriented course on public health genetics. *Health Education & Behavior, 29* (1), 43–60.

Morrison, E. E. (2006). *Ethics in health administration: A practical approach for decision makers.* Sudbury, MA: Jones & Bartlett.

Morrison, E. E., & Furlong, B. (2014). *Health care ethics: Critical issues for the 21st century* (3rd ed.). Burlington, MA: Jones & Bartlett Learning.

National Commission for Health Education Credentialing, Inc. (2010). *Health educator job analysis—2010: Executive summary and recommendations.* Retrieved May 30, 2013, from http://www.nchec.org/credentialing/competency/.

Nelson, W. A. (2005). An organizational ethics decision-making process. *Healthcare Executive, 20* (4), 8–14.

Penland, L. R., & Beyrer, M. K. (1981). Ethics and health education: Issues and implications. *Health Education, 12* (4), 6–7.

Pigg, R. M. (Ed.). (1994). Ethical issues of scientific inquiry in health science education. *The Eta Sigma Gamma Monograph Series, 12* (2), 1-150.

Pigg, R. M. (2006). Conflict and consensus on ethics in publishing. *The Health Education Monograph Series: Foundations of Health Education, 23* (1), 38–41.

Pigg, Jr., R. M. (2010). Three essential questions in defining a personal philosophy. In J. M. Black, S. Furney, H. M. Graf, & A. E. Nolte (Eds.), *Philosophical foundations of health education* (pp. 11–15). San Francisco: Jossey-Bass.

Pozgar, G. D. (2013). *Legal and ethical issues for health professionals* (3rd ed.). Burlington, MA: Jones & Bartlett Learning.

Price, J. H., & Dake, J. A. (2002). Ethical guidelines for manuscript reviewers and journal editors. *American Journal of Health Education, 33* (4), 194–196.

Price, J. H., Dake, J. A., & Islam, R. (2001). Ethical issues in research and publication: Perceptions of health education faculty. *Health Education & Behavior, 28,* 51–64.

Price, J. H., Dake, J. A., & Telljohann, S. K. (2001). Ethical issues regarding service: Perceptions of health education faculty. *American Journal of Health Education, 32* (4), 208–215.

Pritchard, M. S. (2006). *Professional integrity: Thinking ethically.* Lawrence: University Press of Kansas.

Rabinowitz, P. (2013). *The community health toolbox: Ethical issues in community interventions.* Retrieved May 24, 2013, from http://ctb.ku.edu/en/tablecontents/sub_main_1165.aspx.

Reamer, F. G. (2006). *Social work values and ethics* (3rd ed.). New York: Columbia University Press.

Remley, T. P., & Herlihy, B. (2007). *Ethical, legal, and professional issues in counseling* (2nd ed.). Upper Saddle River, NJ: Merrill, Prentice Hall.

Rest, J., Narvaes, D., Bebeau, M. J., & Thoma, S. J. (1999). *Postconventional moral thinking: A neo-kohlbergian approach.* Mahwah, NJ: L. Erlbaum Associates.

Rothschild, M. L. (2000). Ethical considerations in support of marketing of public health issues. *American Journal of Health Behavior, 24* (1), 26–35.

Shaw-Ridley, M., & Ridley, C. R. (2010). The health disparities industry: Is it an ethical conundrum? *Health Promotion Practice, 11,* 454–464.

Shive, S. E., & Marks, R. (2006). The influence of ethical theories in the practice of health education. *Health Promotion Practice, 7* (3) 287–288.

Siegel, M., & Lotenberg, L. D. (2007). *Marketing public health: Strategies to promote social change* (2nd ed.). Sudbury, MA: Jones & Bartlett.

Sperry, L. (2007). *Dictionary of ethical and legal terms and issues: The essential guide for mental health professionals.* New York: Routledge.

Summers, J. (2014). Principles of healthcare ethics. In E. E. Morrison & B. Furlong, *Health care ethics: Critical issues for the 21st century* (3rd ed., pp. 47–63). Burlington, MA: Jones & Bartlett Learning.

Svara, J. (2007). *The ethics primer for public administrators in government and nonprofit organizations.* Sudbury, MA: Jones & Bartlett.

Taub, A., Kreuter, M., Parcel, G., & Vitello, E. (1987). Report of the SOPHE/AAHE joint committee on ethics. *Health Education Quarterly, 14* (1), 79–90.

Telljohann, S. K., Price, J. H., & Dake, J. A. (2001). Selected ethical issues in the teaching: Perceptions of health education faculty. *American Journal of Health Education, 32* (2), 66–74.

The Society of Prospective Medicine Board of Directors (SPM). (1999). Ethics guidelines for the development and use of health assessments. In G. C. Hyner, K. W. Peterson, J. W. Travis, J. E. Dewey, J. J. Foerster, & E. M. Framer (Eds.), *SPM handbook of health assessment tools* (pp. xxii–xxvi). Pittsburgh: The Society of Prospective Medicine.

Thiroux, J. P. (1995). *Ethics: Theory and practice* (5th ed.). Englewood Cliffs, NJ: Prentice-Hall.

Thompson, I., Melia, K., & Boyd, K. (2000). *Nursing ethics* (4th ed.). Edinburgh, Scotland: Churchill Livingstone.

Thurston, W. E., Vollman, A. R., & Burgess, M. M. (2003). Ethical review of health promotion program evaluation proposals. *Health Promotion Practice, 4* (1), 45–50.

Tschudin, V. (2003) *Ethics in nursing: The caring relationship* (3rd ed.). Edinburgh, Scotland: Butterworth Heinemann.

U.S. Department of Health and Human Services (USDHHS). (n.d.). *Health information privacy.* Retrieved May 30, 2013, from http://www.hhs.gov/ocr/privacy.

Westin, A. F. (1968). *Privacy and freedom.* New York: Atheneum.

White, T. I. (1988). *Right and wrong: A brief guide to understanding ethics.* Englewood Cliffs, NJ: Prentice-Hall.

Wiley, D. C. (2002). The ethics of abstinence-only and abstinence-plus sexuality education. *Journal of School Health, 72* (4), 164–167.

Young, M., & Valois, R. F. (2010). Magic, morals, and health: Plus 40 years. *American Journal of Health Education, 41* (1), 18–19.

The Health Education Specialist: Roles, Responsibilities, Certifications, and Advanced Study

Although education about health has been around since the beginning of human intelligence, health education/promotion as a profession is, relatively speaking, an infant. When any infant begins to mature, it takes on its own identity. This chapter chronicles major historical events that have helped shape the identity of health education/promotion since the 1970s. The current identity of health education/promotion is also presented in terms of roles, responsibilities, certification, and accreditation. The importance of advanced study and continuing education in the health education/promotion profession is also discussed.

▷ Quality Assurance and Credentialing

Quality assurance and credentialing often go hand-in-hand. It is important to be familiar with these terms as they apply to health education/promotion. In the business world, the term **quality assurance** means "the planned and systematic activities necessary to provide adequate confidence that the product or service will meet given requirements" (Quality Assurance Solutions, 2010). **Credentialing** is the means by which professions such as health education/promotion demonstrate quality assurance. In other words, credentialing would be the "planned and systematic activities" used to increase confidence that the product or service—in this case, health education specialists—is meeting the requirements of the profession. Credentialing is a process whereby an individual, such as a health education specialist, or a professional preparation program demonstrates that established standards are met. When people or programs meet specific standards established by a credentialing body, they are recognized for having done so. We say, "They earned their credentials," which indicates they are meeting their profession's requirements. Credentialing can take the form of accreditation, licensure, or certification.

Accreditation "is the status of public recognition that an accrediting agency grants to an education institution or program that meets the agency's standards or requirements" (National Transition Task Force on Accreditation in Health Education, 2013). Thus, the health education/promotion program at any particular institution may be accredited by one of several outside agencies discussed later in this chapter. For example, the health education/promotion program at Alpha University could be accredited by Beta Accrediting Group. Such a process takes place after the program at Alpha University creates a self-study document that shows how it meets the Beta Accrediting Group's standards. Accrediting procedures may also include an on-campus visit by representatives from Beta. Throughout the process, factors such as student–teacher ratio, curriculum, and faculty qualifications are closely examined.

Licensure is "the process by which an agency or government [usually a state] grants permission to individuals to practice a given profession by certifying that those licensed have attained specific standards of competence" (Cleary, 1995, p. 39). Licensure applies to most medical professionals, such as doctors, nurses, dentists, and physical therapists. The only health education specialists who are licensed in the United States at the present time are school health education specialists in some states.

Certification "is a process by which a professional organization grants recognition to an individual who, upon completion of a competency-based curriculum, can demonstrate a predetermined standard of performance" (Cleary, 1995, p. 39). Note that certification is granted to an individual, not a program, and it is given by the profession, not by a governmental body. Certification is available for all health education specialists, regardless of specialty area. One who is certified is recognized as a **Certified Health Education Specialist** and may use the initials **CHES** after one's name and academic degree. In fall 2010, an advanced certification became available. Those who obtain this advanced certification are **Master Certified Health Education Specialists** and may use the initials **MCHES** after their names. See **Figure 6.1** for an overview of quality assurance mechanisms available for health education programs in the United States.

▷ History of Role Delineation and Certification

Certification in health education got its formal start around 1978. At that time, individual certification for health education specialists was not available, except for school health education specialists, who had to be licensed or certified in the state where they taught.

Program accreditation was available only for school health and master's level public health professional preparation programs. Many public health programs outside schools of public health, and all community health programs, were not accredited, nor was accreditation available for these programs. This gave rise to a situation in which there were great discrepancies in professional preparation. One program might look different from another program. To say that an individual was a health educator had little meaning. In describing

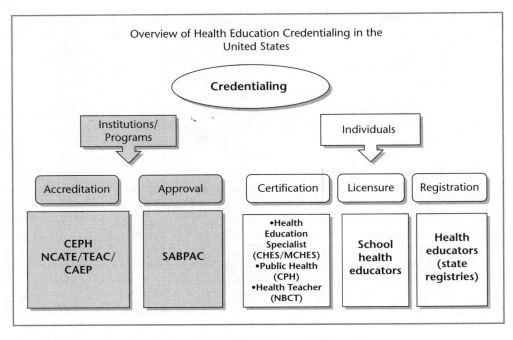

▲ **Figure 6.1** Overview of health education credentialing in the United States

Note: CHES, Certified Health Education Specialist; CAPE, Council for the Accreditation of Educator Preparation; CEPH, Council on Education for Public Health; CPH, Certified in Public Health; MCHES, Master Certified Health Education Specialist; NBCT, National Board Certified Teacher; NCATE, National Council for the Accreditation of Teacher Education; SABPAC, SOPHE/AAHE Baccalaureate Approval Committee; SOPHE, Society for Public Health Education; TEAC, Teacher Education Accreditation Council

From: Cottrell, R. R., Auld, M. E., Birch, D. A., Taub, A., King, L. R., & Allegrante, J. P. (2012). Progress and directions in professional credentialing for health education in the United States. *Health Education and Behavior.* 39(6). 681–694.

the situation, Helen Cleary (see **Figure 6.2**), who was president of the Society for Public Health Education (SOPHE) in 1974, wrote the following:

> What I found in my travels [as SOPHE president] was a profession in disarray. Many, many health educators could neither define themselves nor their role. It was clear that the preparation of most was so varied that there was no common core. There was no professional identity, no sense of a profession. Numbers of competent, bright, young professionals were leaving health education for greener pastures. (Cleary, 1995, p. 2)

As a result of this situation, Cleary began to pursue the idea of credentialing health educators and/or health education programs. To undertake such a project, outside expertise and funding were needed. Thomas Hatch, director of the Division of Associated Health Professions in the Bureau of Health Manpower of the Department of Health, Education and Welfare, expressed an interest in the project. Prior to funding the project, however, he needed assurances that members of the profession would work together to create a credentialing system. Hatch wanted to be certain that those who practiced health education in different settings would have enough in common to develop one set of standards.

In response to Hatch's concern, a conference, known today as the Bethesda Conference on Commonalities and Differences, was held in February 1978 in Bethesda, Maryland. The conference's planning committee was made up of representatives from the eight organizations comprising the Coalition of Health Education Organizations. This planning committee

▶ **Figure 6.2** Helen P. Cleary—
the person most responsible
for establishing certification for
health education specialists

formulated two questions to be answered at the conference: (1) What are the commonalities and differences in the function of health educators practicing in different settings? and
(2) What are the commonalities and differences in the preparation of health educators?
(Cleary, 1995, p. 3).

After much discussion, conference attendees concluded that health education was one
profession and that a credentialing system was necessary. "It was the consensus of the participants that standards were essential if they were to provide quality service to the public and
if they were to survive as a viable profession" (Cleary, 1986, p. 130). Further, the conference
planning committee members were asked to continue as a task force to develop the credentialing system. Thus, the **National Task Force on the Preparation and Practice of Health
Educators** was born (see **Table 6.1**).

TABLE 6.1 **Organizations represented on the National Task Force on the Preparation and Practice
of Health Educators, 1978**

American College Health Association

American Public Health Association, Public Health Education Section

American Public Health Association, School Health Education and Services Section

American School Health Association

Association for the Advancement of Health Education (AAHE)

Conference of State and Territorial Directors of Public Health Education

Society for Public Health Education, Inc.

Society of State Directors of Health, Physical Education and Recreation

In January 1979, funding became available to embark on the project, and **role delineation** for health educators got under way. Alan Henderson was hired as the project director. Under his leadership, a working committee of the task force began the difficult job of defining the health education specialist's role. In describing this process, Cleary (1995) notes, "For the first time in the profession's history, specialists in school health education and in community health education faced each other across the table and learned that each was dealing with similar concepts, but using different terminology and, as well, applying them in different settings" (p. 5).

Once the initial phase of role delineation was completed, the next step was to verify and refine the role of a health educator. Funding for this became available in March 1980. Health education specialists working in all areas of health education were surveyed to verify the role of a health educator. Survey results were positive; there were no significant differences among practitioners in different settings.

In addition to the survey, a conference for college and university health education faculty members was held in Birmingham, Alabama, in February 1981. The conference provided the opportunity for academics to review the initial role delineation work and discuss its potential impact on the field. The planning committee chairman was Warren E. Schaller from Ball State University, and 238 academics from 125 institutions attended.

Many conference participants were happy with the work and direction of the task force, but others were not. Differences of opinion surrounding the health educator as a content expert versus a process expert emerged and probably reflected the different types of professional preparation programs the faculty represented. Although these differences were real, they were not divisive enough to alter the work of the task force.

The third step in the role delineation process involved creating a curriculum framework based on the verified role of a health educator. Initially, the task force decided to develop a curriculum guide, which is a fairly specific set of rules used to develop a curriculum. Little room is left for interpretation because the curriculum must meet the standards established in the guide. Betty Mathews from the University of Washington and Herb L. Jones from Ball State University were recruited to do the actual writing.

After a draft copy of the curriculum guide was developed, it had to be pretested. Eleven regional workshops were held around the country to obtain feedback on the guide. Again, differences surfaced regarding whether health educators were specialists in content or process. Further, some felt entry-level preparation should be at the bachelor's degree level, whereas others believed it should be at the master's degree level. Feedback was also obtained from professional associations and practitioners in the field.

To deal with some of the criticisms and to make the curriculum guide less rigid, it was ultimately transformed into a curriculum framework. A framework merely provides a frame of reference around which a curriculum can be developed. As Cleary (1995) notes, "It does not tell a faculty what to teach or how to teach it. It simply tells them what the students should know when they have completed the program of studies" (p. 9). Marion Pollock was the individual responsible for transforming the curriculum guide into a curriculum framework.

At this juncture, it was important to check with those in the profession to determine if they wanted to continue with the development of a credentialing system and, if so, what kind of system they wanted. The Second Bethesda Conference was held in February 1986, with 99 attendees. Participants were divided into five groups and asked to answer several predetermined questions. When reports from the groups were analyzed, four of the five were in favor of a certification system for individuals and some form of credentialing for professional preparation programs. They recommended that the task force continue to develop the credentialing system.

Over the next two years, the task force continued to work toward the development of a certification system for individual health education specialists. The Professional Examination Service (PES), which developed certification and licensure exams for many other professions, was contracted to assist with this process. Not only was its experience in test development vital to the process, but it was also willing to provide start-up funds to get the process off the ground.

By June 1988, the National Task Force on the Preparation and Practice of Health Education had functioned for 10 years. With the certification of individual health education specialists about to become a reality, it was time to establish a more permanent structure to manage the certification process. As a result, the **National Commission for Health Education Credentialing, Inc. (NCHEC)** was formed to replace the national task force. Today, NCHEC still oversees and administers the health education certification process. NCHEC's mission "is to enhance the professional practice of Health Education by promoting and sustaining a credentialed body of Health Education Specialists. To meet this mission, NCHEC certifies health education specialists, promotes professional development, and strengthens professional preparation and practice" (NCHEC, 2013b).

▷ Individual Certification

When a new certification program is initiated, charter certification is usually available for a limited time. Charter certification allows qualified individuals to get certified on the basis of their academic training, work experience, and references, without taking an exam. After the charter period expires, anyone seeking certification must meet all criteria for certification and pass the examination. The CHES charter certification period began in October 1988 and ended in 1990. When the first exam was held in 1990, 644 candidates passed it to become Certified Health Education Specialists.

The CHES voluntary professional certification program established for the first time a national standard for health education practice. All health education/promotion students are strongly urged to obtain national certification upon graduation (see **Box 6.1**). Certification includes the following benefits (NCHEC, 2013f):

- Establishes a national standard of practice for all health education specialists.
- Attests to the individual health education specialist's knowledge and skills.
- Assists employers in identifying qualified health education practitioners.
- Develops a sense of pride and accomplishment among certified health education specialists.
- Promotes continued professional development for health education specialists.

Currently, eligibility to sit for the CHES exam is based exclusively on academic qualifications. You must "possess a bachelor's, master's or doctoral degree from an accredited institution of higher education; AND (1) an official transcript (including course titles) that clearly shows a major in health education, e.g., Health Education, Community Health Education,

CHES Lauren A. Clark, B.S., CHES, CPST

CURRENT POSITION/TITLE: Injury Prevention Coordinator

EMPLOYER: Riley Hospital for Children

DEGREE/INSTITUTION: B.S., Ball State University, 2010

MAJOR: Health Science

MINORS: Psychology of Human Development, Marketing

My job responsibilities: I coordinate and implement injury prevention programs within the local school systems and throughout the community. My primary focus is on low-income areas that do not have many resources. However, children everywhere can benefit from the variety of services we have to offer. I teach CPR and first aid courses for a variety of children's organizations, churches, daycares, and schools in the area. I also oversee and teach Safe Sitter® classes to children ages 11 to 13. During this 12½ hour course, the students learn the basics of babysitting, how to work with children of different ages and developmental stages, and how to handle emergency situations. These not only are skills they can use now but also are life-long skills that they can use when raising their own children in the future.

With my position, I also have the opportunity to plan and implement programs that teach children about different safety topics such as pedestrian safety, bicycle safety, water safety, sports injuries, and more! Child Passenger Safety is another one of my job responsibilities and is also a passion of mine. Data show that 80 percent of children nationwide are not correctly restrained in vehicles. Without proper restraint, children are put at serious risk should a crash occur. I am certified (CPST) as a technician to perform car seat checks and clinics for parents/guardians who have children in car seats. Beyond all of the programming, one of my most important roles is serving as a resource person for the community. I am regularly contacted by community members with questions regarding injury prevention.

By serving as a resource person, I can answer their questions or help find them additional resources. I am also frequently asked to give presentations at conferences, forums, and community events. At these events, I have the opportunity to impact a large number of individuals who also have a child's best interest at heart.

How I obtained my job: I was finishing up my internship in Indianapolis, IN, and knew that I wanted to stay in the area. I was ecstatic when my internship coordinator contacted my graduating class about a job opportunity available at Riley Hospital for Children. It seemed like a great fit because my career goal was to become a health education specialist and I have always loved working with children and families. I applied for the position online and received a phone call a few weeks later to set up an interview. During the first round of interviews, I was interviewed by two individuals in the department that I work directly with on a day-to-day basis. For my second interview, I was asked to give a presentation on bicycle safety to the entire department, which consisted of eight individuals at the time. Following my presentation, the department members had a chance to interview me. Now, here I am!

What I like most about my job: One thing I considered while applying for jobs was "will I make a difference?" With this position, I have an opportunity to make a difference in the lives of others. I also enjoy the variety that comes with my position. I am constantly implementing different programs within the school systems and community. By doing this, I also have the opportunity to work with different groups and organizations every day. For example, one day I might be teaching CPR and first aid skills to daycare workers in a high-risk area of Indianapolis, and the next day I might be fitting and

BOX 6.1

continued

distributing bicycle helmets to a group of kids at a children's museum. No matter what I am doing day-to-day, I know that I am making a difference in the lives of children.

I am also blessed to work for a company that encourages life-long learning. My department has paid for all of my trainings and certifications. For example, they have sent me to trainings to become a CPR and First Aid Instructor, Safe Sitter® Instructor, Child Passenger Safety Technician, and Playground Safety Inspector. They also encourage me to attend conferences where I can network with other professionals and broaden my expertise.

What I like least about my job: My position is a part of the Trauma Services Department at Riley Hospital for Children. I receive notice every time a child comes into the Emergency Department for a trauma-related injury or incident. It is sad and hard to constantly see children being hurt, disabled, and even killed from situations that could have easily been prevented.

How the Certified Health Education Specialist (CHES) credential has helped me: I believe my CHES certification helped me get the position I have now. Out of the 30+ individuals they interviewed, I was the only one scheduled to take the CHES examination. Others were open to it, but I was the only one that had taken the initiative to sign up and start studying. Not only has my initiative to take the exam helped me, but I also feel like it has made me more qualified for my position. Everything I do at work, I use one or more of the CHES responsibilities and competencies. Without the background knowledge I have gained from my CHES credential, I would not be as confident or successful at what I do.

How my work relates to the responsibilities and competencies of a CHES: Everything I do at work can relate to one or more of the CHES responsibilities and competencies. Based on data and other related information we receive through our trauma registrar, it makes it easy to assess the individual, organizational, and community health needs. I can easily see what types of programs are needed to help reduce injury among our local children. Based on those needs and the interests of the community, I plan and implement injury prevention programs for the children, parents/guardians, and caregivers. For example, if we see a dramatic increase in the number of children injured by bicycle crashes, I know there is a need for education and I can start planning and implementing these types of programs. Evaluation is also the key component of any program I implement. Not only do we want to see how effective our efforts are, we want to improve programs for the future. I am constantly changing programs based on process and impact evaluation methods. Through my programs and on a day-to-day basis, I consistently act as a health education resource person advocating for health and health education. Whether I answer questions, find answers, or find additional resources for individuals in the community, people view me as a reliable resource.

Recommendations for those preparing to become health education specialists: I strongly suggest studying for and taking the CHES exam prior to graduating. Not only are you still in the "studying mode," but it will help you become more prepared for your future career. I would also suggest forming strong relationships with the professors you have now in school. Not only are they a wealth of knowledge, they can serve as a great resource and mentor to you in the future. I still keep in contact with several of my professors. The same goes for your classmates. Once they start their careers as health education specialists, they can all be a great resource to you. This is also a great way to network within the field!

Public Health Education, School Health Education, etc. Degree/major must explicitly be in a discipline of Health Education/Promotion; OR (2) an official transcript that reflects at least 25 semester hours or 37 quarter hours of course work (with a grade 'C' or better) with specific preparation addressing the Seven Areas of Responsibility and Competency for Health Educators" (NCHEC, 2013a).

▷ Graduate Health Education Standards

The roles and responsibilities document, *A Competency-Based Framework for Professional Development of Certified Health Education Specialists* (NCHEC, 1996), defined the skills needed for the entry-level health education/promotion professional. This document provided guidance for professional preparation programs at the bachelor's degree level, but not at the graduate degree level. Although many health education specialists with advanced masters and doctoral degrees had obtained certification, it attested only to the fact that they had entry-level skills. The need existed for an advanced level of certification.

In June 1992, the Joint Committee for Graduate Standards was established. After much work, discussion, and review, the Joint Committee for Graduate Standards developed a draft document that contained additional responsibilities, competencies, and sub-competencies specific to graduate-level preparation (Joint Committee for Graduate Standards, 1996).

In February 1996, 134 health education specialists from more than 100 colleges and universities gathered at the National Congress for Institutions Preparing Graduate Health Educators. At this meeting in Dallas, Texas, the draft document of graduate-level competencies was presented to attendees. After thoroughly discussing and debating these graduate level competencies, recommendations for improvement were presented to the planning committee. Despite some dissension, the general mood was in favor of the graduate-level competencies, and the planning committee was urged to move on with the approval process. After revisions were made, the final version was presented to the AAHE and SOPHE boards of directors, who granted approval in March 1997. These graduate-level competencies served to guide the health education curriculum of professional preparation programs but were not used for individual certification purposes. In fall 2010 an advanced certification became available through NCHEC. Those who obtain this advanced certification are designated Master Certified Health Education Specialists (MCHES). A graduate degree is not required to obtain the MCHES designation; rather, MCHES indicates that an individual is practicing advanced-level competencies.

▷ Competencies Update Project

Since the initial Role Delineation Project began more than 30 years ago, health education/promotion has evolved and matured. Changes in the profession created a need to re-verify the competencies and sub-competencies of a health education specialist. The **Competencies Update Project (CUP)** began in 1998 and was completed in 2004 (Gilmore, Olsen, Taub & Connell, 2005). The majority of the CUP work was conducted by

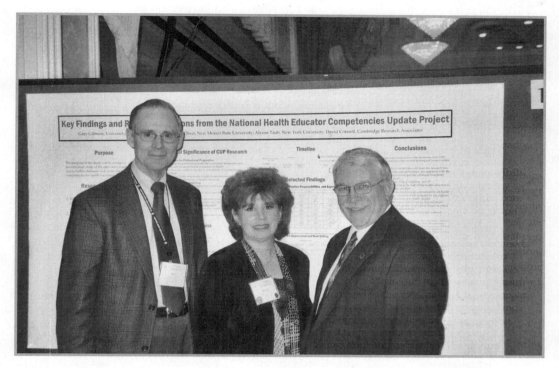

▲ **Figure 6.3** CUP Steering Committee. From left, Gary Gilmore, chair; Alyson Taub; and Larry Olsen.

a three-person steering committee comprised of Gary Gilmore, chair; Alyson Taub; and Larry Olsen (see **Figure 6.3**). The profession owes a deep debt of gratitude to these individuals for the time and effort they invested in this project.

▷ Health Education Job Analysis 2010

The National Commission for Certifying Agencies (NCCA) accredits professional credentials offered by certifying agencies. To obtain a "gold standard" endorsement from NCCA, an accrediting agency must follow recognized best practices. One of these best practices is updating the job analysis for the agency's field every five years.

In August 2008, the NCHEC received a "gold standard" endorsement from NCCA for the CHES credential. In May 2013, the NCCA granted re-accreditation for the CHES credential and the MCHES credential was granted its initial accreditation (NCHEC, 2013c). To meet the five-year update requirement, NCHEC along with AAHE and SOPHE commissioned the 2010 job analysis study (AAHE, NCHEC, & SOPHE, 2010). This study was needed to update the health education competencies, last revised in 2005 by the CUP project. Results of the study were released in 2010, called the Health Education Job Analysis 2010 model (*HEJA 2010* model). The areas of responsibility remained essentially the same as in the initial

TABLE 6.2 **Comparison of areas of responsibility (1985–2010)**

Entry-Level Framework (1985)	Graduate-Level Framework (1999)	CUP Model (2006)	HEJA Model (2010)
I. Assessing individual and community needs for health education	I. Assessing individual and community needs for health education	I. Assessing individual and community needs for health education	I. Assess needs, assets, and capacity for health education
II. Planning effective health education programs	II. Planning effective health education programs	II. Plan health education strategies, interventions, and programs	II. Plan health education
III. Implementing health education programs	III. Implementing health education programs	III. Implement health education strategies, interventions, and programs	III. Implement health education
IV. Evaluating effectiveness of health education programs	IV. Evaluating effectiveness of health education programs	IV. Conduct evaluation and research related to health education	IV. Conduct evaluation and research related to health education
V. Coordinating provision of health education services	V. Coordinating provision of health education services	V. Administer health education strategies, interventions, and programs	V. Administer and manage health education
VI. Acting as a resource person in health education	VI. Acting as a resource person in health education	VI. Serve as a health education resource person	VI. Serve as a health education resource person
VII. Communicating health and health education needs, concerns, and resources	VII. Communicating health and health education needs, concerns, and resources	VII. Communicate and advocate for health and health education	VII. Communicate and advocate for health and health education
	VIII. Applying appropriate research principles and techniques in health education		
	IX. Administering health education programs		
	X. Advancing the profession of health education		

Note: CUP, Competences Update Project.

From National Commission for Health Education Credentialing, Inc. (NCHEC), Society for Public Health Education (SOPHE), American Association for Health Education (AAHE). (2010a). *A Competency-based Framework for Health Education Specialists—2010*. Whitehall, PA: Author. By permission.

entry-level framework and the CUP project with only minor wording changes. This can be seen in **Table 6.2**. The fact that the responsibilities have remained fairly consistent with only minor wording changes confirms the previous work of the role delineation project and the CUP project.

The important point here is that the health education/promotion profession has and continues to carefully and systematically review and validate the competencies of a health education specialist. The CHES exam is based on these standards, and the health education/promotion curricula of professional preparation programs should be grounded on them as well.

▷ Health Education Specialist Practice Analysis

For the NCHEC to maintain accreditation for the CHES and MCHES credentials, the profession of health education/promotion must conduct an analysis of the practice of the health education specialists every five years. At the time this book went to press, NCHEC, and its partners SOPHE and ProExam, were beginning the work for the Health Education Specialist Practice Analysis (HESPA). The 18-month project began in Spring 2013 (NCHEC, 2013e). It is estimated that the next set responsibilities, competencies, and sub-competencies will be released in early 2015.

▷ International Efforts in Quality Assurance

Outside the United States, efforts to ensure quality in health education/promotion have also occurred. According to Allegrante, Barry, Auld, Lamarre, and Taub (2009), Canada, Australia, New Zealand, member states of the European Union and Council of Europe, Spain, Japan, Israel, the People's Republic of China, India, and Taiwan have all endeavored to improve health education or health promotion practice.

In an effort to promote international exchange and understanding related to the core competencies of health education/promotion and various credentialing mechanisms, a working group of 26 health education/promotion scholars and leaders from around the world met at the National University of Ireland in the summer of 2008. This meeting, now known as the Galway Consensus Conference, was a first effort to identify and codify agreement around quality assurance and credentialing on an international basis.

At this conference, the Domains of Core Competencies were developed (Allegrante, Barry, Airhihenbuwa et al., 2009). The domains are broader than competencies, but using these broad domains, competencies and credentialing systems can be developed by nations around the world. The Domains of Core Competencies align nicely with the NCHEC Responsibilities of a Health Education Specialist (NCHEC, 2013d). Several of the Domains are exactly the same as the NCHEC responsibilities including, assessing, planning, implementing, evaluating, and advocacy. Three Domains, catalyzing change, leadership and partnerships, are not identified as one of the seven major NCHEC Responsibilities, but would still be considered important skills that would actually be delineated at the competency or sub-competency level by NCHEC.

Since the Galway Consensus Conference, a new round of efforts to enhance professional preparation standards and credentialing have emerged in North America, throughout Europe, and in other regions and countries of the world such as Australia, Canada, Latin American, and New Zealand (Allegrante, Barry, Auld & Lamarre, 2012). In Europe, professional standards for health promotion have been developed, reviewed, and are ready for implementation (Speller, Parish, Davison, & Zilnyk, 2012).

▷ Program Accreditation

"Accreditation is a process by which a recognized professional body evaluates an entire program against predetermined criteria or standards" (Cleary, 1995). In most cases, colleges and universities that train students to enter a given profession are accredited by a recognized professional body that operates independently of the school. If a program does not meet the standards of the recognized professional body, it can lose its accreditation. A nonaccredited program might have difficulty recruiting new students, placing program graduates in jobs, and may be restricted in its participation in the profession. Therefore, accreditation helps ensure that all students entering the profession have similar training and preparation.

In health education/promotion, accreditation is available through four accrediting bodies. Health education/promotion programs that are affiliated with a college of education and train students for positions in school health may be accredited through the National Commission for the Accreditation of Teacher Education (NCATE) or the Teacher Education Accreditation Council (TEAC). When this text was written, TEAC and NCATE were in the process of merging into one new organization called the Council for Accreditation of Educator Preparation (CAEP) (CAEP, 2013).

The Council on Education for Public Health (CEPH) accredits schools of public health and graduate public health programs (CEPH, 2013b). In the past, undergraduate public health programs in the same unit as a Master of Public Health (MPH) degree program could be accredited along with the MPH program. Beginning in January 2014, freestanding undergraduate programs (those not affiliated with a graduate program) could also be accredited through CEPH. Undergraduate programs in school health or public/community health that are not affiliated with an MPH program may elect to obtain approval through the SOPHE/AAHE. This is done through the SOPHE/AAHE Baccalaureate Program Approval Committee (SABPAC) process. As of June 2013, 21 institutions had voluntarily chosen to undergo the SABPAC approval process and received program approval (SOPHE/AAHE, 2013).

Having four accreditation-approvals available is considered by many a weakness in the profession. As Cleary (1995) noted, "There were (and are) huge gaps and great discrepancies in the accreditation/approval process" (p. 16). Professional preparation is not at all uniform in the profession (Cleary, 1986). Some programs focus more on content, such as drugs, sexuality, stress, and physical fitness, whereas other programs emphasize process courses, such as planning, implementing, and evaluating. Some programs stress individual behavior change, and others stress population-based approaches to change. In 1987, the National Task Force on the Preparation and Practice of Health Educators attempted to develop a registry of health education programs. This effort, however, had to be abandoned. There was too much variety in faculty, administrative arrangements, courses, and philosophies of the various professional preparation programs to agree on criteria for inclusion in the registry (Cleary, 1995). There were 273 programs listed in the 2009 edition of the AAHE *Directory of Institutions Offering Undergraduate and Graduate Degree Programs in Health Education* (M. Goldsmith, personal communication, August 3, 2010). Most of these programs were neither approved nor accredited, and there was no professional body monitoring their efforts. This clearly indicates a lack of consistency and quality control in the profession. Further, with the demise of AAHE there is no longer a current listing of institutions offering health education degrees, so no follow-up has been done to update the status of these programs. SOPHE is considering taking on this task in the future.

▷ Accreditation Task Forces

Accreditation has been a major focus for the health education/promotion profession since 2000. In January 2000, the SOPHE and AAHE co-sponsored a meeting in Dulles, Virginia, to explore the issue of accreditation. Twenty-four professionals who were broadly representative of health education/promotion professional preparation programs or other stakeholders were invited to attend. Meeting participants reached consensus that a "coordinated accreditation system" was needed.

As a result of this meeting, the SOPHE/AAHE National Task Force on Accreditation in Health Education was established and charged to (1) "gather background information and refine plans for a comprehensive, coordinated quality assurance system that meets commonly accepted standards of accreditation, and (2) develop processes for ensuring profession-wide involvement in the discussion and design of such a system to foster its adoption and utilization" (SOPHE, 2000, p. 5).

After a comprehensive study of the issue, the task force completed its work in the spring of 2004 and submitted its final report to the AAHE and SOPHE boards of directors (Allegrante et al., 2004). In this report, four principles were given to guide the profession:

1. Health education is a single profession, with common roles and responsibilities.

2. Professional preparation in health education provides the health education specialist with knowledge and skills that form a foundation of common and setting-specific competencies.

3. Accreditation is the primary quality assurance mechanism in higher education.

4. The health education profession is responsible for assuring quality in professional preparation and practice (Allegrante et al., 2004, p. 676).

On the basis of these four principles, the task force developed eight important recommendations that were included within the study's final report. Since the release of the report, many of the recommendations have been or are being implemented. Below is a summary of the seven recommendations, followed by a comment on the progress that has been made on each recommendation:

1. Accreditation should replace approval as the accepted quality assurance mechanism for health education professional preparation. (This is nearly accomplished. CEPH is now accepting accreditation applications from freestanding undergraduate programs. SABPAC will serve those programs currently in the approval process and will then be phased out.)

2. The National Council for the Accreditation of Teacher Education (NCATE) should be the accrediting body for school health education programs and the Council on Education for Public Health (CEPH) should be the accrediting body for community/public health education programs. (NCATE is merging into a new organization –CAEP– but it will be the accrediting body for school health education and CEPH has accepted the responsibility to serve as the accrediting body for undergraduate community/public health education programs.)

3. Future accreditation should be based upon the best practices of existing accreditation systems. (This is being accomplished.)

4. Students prepared in health education at the graduate level should meet *all* health education competencies with graduate-level proficiency. (This recommendation has been met. To achieve the MCHES designation, all competencies must be met in addition to additional advanced level competencies.)

5. Separate designations should be developed to identify undergraduate level practitioners from graduate level practitioners. (The NCHEC certification process designates those with entry-level skills [CHES] and those with advanced skills [MCHES].)

6. Undergraduate and graduate certification of individual health education specialists should be provided by NCHEC. In order to be eligible for CHES and MCHES certification, students must be graduates from schools/programs that are accredited. (NCHEC is the entity responsible for certifying entry-level and advanced level health education specialists. NCHEC has agreed in principle to only certify students from accredited programs and will move to implement this recommendation when accreditation is widely available and enough time has expired to allow programs to transition to the new accreditation process.)

7. The results of the Task Force should be shared with those professional associations that include public/community health education specialists as members. (Numerous articles have been written in professional journals and presentations made at professional meetings regarding the task force recommendations. In addition, there is a website with current news from the Task Force; see Weblinks.)

8. Implementation of the Task Force results will require a profession-wide effort and resources from stakeholders for an extended period of time. (This has occurred as the Task Force continues to function and has successfully lobbied for many of the changes noted above.)

Both the AAHE and SOPHE boards accepted the final report and then instituted a second committee to transition from the National Task Force recommendations to an implementation phase of the process. Dr. David Birch, Southern Illinois University (now University of Alabama), and Dr. Kathleen Roe, San Jose State University, co-chaired this committee called the National Transition Task Force on Accreditation in Health Education.

The work of this task force culminated in a three-day meeting of health education/promotion professional preparation programs in Dallas, February 23–25, 2006 (Taub, Birch, Auld, Lysoby, & King, 2009). At this "Third National Congress on Institutions Preparing Health Educators," accreditation issues were presented, discussed, and debated. Some attendees felt accreditation should move forward as quickly as possible. Others seemed reluctant to move in the direction of accreditation and wanted more discussion and debate. Several small programs expressed concern that they would not be able to meet accreditation requirements. Some present were concerned that the CEPH was being considered as the accreditation body and that using CEPH would push all health education/promotion programs to become public health programs. Others felt that if the roles and responsibilities identified by the CUP were used as the basis of accreditation, CEPH would be a suitable accrediting body. At the end of the conference, most participants supported the initiation of a coordinated accreditation system (Taub et al., 2009).

To follow up the work of the National Transition Task Force and the Third National Congress, a third task force was initiated late in 2006. This task force, co-chaired by Dr. David Birch and Dr. Randy Cottrell, was named the National Implementation Task Force for Accreditation in Health Education. It is still functioning today with the charge to continue preparing the health education/promotion profession for accreditation (Cottrell et al., 2009, 2012).

Much progress has been made in meeting the recommendation of the first National Task Force on Accreditation in Health Education (Cottrell, Auld, et al., 2012). Advanced certification for health education specialists began in fall 2010 with initial testing in 2011. At the time this text was written, CEPH had distributed guidelines or criteria for accrediting free-standing undergraduate public/community health education programs (CEPH, 2013a). First applications were accepted in January 2014. Also, NCHEC agreed, in principle, that it will only certify health education specialists who graduate from accredited programs. The implementation of this recommendation will, however, have to wait until there are a sufficient number of accredited undergraduate public/community programs and a sufficient number of graduates from these programs to support the continued operations of NCHEC.

▷ Responsibilities and Competencies of Health Education Specialists

The skills needed to practice health education/promotion are clearly delineated as responsibilities, competencies, and sub-competencies. **Responsibilities** essentially specify the overall scope of practice for health education specialists. They provide a general idea of what health education specialists do, but do not provide the detail necessary to practice health education/promotion.

Under each responsibility there are four to seven **competencies**. A competency "reflects the ability of the student to understand, know, etc." (National Commission for Health Education Credentialing, 1996, p. 12). Each competency is further broken down into four to fourteen **sub-competencies**. A sub-competency "reflects the ability of the student to list, describe, etc." (NCHEC, 1996, p. 12). All health education specialists should be able to demonstrate at least minimal skills to meet all of the competencies and sub-competencies of a health education specialist.

The responsibilities, competencies, and sub-competencies of health education specialists were first described in the *Framework for the Development of Competency-Based Curricula for Entry Level Health Educators* (National Task Force on the Preparation and Practice of Health Educators, 1985). This document was later modified and reformatted based on the results of the CUP project, previously discussed in this chapter. The *Competency-Based Framework for Health Educators—2006* (NCHEC, SOPHE, & AAHE, 2006) combined the 1985 Entry-Level Framework responsibilities and the 1999 Graduate-Level Framework responsibilities into one set of seven responsibilities. These responsibilities were applicable to all health education specialists regardless of degree held, years of experience, or work setting.

The Health Education Job Analysis 2010 model (*HEJA 2010* model) is the most recent update of health education roles, responsibilities, competencies, and sub-competencies.

TABLE 6.3 **HEJA 2010 model hierarchical approach**

Level of Practice	Sub-Competencies
Entry-Level (less than 5 years of experience; baccalaureate or master's degree)	162 entry-level sub-competencies
Advanced 1 (5 or more years of experience; baccalaureate or master's degree)	162 entry-level sub-competencies **PLUS** Advanced 1 sub-competencies
Advanced 2 (doctorate and 5 or more years of experience)	162 entry-level sub-competencies **PLUS** Advanced 1 sub-competencies **PLUS** Advanced 2 sub-competencies

Note: Information regarding the Advanced 1 and Advanced 2 sub-competencies had not been released at the time of this writing but should be released in future NCHEC reports to the profession.

From National Commission for Health Education Credentialing, Inc. (NCHEC), Society for Public Health Education (SOPHE), American Association for Health Education (AAHE). (2010a). *A Competency-Based Framework For Health Education Specialists—2010*. Whitehall, PA: Author. By permission.

It has 39 competencies within seven major areas of responsibility. The areas of responsibility remain essentially the same as those in the initial entry-level framework and the CUP project, with only minor wording changes (see **Table 6.3**). However, the total number of sub-competencies in the HEJA 2010 model is now 223, compared to 163 in the CUP framework. Additional sub-competencies are identified in areas related to ethics, partnership development, training, consultative relationships, influencing policy, and promoting the health education/promotion profession. Of the 223 sub-competencies, 162 are designated as entry-level competencies, and 61 are designated as advanced-level competencies (AAHE, NCHEC, & SOPHE, 2010).

The *HEJA 2010* document should be used by health education/promotion students on a regular basis during their professional preparation program (see Appendix B). The NCHEC (1996) suggested that the competencies be used "as a personal inventory to assess progress toward becoming a health educator; that is to determine which competencies and sub-competencies have been mastered. It is suggested that the student assess his or her progress at intervals during the student's course of study and do a final review at the completion of the health education program" (p. 7). Students who are diligent in monitoring their progress and who can perform the competencies and sub-competencies have a much greater chance of passing the credentialing exam to become a CHES.

Because the seven major responsibilities identified in the *HEJA 2010 model* are the core of what a health education specialist does, it is important to have a basic understanding of them. The following sections briefly describe each responsibility.

Responsibility I: Assess Needs, Assets, and Capacity for Health Education

The first major area of responsibility listed for health education specialists involves assessing needs, assets, and the capacity for health education/promotion. This responsibility provides the foundation for program planning (Bensley & Brookins-Fisher, 2009). In fact, "Conducting a needs assessment may be the most critical step in the planning process..." (McKenzie, Neiger,

& Thackeray, 2013, p. 72). A **needs assessment** is a process that helps program planners determine what health problems might exist in any given group of people, what assets are available in the community to address the health problems, and the overall capacity of the community to address the health issues. Other terms used to describe this process include *community analysis, community diagnosis*, and *community assessment* (McKenzie et al., 2013).

In a needs assessment, "**Capacity** refers to both individual and collective resources that can be brought to bear for health enhancement" (Gilmore, 2012, p. 9). More specifically, assessing capacity identifies the assets—skills, resources, agencies, groups, and individuals—that can be brought together in a community to solve problems and empower a community. According to the World Health Organization **community empowerment** "refers to the process by which people gain control over the factors and decisions that shape their lives. It is the process by which they increase their assets and attributes and build capacities to gain access, partners, networks and/or a voice, in order to gain control" (World Health Organization, 2013). For that reason, it is critical to include members of the community on any planning team.

All health education specialists, regardless of the setting in which they are employed, must have the skills to assess the needs and capacity of those groups or individuals to whom their programs are directed. For example, a school health education specialist needs to base curriculum on the needs of the students, a health education specialist in the corporate setting needs to plan programs based on the needs of the company's employees, and public health education specialists should base their health education/promotion efforts on the needs of the community they serve.

Health education/promotion programs should not be based on the whim of the health education specialist or any small group of decision makers. Resources are too valuable to waste on programs that do not address the needs of the population being served. As McKenzie et al. (2013) notes, "...failure to perform a needs assessment may lead to a program focus that prevents or delays adequate attention directed to a more important health problem" (p. 72). Conversely, "We know our health education programs are on target when we base them on accurate needs assessment data and a careful interpretation of their meaning" (Doyle & Ward, 2001, p. 124). Ultimately, a well-conceived and well-conducted needs assessment determines if a health education/promotion program is justified. It also defines the nature and scope of a program (Gilmore, 2012).

To conduct a needs assessment, health education specialists should know how to locate and obtain valid sources of information related to their specific population(s) with similar characteristics. For example, this may entail a literature review or accessing information from local, county, or state health departments. In addition to examining pre-existing information, called **secondary data**, it may be necessary for health education specialists to gather data of their own, known as **primary data**. They may have to conduct mail, electronic, and/ or telephone surveys; hold focus group meetings (see **Figure 6.4**); and/or use a nominal group process. After all this information is collected, the health education specialist must be able to analyze the data and determine priority areas for health education/promotion programming.

The following example demonstrates the importance of a needs assessment. A health education internship student was placed with the Shriners Hospital for Burned Children in Cincinnati, Ohio. The hospital identified a problem with children being burned around campfires during the summer months and asked the student to develop a fire safety program for young campers. Fortunately, the site supervisor required the student to conduct

▲ **Figure 6.4** A group of health education specialists meeting to discuss information gathered during the assessment phase that will be used to guide the planning phase

a needs assessment before planning the program. After conducting focus groups, interviewing camp counselors, and reviewing the literature, it was concluded that campers were the wrong group to target with the program. Instead, a program for the camp leaders and counselors was needed. If the needs assessment had not been done, valuable time and resources would have been spent developing a program for the wrong audience.

Responsibility II: Plan Health Education

Planning involves more than just determining a location and time for a health education/promotion program. Planning begins by reviewing the health needs, problems, concerns, and capacity of the priority population obtained through the needs assessment. Early in the planning process, it is important to recruit interested stakeholders, such as community leaders, representatives from community organizations, resource providers, and representatives of the community population, to support and help develop the program. Without the help of these stakeholders, it may be impossible to develop effective programs. To be effective in the planning process, the health education specialist should have strong written and oral communication skills, leadership ability, and the expertise to help diverse groups of people to reach consensus on issues of interest.

As part of the planning process, health education specialists must be competent to develop goals and objectives specific to the proposed health education/promotion program. These goals and objectives are the foundation on which the program is established. Writing specific and measurable objectives is critical. No health education/promotion program should be initiated without objectives, or considered complete until an evaluation of the objectives is conducted. Writing good objectives is a skill you can only obtain through guided practice and experience. After program goals and objectives are written, the next step is to develop appropriate interventions that will meet these goals and objectives.

Consider the following example of the planning process. A health education specialist, who is working in the university health service wellness center, analyzes the results of a recently conducted needs assessment. Next, the health education specialist recruits a variety of individuals to develop a plan for the university. This group includes representatives of the Greek system, student life organization, resident life (dorms), athletics, health education/promotion program, provost's office, campus security, and local chamber of commerce. Together, they review the needs assessment data and agree that alcohol-related incidents are a health problem on campus that needs to be addressed.

First, the planning group uses existing baseline data on alcohol-related incidents to establish written objectives for the overall program. Next, they plan a variety of strategies to increase awareness of alcohol-related problems, modify alcohol-drinking behaviors, and reduce the number of reported alcohol incidents on campus. They organize a campus-wide alcohol awareness day, and they devise strategies with local bar owners to reduce excessive drinking. They also establish an agreement with campus security and the provost to refer any student involved in an alcohol-related incident to a mandatory alcohol education program that they will develop. In addition, they create posters and flyers promoting responsible drinking, train a bevy of peer student leaders to speak to dorm and Greek groups, and plan a variety of nonalcohol alternative events for the campus community. For each and every strategy, they write specific objectives, establish implementation timelines, assign tasks to committee members, and establish a budget. If the planned strategies are successful, the program objectives will be met.

An important aspect of planning includes observing the **Rule of Sufficiency**. This rule states that any strategies chosen must be sufficiently robust, or effective enough, to ensure the stated objectives have a reasonable chance of being met. For example, in the preceding scenario, do you think the primary objective (e.g., reduce the number of alcohol-related incidents on campus by 20 percent) has a reasonable chance of being reached if all the listed program strategies are implemented? On the other hand, if the only strategy used was to hand out a pamphlet on alcohol abuse to students, the intervention will not be robust enough to achieve the stated objective. In that case, the Rule of Sufficiency would not be met. Either the intervention strategies need to be enhanced, or the program should not be implemented. Time and resources are wasted if interventions are not effective enough to create the desired change. Further, if interventions fail to meet their objectives, then both the reputation of the health education specialist and the health education/promotion profession suffer.

Responsibility III: Implement Health Education

After a needs assessment is conducted and analyzed, objectives are written, and intervention strategies are developed, it is time to implement the program. For many health education specialists, implementation is the most enjoyable of the responsibilities because it involves putting the program into action.

To successfully implement a program, the health education specialist must have a thorough understanding of the people in the priority population. What is their current level of understanding regarding the issue at hand? What will it take to get the people to participate? Do they need financial assistance or child care? What time of the day should the program be offered? What location(s) would be most convenient? Although some of these questions can be answered from the initial needs assessment, it may also be necessary to obtain additional information about the priority population before proceeding with implementation.

When conducting various health promotion and education programs, it is important for the health education specialist to be comfortable using a wide range of educational methods or techniques. In school health, for example, it is not enough to simply lecture to students about "proper" health behaviors. A successful health education specialist uses many teaching strategies such as brainstorming, debate, daily logs, position papers, guest speakers, problem solving, decision making, demonstrations, role playing, drama, music, and current events. In community health, most programs require going beyond developing and distributing a simple pamphlet on a given health topic. Again, a wide variety of strategies should be used, including television, radio, newspapers, billboards, celebrity spokespersons, behavioral contracting, community events, contests, incentives, support groups, and many more. As a general rule, health education specialists should always use multiple intervention activities when planning and implementing programs.

Health education specialists should also include population-based approaches to create health-improvement changes. Instead of focusing on individuals, population-based approaches focus on policies, rules, regulations, and laws to modify behaviors of a priority group or population. For example, instead of working one-on-one with individuals to enhance exercise levels, it might be more effective to work toward funding new walking and biking trails, having bike racks available at bus stations, initiating a city-wide walk/bike-to-work day, advocating for improved pedestrian safety laws, and so forth.

After a program is in place and operating, the responsibility of the health education specialist is not over. The health education specialist should continue to monitor the program to make certain everything is going as planned. If problems are noted, it may be necessary, even while the program is in progress, to revise the objectives or the intervention activities.

When implementing program strategies or interventions, health education specialists may need to apply a variety of sub-competencies such as presentation skills, group facilitation skills, pretest/posttest administration, data collection, and technology utilization, all of which must be demographically and culturally sensitive. During the intervention phase, a health education specialist typically has the most contact with the public. The Code of Ethics for health education specialists (see Appendix A) should be strictly followed, and one should always dress and act in an appropriate professional manner.

Responsibility IV: Conduct Evaluation and Research Related to Health Education

Accurate evaluations must be conducted to measure the success of health education/promotion programs. These evaluations help reveal whether or not implemented programs are meeting their specified objectives. Programs not properly evaluated may be wasting valuable time, money, and other resources. Further, an unevaluated program cannot "prove its worth." So, it may risk being cut back or even eliminated when resources are short and downsizing occurs.

To conduct an effective evaluation, the health education specialist must first establish realistic, measurable objectives. As previously mentioned, this is an important part of the planning process. After objectives are in place, the health education specialist must develop a plan that will accurately assess if the program objectives have been met. Depending on the setting, this process may involve developing and administering tests, conducting surveys, observing behavior, tracking epidemiological data, or other methods of data collection. Evaluation plans can be simple or extremely sophisticated, depending on the program being evaluated, the expectations of the program planners, and the requirements of the funding agents.

After data is collected, it must be analyzed and interpreted. Reports are then developed and distributed to the appropriate parties. Ultimately, the evaluation results should be used to modify and improve current or future program efforts. In some cases, evaluation results may indicate that a program needs to be discontinued and funding redirected to other, more productive efforts. Health education specialists must have the fortitude to make these difficult decisions when needed.

In addition to evaluation, research is a vital activity for any profession, including health education/promotion. A profession moves forward and improves in large part as a result of the quality of its research and the new information it generates. **Health education research** can be defined as "a systematic investigation involving the analysis of collected information or data that ultimately is used to enhance health education knowledge or practice, and answers one or more questions about a health-related theory, behavior or phenomenon" (Cottrell & McKenzie, 2011, p. 2). Although more complex research skills are required at advanced levels, entry-level health education specialists should be able to read, synthesize, and use research results to improve their practice.

Responsibility V: Administer and Manage Health Education

A great deal of administration, management, and coordination is needed to bring a health education/promotion program to fruition. Even though some administrative tasks may be performed by entry-level health education specialists, administration and management responsibilities are generally handled by professionals at more advanced levels of practice. For example, experienced health education specialists often become program managers or staff supervisors. "Good management and supervisory skills require training in a variety of organizational, psychological and business environments. Good management incorporates effective 'people skills' and knowledge of budgeting, task assignments and performance evaluation" (NCHEC, SOPHE, & AAHE, 2006, p. 33).

Health education specialists must facilitate cooperation among personnel, both within programs and between programs. Some public school systems, for example, have initiated coordinated school health programs. This involves coordinating the activities and services of school nurses, counselors, psychologists, food service personnel, physical educators, health education specialists, teachers, administrators, support staff, parents, and public health agencies. The ultimate goal is to develop both curricular and extracurricular programs to improve the health status of students, faculty, staff, and the community as a whole. Further, health education specialists in school settings may serve as curriculum coordinators or project directors and can be responsible for managing grants and program budgets.

Similar examples can be seen in the community setting. For example, a health department decides to apply for grant funds to reduce the incidence of tobacco use in its community. The health education specialist may form a coalition by bringing together individuals or groups with a vested interest in reducing tobacco use. Coalition members might include representatives from the American Cancer Society, American Lung Association, American Heart

Association, local medical society, local dental association, public health department, public school system, and YMCA/YWCA. Coordination and integration of the services offered by these various groups would be critical to the successful development of a grant proposal and ultimately to the success of the funded program. It may even be necessary for the health education specialist to conduct or coordinate in-service training programs to ensure that all coalition members have similar knowledge related to tobacco prevention programs. Obviously, administrative and management skills are needed throughout this entire process.

Responsibility VI: Serve as a Health Education Resource Person

Health education specialists are often called to serve as resource persons. It is not unusual for a student to seek out the health teacher for assistance when having a health-related problem. In the corporate setting, health education specialists get questions about a wide range of topics, including nutritional supplements, cancer signs and symptoms, the best type of shoe to wear for jogging, and many more.

Because it is impossible for health education specialists to know all the information that could be needed in a given position, they must have the skill to access resources they need. It may be necessary to visit the library; use computerized health retrieval systems; access health databases; find information on specific diseases; obtain local, regional, state, and national epidemiological data; and so on. It is critical that the health education specialist be able to differentiate valid information from questionable, misleading, false or fraudulent information. As part of this resourcing process, it may also be necessary for health education specialists to select or develop their own effective educational resources for distribution to their priority populations.

Consider, for example, the entry-level health education specialist who was hired by a large metropolitan hospital. Her duties included developing health education/promotion programs for the community and resource materials for patients. Her first assignment was to develop educational materials on the problem of incontinence in older adults. This subject had not been covered in her professional preparation program. However, because of the skills she had previously learned, she was able to locate a variety of resources on the topic, evaluate their validity, select relevant information, and then develop an educational pamphlet and video on the topic.

Being able to simply retrieve information is not enough. Health education specialists must be able to establish effective consultative relationships with people who seek assistance, whether they are students, clients, employees, or other health education specialists. Health education specialists must instill confidence and communicate effectively in a nonthreatening manner. In some situations, health education specialists may decide to market their skills to individuals or groups, as resource consultants. They may even decide to focus their career entirely as a resource person.

Responsibility VII: Communicate and Advocate for Health and Health Education

Health education specialists must interact with various groups of people, including other health professionals, consumers, students, employers, employees, and fellow health education specialists. They must be skilled in written communication, oral communication, and mass media use including social media. Health education specialists need to feel comfortable working with individuals, small groups, and large groups, as the situation warrants. In essence, communication is the primary tool of the health education specialist.

It is often necessary for health education specialists to serve as communication filters between medical doctors/researchers and students or clients. Health education specialists must be able to "translate" difficult scientific concepts so that constituents can understand the information necessary to improve and protect their health. For example, a physician may tell a patient to start an exercise program, reduce fat in the diet, or manage stress better. Although many patients have a general idea of what these recommendations mean, they may not have the knowledge or skills to implement them. Most physicians cannot take the time to teach patients how to incorporate these changes into their lifestyles. Health education specialists can communicate detailed information on exercising safely, teach the client to recognize high-fat foods by reading food labels, and instruct the patient in progressive neuromotor relaxation. This may involve conducting one-on-one instruction, developing a videotape for patients to watch, creating brochures for distribution to patients, teaching classes, or coordinating support groups.

Beyond communicating health information, Responsibility VII requires health education specialists to "advocate" for health and health education/promotion. This means they should initiate and support legislation, rules, policies, and procedures that will enhance the health of the populations with which they work. Health education specialists should be involved in supporting nonsmoking laws, mandatory helmet laws, seatbelt laws, antidrug policies, rules to prevent selling "junk foods" in school cafeterias, initiatives to develop walking/biking trails, gun safety laws, and so forth.

Further, health education specialists should "advocate" for their profession. They should educate potential employers about the value of hiring professionally trained and degreed health education specialists with CHES status. When health education specialists hold positions with hiring authority, they should advertise for and hire degreed and certified health education specialists. It is important that health education specialists talk to legislators, policy makers, personnel directors, allied health workers, coworkers, family, and friends about the value of health education/promotion. They should join health education professional associations and support national initiatives designed to move the profession forward. These include the development of National Health Education Standards and the current initiatives for program accreditation and unification of the professional associations. Although advocating for the profession may seem awkward and somewhat akin to "blowing one's own horn," if health education specialists do not promote their profession, who will?

Summary of Responsibilities and Competencies

The responsibilities, competencies, and sub-competencies required for health education specialists do not function independently; they are highly interrelated. All of the responsibilities demand excellent communication skills. Conducting an accurate needs assessment requires research skills to identify and gather appropriate resources. Planning should be based on a valid and reliable needs assessment. When implementing programs, be prepared to serve as a resource person when asked. Evaluation relies on goals and objectives established during the planning process. Coordinating people and administering programs are necessary in planning, implementing, and evaluating programs.

It is not enough to be proficient in one, two, or even six of the responsibility areas. All seven responsibilities are critical for effective health education/promotion to take place. It is beyond the scope of this book to teach the reader how to do these tasks. Rather, it is the intent of this text to familiarize readers with the responsibilities, competencies, and skills they will be taught in later classes and ultimately practice in their employment settings.

▷ Multitasking

It is often necessary for health education specialists to use several competency-related skills simultaneously. This requires **multitasking**: the skill of coordinating and completing multiple projects at the same time. In college, health education/promotion students are often given a project at the beginning of a term. There is a specific amount of time to complete the project, and when the term ends the project is completed. In the work world, things do not function this way. Health education specialists work on multiple projects at the same time, and each project is usually in a different stage of completion.

Organization is the key to successful multitasking. For example, one health education/promotion internship student used a visual concept to help her stay organized while working on multiple projects. Using a bulletin board, unfinished projects and tasks were represented by floating balloon images. Once completed, these "balloons" were placed at the bottom of the bulletin board in the hand of a stick figure that represented the health education specialist. Other effective tools for multitasking include spreadsheets, timelines, and "to do" lists. With use of a smartphone, such lists can be readily at one's fingertips for referencing and updating.

▷ Technology

As in most professions, health education specialists must be familiar with and comfortable using computers and other forms of technology. Because computer software and hardware are constantly changing, it is important to keep up to date on the latest technological aids. Entry-level health education specialists are expected to have required technology skills by the time they enter their internships and certainly by the time they accept their first position. See **Box 6.2** for a list of entry-level computer skills.

Social networking is another aspect of technology that needs to be fully explored and used by health education specialists. Social networking involves connecting to individuals (or organizations) that are tied (connected) by one or more specific types of interdependency, such as friendship, kinship, common interest, financial exchange, occupational or professional interests, or beliefs. Facebook, Myspace, LinkedIn, Twitter, Instagram, YouTube, and Blogger are just a few examples of social networking sites that may be of value to health education specialists. These social networking services can be used by health education specialists to connect people with similar health interests, such as losing weight or reducing stress. They can also be used to link people who have a common cause, such as passing nonsmoking legislation. In addition, they are helpful for sending information or updates about programs sponsored by a given health agency. The possible uses for social networking in health education are limited only by one's imagination and creativity.

▷ Role Modeling

Being a healthy role model is not listed anywhere in the roles and responsibilities of a health education specialist, but it has been discussed and debated extensively in the profession (Davis, 1999; Bruess, 2003). Some people feel that health education specialists should not be expected to be healthy role models. This expectation may discriminate against professionals

> **BOX 6.2**
>
> ## Entry-Level Technology Skills (Not Prioritized)
>
> - Basic word processing/text editing skills including use of writing tools such as spell checkers, electronic thesaurus, etc.
> - Basic to advanced electronic spreadsheet use, beginning with elementary worksheets and progressing to more sophisticated "what-if" analyses
> - Introductory statistical analysis software and data entry (assuming that statistics applications are also learned)
> - Preparing effective PowerPoint presentations
> - Critiquing components of computer-assisted health education software (health assessments to computer-assisted instruction)
> - Electronic retrieval of quality health information—search engines, databases, and indexes of health literature
> - Electronic health information media literacy, including evaluating the quality of health Web sites
> - Using a Web page editor to design and develop effective health-based Web pages. This would include skills needed to upload pages to a server and then marketing the site to specific Internet audiences
> - Professional e-mail and discussion list etiquette
> - Use of common technological innovations in health education/promotion such as digital video/photography, scanners, personal digital assistants, and computer-assisted interviews, and surveys
> - Use of various social media formats in communication with clients
> - Preparing videos and uploading them to the Internet
>
> Source: Modified from an initial list provided by Dr. Ernesto Randolfi, Montana State University–Billings. Posted to HEDIR Listserve, 2002.

who suffer from disease conditions that cause obesity or preclude a regular exercise regimen. Others think that being a healthy role model puts too much pressure on health education specialists, especially because there is no accepted definition for what "healthy" means. On the other hand, many in the profession believe that being a healthy role model is important to effectively carry out the responsibilities of the profession. Some even argue that ethically, health education specialists must be role models.

The authors of this text tend to believe that role modeling is an important aspect of being a health education specialist. The purpose of presenting this issue is to stimulate health education/promotion students to enter the debate. Do you feel health education specialists should be role models? Do you think health education specialists who are not role models will be less effective in their work? What does it mean to be a role model? Are you a role model now? Do you want to be a role model in the future?

▷ Advanced Study in Health Education

After receiving a bachelor's degree in health education/promotion, students should not stop the educational process. At the very least, health education specialists should continue to learn on their own. One way of doing so is to participate in one or more professional associations (see Chapter 8). Such memberships allow the opportunity to read professional publications and attend state, regional, and national meetings of the associations.

If you are a CHES, an average of 15 continuing education contact hours are *required* each year (75 across five years) to maintain certification. These may be obtained by reading professional journals and submitting responses to questions on selected articles, by attending various professional meetings and workshops, by taking additional coursework, or by participating in other professional development activities.

At some point, health education specialists with a bachelor's degree should consider getting a master's degree. In some areas of the country and in some health education/promotion settings, such as medical care and worksite health education/promotion, the master's degree is often considered the entry-level degree. In other words, to be considered for employment in these settings, the health education specialist must hold an appropriate master's degree (see **Box 6.3**).

BOX

6.3

Practitioner's Perspective

GRADUATE LEVEL STUDY Jovanni V. Reyes, M.S., CHES

CURRENT POSITION/TITLE: Graduate Research/ Teaching Assistant
EMPLOYER: Texas A&M University
DEGREE/INSTITUTIONS: B.S., Health, Texas A&M University, College Station TX; M.S., Health Education, Texas A&M University, College Station TX
UNDERGRADUATE MAJOR: Health (Emphasis: Allied Health)
GRADUATE MAJOR: Health Education

Background: I was born and raised in a low-socioeconomic status (SES) part of Dallas, Texas, and am the first person in my immediate and extended family to pursue an education after high school. Although my family could never provide funds for my collegiate expenses, I have worked exceptionally hard to acquire awards and resources that will help me further my education. It was in my undergraduate course, "Race, Ethnicity and Health," where I first became interested in the issues of health disparities, health education and health promotion. I began to realize that I could relate to many of the issues that were discussed. Raised in a low-socioeconomic neighborhood, I have witnessed firsthand the inequalities that minorities experience due to lack of access to quality health care services. These experiences have provided me with a heightened awareness of the actual health issues among minority communities. My research interests include: minority health, health disparities, sexual/reproductive health, adolescent risk behaviors, impact of violence on health, and adultification

and its impact on health. My current research focuses on the topic of teen pregnancy within minority populations and how the issue in turn affects quality of life. I was raised in a neighborhood where teen pregnancy was the norm. Every year, I saw more and more young pregnant adolescent girls struggling through life, experiencing the consequence of lack of access to information and services. Health issues that are highly prevalent among minorities surround me and I feel it is my job to educate people about prevention and treatment. I feel obligated to further my education for the sake of my family and my community. I want to gain as much knowledge as I can so that I can give back to my community. One of the reasons why I chose to further my education is to show both my family and the people of my community that it can be done. With hard work and determination, even children raised in a violence-filled low-socioeconomic neighborhood can defy statistics and be whatever they want to be. I am currently pursuing a terminal research degree in health education with a focus on minority health and health disparities. I am continuing graduate school because I desire to learn more about health education/promotion and health behaviors and how they affect the world around me. This is my inspiration towards becoming a health disparity researcher and educator. My goal is to help fill gaps within the

BOX 6.3 *continued*

research related to health disparities, and by filling the gaps, I wish to help in eliminating the current inequalities.

Overall impression of graduate school: Being that I was the first in my entire extended family to pursue graduate school, I have to admit that at first the idea was extremely intimidating. I literally had no guidance from family or friends due to the simple fact that I was the only person I knew who had ever chosen to continue school after a bachelor's degree. The first week was tremendously nerve wrecking and it was then that a few professors pulled me aside to talk with me about my transition into graduate school. After talking with them and giving them part of my background I could see that the professors were truly there to support me in my educational endeavor. I remember one of my professors made us call her by her first name because not only was she our mentor and teacher but from that day on we were her colleagues. The idea that everyone (i.e., faculty, students and staff) is working together to both promote health and support each other was mind-blowing to me.

What I liked most about graduate school: Graduate school not only opened endless doors of opportunities for me but it also helped me become a better health educator and helped me better understand things around me. Sitting in three-hour classes with my fellow colleagues leads to interesting, and sometimes controversial, conversations. This was my favorite part of graduate school, everyone having an actual conversation and voicing their opinion about various topics. As an undergraduate, some professors limited discussions or avoided certain topics in fear that the conversation would cause some type of riot. The courses I took in my graduate studies were primarily open discussions of different opinions, which often lead to a better understanding of different cultures, races, ethnicities, SES, etc. The more we, as health education specialists, get to

know other people, the better we're prepared to educate them.

What I liked least about graduate school: During graduate school, there is definitely going to be an overwhelming number of projects and research opportunities. Initially, I wanted to get as much experience as I could and was really tempted to jump on as many projects as possible. After several talks with a few professors, I began to realize that although numerous opportunities will arise, I only have so many hours in a day. Professors are always going to be working on interesting research projects but it is important to only "bite off as much as you can chew." The idea of restricting myself from amazing research was devastating to me. In spite of this, when I was finally able to focus on a specific project, I began to see where my passion was. There is always going to be a million really cool research projects but there are only so many that you can really become passionate about.

Recommendations for Health Education students considering graduate study: My overall advice to students is to never fear the future. The idea of graduate school can be intimidating and scary but what students need to know is that the people they meet and network with, are there to support them in whatever they choose to do in life. Students usually don't jump for joy when someone recommends that they stay in school a few more years but graduate school isn't only about sitting in a classroom and gaining new knowledge, it's about applying the knowledge you know to the outside world. It's about making a difference. It's the beginning of a new journey and along the way you acquire new skills, network with new people, and all of it is beneficial not only to you as an educator but also as a person. Don't be afraid to get out there and push your limits.

In school settings, the master's degree brings additional financial rewards and, in some states, progress toward more permanent teaching certificates or licences. It is usually advised, however, not to complete a master's degree in teaching prior to obtaining your first teaching position. Hiring a new teacher with a master's degree, versus one with a bachelor's degree, is more expensive for a school district. This factor may put a person with a master's degree at a disadvantage in the hiring process.

In community or public health settings, the master's degree may bring additional financial rewards, as well as promotions within the agency. It may also open the door to higher-level positions with other public health agencies or public health departments.

▷ Master's Degree Options

There are multiple types of master's degrees. Typical choices include a Master's of Education (**M.Ed.**), Master's of Science (**M.S.**), Master's of Arts (**M.A.**), Master's of Public Health (**M.P.H.**), and Master's of Science in Public Health (**M.S.P.H.**) (Bensley & Pope, 1994). Some colleges and universities may offer only one degree option, while others may offer more than one.

The M.Ed. degree is typically found in institutions where the health education/promotion program is located in a College of Education or Teacher's College. Although many students in these programs focus on school health, this does not mean that everyone who obtains this degree must pursue a career in public schools. Some colleges and universities offer M.Ed. degrees, which emphasize areas such as community health and corporate health promotion.

The M.S. and M.A. degrees are usually found in universities in which the health education/promotion program is located in colleges other than education. Because there is no accepted accreditation for these programs, schools have much flexibility to develop programs that meet the needs of the local job market. These degrees offer a variety of emphasis areas, including public health, community health education/promotion, and corporate health promotion.

When considering differences between the M.S., M.A., and M.Ed. degrees, remember that the M.S. may be the more scientific or research-oriented degree, whereas the M.A. and M.Ed. may be more practitioner oriented. This distinction, however, is not always true. Prospective students need to carefully examine the stated mission and degree requirements for any graduate-level health education/promotion program.

As their names imply, the M.P.H. and M.S.P.H. are degree choices for those wishing to work in the field of public health. At one time working in the field of public health meant one would work in a city, county, or state public health department. The definition of public health, however, has been greatly expanded and now includes many other sites including voluntary agencies, public schools, worksites, hospitals, and so forth. The M.S.P.H. degree is typically more research oriented than the M.P.H. degree; otherwise, the degrees are similar. The M.P.H. can be awarded in a variety of specialty areas such as nursing, dietetics, or epidemiology. The M.P.H. with an emphasis in health education/promotion is the degree of most interest to health education specialists. It is similar and often identical to an MS or MA degree in community health education.

Most M.P.H. degree-granting colleges and universities are accredited by the CEPH. Thus, the requirements to obtain an M.P.H. are more standardized than the requirements to obtain the M.S., M.A., or M.Ed. degrees, which typically are not accredited by any professional body. Resulting in part from accreditation, the M.P.H. degree may enjoy a higher status and more credibility than other health education/promotion degree designations. To obtain M.P.H. accreditation, the curriculum must contain five specific areas of knowledge: biostatistics, epidemiology, health services administration, social and behavioral sciences, and environmental health.

The M.P.H. in health education/promotion has the reputation of being a more prestigious degree than the M.S., M.A., or M.Ed. There are, however, more health education specialists with M.S., M.A., or M.Ed. degrees than there are with the M.P.H. degree. The 2009 AAHE directory lists 96 institutions that provide master's-level non-M.P.H. health education/promotion degrees (M. Goldsmith, personal communication, August 3, 2010). Many of the institutions that offer non-M.P.H. health education/promotion degrees are now also offering the M.P.H. degree.

As of June 2013 there were 48 accredited schools of public health (up from 38 in 2007) and 88 accredited graduate public health programs (up from 68 in 2007) (CEPH, 2013c). Not all of these public health programs, however, provide a concentration in health education/promotion. From one college to another, there are great variations in degree concentration options. Carefully examine program requirements and master's degree options within the context of your future career goals.

▷ Selecting a Graduate School

Determining which college or university to attend is a decision that goes hand-in-hand with deciding which degree to pursue. In terms of practicality, factors such as cost, location, and size must be considered (Cottrell & Hayden, 2007). There is no current listing for non-CEPH accredited community health education programs. AAHE used to maintain a list of all health education professional preparation programs, but with AAHE no longer in existence, that list is not up to date. SOPHE is considering developing a list of all health education professional preparation programs, but has yet to do so. The best advice for students at this time is to look on the Web sites of various universities of interest to see what programs they offer. A good, current list of CEPH-accredited schools and programs in public health can be found online at the CEPH's Web site, http://www.ceph.org. Students will still need to look at each CEPH approved program's Web site to determine which offer a specialization in health education.

College or university reputation is an important factor to consider when selecting a health education/promotion graduate program. There is a definite hierarchy among colleges and universities in the United States. Graduating from one of the more prestigious institutions may lend instant credibility to the graduate degree and enhance job opportunities.

Next, consider the reputation of the health education/promotion program at a given institution. To learn about various programs, bachelor's-level health education specialists can talk to other professionals in the field whom they admire and trust. A visit or call to current or former college professors may also be a good source of information. Contacting recent graduates from a program is also a good way to learn about a particular program and may help in the decision-making process (Cottrell & Hayden, 2007).

After narrowing your list to several programs, carefully review each program's admission requirements and application forms. These can usually be found online and most universities now have electronic applications. If you need more information about program curricula, or application procedures contact the program administrator for such information.

▷ Admission Requirements

As an undergraduate health education/promotion student, it is not too early to be concerned about admission requirements to graduate school. Although admission requirements vary greatly from one university to another, the undergraduate grade point average (GPA) has traditionally been important. In general, a student should strive to achieve an overall undergraduate GPA of at least a 3.0 on a 4.0 scale to be considered by most graduate programs. Some institutions do not specify a minimum GPA (Bensley & Pope, 1994). Instead, they tend to use more individual and subjective criteria in their admission process. In either case, it is important for new health education/promotion students to attempt from the first term of their freshman year to achieve the best grades possible. Too often, low grades in the first two years of college prevent otherwise good students from being accepted into the master's degree program of their choice.

In addition to GPA requirements, most graduate programs require a completed application form, a letter of application, and several letters of reference. To be considered for admission, some programs also require students to submit scores from a standardized performance test such as the Graduate Record Exam or Miller Analogy Test. These scores may be a major component in the decision-making process, or they may simply be used in conjunction with other applicant information to provide a more well-rounded view of the prospective student.

▷ Financing Graduate Study

Funding a graduate degree may not be as burdensome as funding undergraduate education. Many colleges and universities award assistantships or fellowships to graduate students on a competitive basis. Typically, these graduate awards pay all or part of the graduate tuition and provide students with a monthly stipend to cover living expenses during their graduate studies. In return, students agree to work for the health education/promotion program.

If the award is a **graduate teaching assistantship** (or fellowship), the student teaches a specified number of undergraduate courses each term. These are usually introductory health education/promotion courses that meet general university requirements, or they are the first courses for health education/promotion majors. If the award is a **graduate research assistantship** (or fellowship), the student usually works closely with one or more faculty members on a particular research project. Students might be assigned to do literature reviews, assist with data collection, enter data into the computer, or a host of other research-related activities (Cottrell & Hayden, 2007).

Graduate assistantships and fellowships not only provide an excellent alternative for funding graduate education but also provide valuable health education/promotion work experience for the student. Further, a graduate assistantship may provide an advantage in the job market after the degree program is completed.

Summary

Since the late 1970s, many people have dedicated much time and hard work to defining and developing the roles and responsibilities of a health education specialist. The initial stages of this work were known as the Role Delineation Project. Eventually, a set of responsibilities, competencies, and sub-competencies were agreed on for health education specialists, regardless of whether they ultimately wished to work in schools, communities, clinics, or corporate settings. These responsibilities, competencies, and sub-competencies encouraged college and university professional preparation programs to develop their curricula based on a standardized set of skills for teaching all health education/promotion students. These standards were also the basis for establishing individual certification within the profession.

In 1997, three additional responsibilities with accompanying competencies and sub-competencies were identified for graduate preparation in health education/promotion. With the completion of the CUP in 2005, the initial seven responsibilities and the three graduate responsibilities were united into seven revised responsibility areas that are now common to all health education specialists regardless of setting, degree, or experience. In 2010, the results of the Health Education Job Analysis study were released, which increased the number of competencies to 39 and sub-competencies to 223. All health education/promotion professional preparation programs should now be training students based on the HEJA 2010 standards. At this writing, work on another job analysis has begun and the results should be available in 2015.

Continued study in health education/promotion is necessary to stay current with health information and new techniques for conducting health education/promotion programs. All health education specialists should read professional journals, join one or more professional associations, and take an active role in their functioning. CHESs and MCHES must obtain continuing education credits to maintain their certification. Most bachelor's-level health education specialists should consider a master's degree at some point in their career. Decisions concerning graduate study should not be taken lightly. Undergraduate health education/promotion students need to be aware of the admission requirements for graduate school and work toward meeting those requirements. Graduate assistantships or fellowships provide an excellent alternative to fund graduate education.

Review Questions

1. Define *credentialing* and explain the differences among certification, licensure, and accreditation.

2. Outline the major events of the Role Delineation Project. How does the CUP relate to role delineation? What is the significance of the CUP? How does the HEJA 2010 relate to role delineation and what is its significance?

3. Review the "Responsibilities and Competencies for Entry-Level Health Educators" (Appendix B). Do you think they are more focused on health content or the process skills needed to be a health education specialist? Defend your position and explain why you believe the health education/promotion profession has moved in this direction.

4. Identify two ways health education specialists can stay up to date in the field.

5. What are the differences among the following academic degrees: M.A., M.Ed., M.S., M.P.H., and M.S.P.H.?

6. What technology skills are important for current and future health education specialists?

7. Briefly describe the process for applying to graduate school and discuss the potential benefits of serving as a graduate assistant.

▷ Case Study

Anita considers herself a school health education specialist. She graduated from college with a major in health education/promotion and an emphasis in school health. She is licensed by the state in which she lives to teach health education in the schools. She is also a CHES and has been vocal in advocating that all school health education specialists should be CHESs. Anita has been asked to provide a 30-minute presentation to an audience that will be mostly school health education specialists. Your task is to help Anita develop the main points of her presentation. Why should school health education specialists become CHESs? Also, be the devil's advocate. What arguments will she likely hear from those who are not certified and do not feel certification is important? How can she respond to these arguments? (Note: This same case study can be replicated with Anita being a community health education/promotion specialist, worksite health education/promotion specialist, or clinic/hospital health education/promotion specialist.)

▷ Critical Thinking Questions

1. If Helen Cleary and her contemporaries had not begun the Role Delineation Project, and if there were no certification (CHES) available to health education specialists, how do you think the profession would be different today? Think in terms of professional preparation, recognition, employment opportunities, and so on.

2. Suppose that an accreditation system were developed and implemented that required all health education/promotion professional preparation programs to meet the same guidelines and standards. How do you think such a system would impact the profession? What do you see as the potential positive outcomes and the potential negative outcomes of such accreditation? Do you feel that only students graduating from accredited programs should be allowed to sit for the certification exam?

3. Review the National Health Education Competencies that resulted from the HEJA 2010 model (see Appendix B). Do you feel they accurately represent professional practice? Why or why not? What changes do you think should be made in terms of eliminating competencies, adding competencies, or moving sub-competencies from one level to the other?

▷ Activities

1. Read each competency and entry-level sub-competency of a health education specialist (see Appendix B). Score each competency and sub-competency using the following scale:

   a. I currently have the skill to meet this competency/sub-competency.

   b. I am uncertain if I have the skill to meet this competency/sub-competency.

   c. I do not have the skill to meet this competency/sub-competency.

   After rating each competency and sub-competency, make a list of things you can do to enhance your skills. Keep this table, and periodically reevaluate your skills throughout your program of study.

2. Identify one or more universities you may wish to attend for graduate school, go online, and read about the program, its curriculum, degrees offered, financial aid and graduate assistant opportunities, and application procedures.

3. Make an appointment with a professor at your school to talk about graduate school. Ask about schools the professor attended and the degrees earned. Finally, ask for advice on what degree to earn and what school to attend.

▷ Weblinks

1. **http://www.nchec.org/**

   National Commission for Health Education Credentialing (NCHEC)

   Use this Web site to learn more about becoming a CHES. The site provides helpful information about health education certification including application procedures.

2. **http://www.ceph.org/**

   Council on Education for Public Health

   The council is responsible for accrediting programs in public health. A complete list of accredited schools and programs of public health can be found at this site. This site can help identify accredited public health education graduate programs to which one may want to apply.

3. **http://www.healthedaccred.org/**

   National Implementation Task Force for Accreditation in Health Education

   This Web site provides information about the history of the Accreditation Task Forces, the benefits of accreditation, current quality assurance providers, SABPAC, and more.

References

Allegrante, J. P., Airhihenbuwa, C. O., Auld, M. E., Birch, D. A., Roe, K. M., & Smith, B. J. (2004). Toward a unified system of accreditation for professional preparation in health education: Final report of the National Task force on Accreditation in Health Education. *Health Education & Behavior, 31* (6), 668–683.

Allegrante, J. P., Barry, M. M., Airhihenbuwa, C. O., Auld, M. E., Collins, J. L., et al. (2009). Domains of core competency, standards, and quality assurance for building global capacity in health promotion: The Galway Consensus Conference Statement. *Health Education & Behavior, 36* (3), 476–482.

Allegrante, J. P., Barry, M. M., Auld, M. E., Lamarre, M., & Taub, A. (2009). Toward international collaboration on credentialing in health promotion and health education: The Galway Consensus Conference. *Health Education & Behavior, 36* (3), 427–438.

Allegrante, J. P., Barry, M. M., Auld, M. E., & Lamarre, M. (2012). Galway revisited: Tracking global progress in core competencies and quality assurance for health education and health promotion. *Health Education & Behavior.* 39 (6), 643–647.

American Association for Health Education (AAHE), National Commission for Health Education Credentialing (NCHEC), & Society for Public Health Education (SOPHE). (2010). Health Educator Job Analysis—2010: Executive Summary and Recommendations. Retrieved August 19, 2013, from http://www.nchec.org/_files/_items/nch-mr-tab2-169/docs/health%20educator%20job%20analysis%20ex%20summary-final-2-19-10.pdf.

Bensley, L. B., Jr., & Pope, A. J. (1994). A study of graduate bulletins to determine general information and graduation requirements for master's degree programs in health education. *Journal of Health Education, 25* (3), 165–171.

Bensley, R. J., & Brookins-Fisher, J. (2009). *Community health education methods: A practical guide* (2nd ed.). Boston: Jones and Bartlett Publishers.

Bruess, C. (2003). The importance of health educators as role models. *American Journal of Health Education, 34* (4), 237–239.

Cleary, H. P. (1986). Issues in the credentialing of health education specialists: A review of the state of the art. In William B. Ward (Ed.), *Advances in health education and promotion,* (pp. 129–154). Greenwich, CT: Jai Press, Inc.

Cleary, H. P. (1995). *The credentialing of health educators: An historical account 1970–1990.* New York: The National Commission for Health Education Credentialing, Inc.

Cottrell, R. R., Auld, M. E., Birch, D. A., Taub, A., King, L. R., et al. (2012). Progress and directions in professional credentialing for health education in the United States. *Health Education and Behavior 39* (6), 681–694.

Cottrell, R. R., & Hayden, J. (2007). The why, when, what, where and how of graduate school. *Health Promotion Practice 8* (1), 16–21.

Cottrell, R. R., Lysoby, L., Rasar King, L., Airhihenbuwa, C. O., Roe, K. M., et al. (2009). Current developments in accreditation and certification for health promotion and education: A perspective on systems of quality assurance in the United States. *Health Education & Behavior, 36* (3), 451–463.

Cottrell, R. R., & McKenzie, J. F. (2011). *Health promotion and education research methods.* Boston: Jones and Bartlett Publishers.

Council on Education for Public Health. (2013a). *Criteria.* Available at: http://ceph.org/assets/SBP-criteria.pdf.

Council for Accreditation of Educator Preparation. (2013b). *Home.* Available at: http://caepnet.org/.

Council on Education for Public Health. (2013c). *U.S. Schools of Public Health and Graduate Public Health Programs Accredited by the Council on Education for Public Health.* Available at: http://ceph.org/accredited/.

Davis, T. M. (1999). Health educators as positive health role models. *Journal of Health Education, 30* (1): 60–61.

Doyle, E., & Ward, S. (2001). *The process of community health education and promotion.* Mountain View, CA: Mayfield Publishing.

Gilmore, G. D. (2012). *Needs and capacity assessment strategies for health education and health promotion.* Boston: Jones and Bartlett.

Gilmore, G. D., Olsen, L. T., Taub, A., & Connell, D. (2005). Overview of the National Health Educator Competencies Update Project, 1998–2004. *American Journal of Health Education, 36* (6), 363–370.

Joint Committee for Graduate Standards. (1996). *National Congress for Institutions Preparing Graduate Health Educators.* Program Booklet, 1.

McKenzie, J. F., Neiger, B. L., & Thackeray, R. (2013). *Planning, implementing & evaluating health promotion programs* (6th ed.). Boston: Pearson Education, Inc.

National Commission for Health Education Credentialing. (1996). *A competency-based framework for professional development of certified health education specialists.* New York: National Commission for Health Education Credentialing.

National Commission for Health Education Credentialing. (2013a). *Eligibility for the CHES exam.* Retrieved August 19, 2013, from http://www.nchec.org/exam/eligible/ches/.

National Commission for Health Education Credentialing. (2013b). *Mission and Purpose.* Retrieved August 19, 2013, http://www.nchec.org/aboutnchec/mission/.

National Commission for Health Education Credentialing. (2013c). *NCHEC receives distinguished recognition from NCCA*. Retrieved August 19, 2013, http://www.nchec.org/_files/_items/nch-mr-tab2-225/docs/ncca%20press%20release.pdf.

National Commission for Health Education Credentialing. (2013d). *Responsibilities and Competencies for Health Education Specialists*. Retrieved September 28, 2013, http://www.nchec.org/credentialing/responsibilities/

National Commission for Health Education Credentialing. (2013e). The next health education job analysis is underway. *NCHEC News 24* (2): 3.

National Commission for Health Education Credentialing. (2013f). *Why certify? Credentialing and benefits of certification*. Retrieved August 19, 2013, http://www.nchec.org/credentialing/credential/.

National Commission for Health Education Credentialing, Society for Public Health Education, & American Association for Health Education. (2006). *A competency–based framework for health educators—2006*. NCHEC: Whitehall, PA.

National Task Force on the Preparation and Practice of Health Educators. (1985). *Framework for the development of competency-based curricula for entry level health educators*. New York: National Commission for Health Education Credentialing, Inc.

National Transition Task Force on Accreditation in Health Education. (2013). *What is Accreditation?* Retrieved August 19, 2013, from http://www.healthedaccred.org/docs/home/Benefits%20of%20accred.pdf.

Quality Assurance Solutions. (2010). *Quality assurance definition*. Retrieved August 19, 2013, http://www.quality-assurance-solutions.com/Quality-Assurance-Definition.html.

Society for Public Health Education. (2000). Future directions for quality assurance of professional preparation in health education. *News & Views, 27* (3).

SOPHE/AAHE. (2013). *SOPHE/AAHE bacalaureatte approved programs in community health education*. Retrieved August 19, 2013, http://www.healthedaccred.org/docs/10_sabpac/SABPAC%20Approved%20Programs_march2013.pdf.

Speller, V., Parish, R., Davison, H., & Zilnyk, A. (2012). Developing consensus on the CompHP professional standards for health promotion in Europe. *Health Education & Behavior, 39* (6), 663-671.

Taub, A., Birch, D. A., Auld, M. E., Lysoby, L., & King, L. R. (2009). Strengthening quality assurance in health education: Recent milestones and future directions. *Health Promotion Practice, 10* (2), 192–200.

World Health Organization (2013). Track 1: Community Empowerment. Retrieved August 19, 2013, http://www.who.int/healthpromotion/conferences/7gchp/track1/en/.

The Settings for Health Education/Promotion

Today, most Americans live a healthier and longer life than ever before. Despite this fact, it is clear that many, if not most, Americans are not living at their optimal level of health. Hereditary, environmental, societal, and behavioral factors predispose too many U.S. citizens to disease, suffering, disability, and premature death. Health education specialists are professionally trained to help individuals and communities reduce their health risks. According to the U.S. Department of Labor Bureau of Labor Statistics (2013), there were 63,400 health education specialists employed in the United States in 2010 earning a median annual wage of $45,830 or a median hourly wage of $22.03. The job outlook for 2010–2020 is for health education positions to grow at a "much faster than average" rate. The challenge for health education specialists is to help people reduce their risk for disease and death and increase the probability of a long, happy, and productive life.

To meet this challenge, health education specialists conduct programs in a variety of settings (National Commission for Health Education Credentialing [NCHEC], 2013). The use of multiple settings is important because it allows health education specialists to reach the greatest number of people in the most convenient, efficient, and effective ways possible.

Although the goals of health education/promotion and the skills needed to carry out the responsibilities are nearly the same in all settings (English & Videto, 1997), the actual duties of a specific job may differ greatly from setting to setting.

Professional preparation programs in health education/promotion should prepare students to meet the various competencies and sub-competencies of a health education specialist and thus prepare students for employment in one or more of four major settings. These settings are schools, hospitals/clinics, public/community health agencies, and business/industry. On obtaining advanced degrees, students from any of these settings may seek employment as college or university health education faculty. In addition, health education specialists can work in a variety of nontraditional employment areas.

This chapter discusses each of the four major settings for health education/promotion. After a short introduction to the setting, a description of one day in the career of a health education specialist from that particular setting is presented. This is designed to give the reader a general idea of what a workday is like. Because of the great diversity in duties from one health education specialist to another even within the same setting, it is impossible to say that this is a typical day. For most health education specialists, there is no such thing as a typical day. Following this is a section that describes additional responsibilities that might be assigned to health education specialists in the setting. Again, this is not intended to be an exhaustive list but rather to further the reader's understanding of job responsibilities in that setting. Finally, each section ends with a listing of some advantages and disadvantages for that setting. As students become interested in one or more settings they are encouraged to contact, interview, and job shadow health education specialists working in those settings.

▷ School Health Education/Promotion

School health involves "all the strategies, activities, and services offered by, in, or in association with schools that are designed to promote students' physical, emotional, and social development" (American School Health Association, 2013). **School health education/promotion,** as the name implies, primarily involves instructing school-age children about health and health-related behaviors. The initial impetus for school health stemmed from the terrible epidemics of the 1800s and the efforts of the Women's Christian Temperance Movement to promote abstinence from alcohol in the early 1900s. Many states mandated school health education/promotion to inform students about these health hazards. Unfortunately, these mandates have seldom been strictly enforced. Further, teachers often have been underqualified, with only an academic minor or a few elective courses to prepare them for the health classroom. Frequently they hold a dual certification in health education/promotion and physical education with the majority of their professional preparation being in physical education. As a result, the quality of school health programs often has been compromised (Breckon, Harvey, & Lancaster, 1998; Naidoo & Wills, 2000).

Despite these limitations, the potential for school districts and health instruction programs in particular to impact students is tremendous. Jalloh (2007) noted that "school-based health education is an opportunity waiting to be taken advantage of; an opportunity for you to discover the best way to influence positive health-related change in the lives of youth and to maximize the use of some education dollars to achieve synergistic health and education goals" (p. 18). It is easier and more effective to establish healthy behaviors in childhood than it is to change unhealthy behaviors in adulthood. The goal of health education/promotion in schools is to help students adopt and maintain healthy behaviors (Joint Committee on National Health Education Standards, 2007). Each school day provides the opportunity to reach 49.8 million students. The 98,800 schools in the United States (National Center for Educational Statistics, 2013) should provide a laboratory where students can eat healthy foods, participate in physical activity, and learn how to take care of their health and well-being. School health programs have demonstrated effectiveness when they are well planned, sequential, provided significant time in the curriculum, and taught by a trained health education specialist (Fisher, Hunt, Kann, Kolbe, Patterson, et al., 2003).

The sophistication of school health education/promotion programs has increased dramatically over the years. Today's school health education specialist needs to be well trained and prepared to deliver a comprehensive and demanding curriculum. Comparing the 1922 "Rules of Good Health" with the 2007 National Health Education Standards (Joint Committee on National Health Education Standards, 2007) clearly illustrates this point (see **Tables 7.1** and **7.2**).

TABLE 7.1 **Rules of Good Health—1922**

1. Take a full bath more than once a week.
2. Brush teeth at least once a day.
3. Sleep long hours with window open.
4. Drink as much milk as possible, but no coffee or tea.
5. Eat some vegetables or fruit every day.
6. Drink at least four glasses of water a day.
7. Play part of every day outdoors.
8. Have a bowel movement every morning.

Source: "Rules of the Health Game" in Milk and Our School Children, U.S. Dept. of the Interior, Bureau of Education, Health Education, No. 11 (1922).

TABLE 7.2 **National Health Education Standards**

1. Students will comprehend concepts related to health promotion and disease prevention to enhance health.
2. Students will analyze the influence of family, peers, culture, media, technology, and other factors on health behaviors.
3. Students will demonstrate the ability to access valid information and products and services to enhance health.
4. Students will demonstrate the ability to use interpersonal communication skills to enhance health and avoid or reduce health risks.
5. Students will demonstrate the ability to use decision-making skills to enhance health.
6. Students will demonstrate the ability to use goal-setting skills to enhance health.
7. Students will demonstrate the ability to practice health-enhancing behaviors and avoid or reduce health risks.
8. Students will demonstrate the ability to advocate for personal, family, and community health.

Source: Reprinted with permission from the American Cancer Society. *National Health Education Standards: Achieving Excellence, Second Edition.* Atlanta, GA: American Cancer Society, 2007. http://www.cancer.org/bookstore.

When the school health education/promotion component is made part of a broader, district-wide approach known as a **coordinated school health program**, the potential to impact students in a positive way is even greater. Allensworth and Kolbe (1987) were the first to envision a comprehensive and coordinated school health program. They defined it as

> an integrated set of planned, sequential, school-affiliated strategies, activities, and services designed to promote the optimal physical, emotional, social, and educational development of students. The program involves and is supportive of families and is determined by the local community based on community needs, resources, standards and requirements. It is coordinated by a multidisciplinary team and accountable to the community for program quality and effectiveness. (p. 60)

In other words, a coordinated school health program coordinates and integrates various aspects of a school district to best impact the health of the students, faculty, staff, administration, and community as a whole. This includes food services, nursing services, school counseling and psychology, health instruction, physical education, administration, school environment, community involvement, and faculty/staff wellness (Centers for Disease Control and Prevention [CDC], 2013b).

A health education specialist choosing to work in the school setting will find a challenging and rewarding career. Given the number of school districts in the United States, it is obvious that a large number of people teach health education/promotion in the schools. Unfortunately, many of these people are not health education specialists. Some school districts have used biology, physical education, home economics or family life, and consumer science teachers to teach health. Even when certified health education teachers are employed, they may have only a minor in health education/promotion and are not fully prepared. A further problem confounding the employment situation in the schools is that the requirement for health education/promotion is usually less than for other academic subjects. Students typically need only one or two semesters of health education/promotion to graduate from high school, whereas they probably are required to complete four years of English. With such a minimal requirement, the number of health teachers needed and the resulting demand for health teachers are lower than in other teaching fields. The bottom line is that, in many parts of the country, it is difficult to obtain a job in school health.

Those students who are really committed to being outstanding health teachers, however, should not be deterred from this career path. With time, dedication, networking, and perseverance, those who really want to teach health in the schools can usually find employment. Substitute teaching, coaching, and volunteering are good ways to make oneself known in a school district and increase the likelihood of eventual employment. Students are encouraged to talk to their own professors to determine the job market for school health education/promotion in their area.

Beyond teaching in the classroom, the school health education specialist should also take a leadership role in advocating for and the development of school health policy. Policies are written statements that guide the school district related to many health issues (McKenzie, Pinger, & Kotecki, 2012). For example, a school district may have policies related to tobacco use on school property, the food and snack items available in the cafeteria (see **Figure 7.1**), safety measures, violence, suicide, staff wellness programs, community advisory committees, and many more issues. Further, once policy is developed, it needs to be carefully

▶ **Figure 7.1** Food service is one component of a coordinated school health program.

implemented and then monitored. Policy work is not easy, but it is extremely important for a school district (McKenzie et al., 2012). It is often the policy work that provides the most visibility to a coordinated school health education program and individual school health education specialists. When school boards, administrators and the community know about and are proud of the health education program, that program is a success.

A Day in the Career of a School Health Education Specialist

At 5:45 A.M. the alarm goes off, and Ms. Bell's day starts. Ms. Bell teaches seventh- and eighth-grade health at a junior high school in a suburban school district. After going through the normal morning routine, she arrives at the school building around 7:00 A.M. There is a half-hour before homeroom, so she picks up her mail and duplicates a test that she prepared the night before for her eighth-grade health class. Essentially, homeroom involves administrative responsibilities and a considerable amount of paperwork.

In homeroom she takes attendance, gets a lunch count, listens to announcements over the loudspeaker, and collects money from a fruit sale fund-raiser. The fruit sale is being conducted by the PTA to raise money for new computers in the school. The PTA used to sell candy, but because of a new district policy that Ms. Bell and the Coordinated School Health team advocated for, candy sales are no longer allowed as fund raisers.

At 7:45 A.M. the first period starts. This school has eight 50-minute periods, with only 4 minutes between periods. In the first three periods, Ms. Bell teaches seventh-grade health. Today's lesson is on refusal skills related to alcohol and drug use. Ms. Bell has written three scenarios that students could find themselves in. The scenarios are open ended, so after each one Ms. Bell leads a discussion on how to use refusal skills to get out of a bad situation. She then asks students to role-play the situations to gain further practice in using refusal skills. Unfortunately, only two of her three classes will get this lesson today. The second-period class is one day behind because of an assembly that was held a week ago. Ms. Bell has to find a way to catch this group up with the rest of the classes.

Ms. Bell's fourth period is divided in half. The first half, she has lunch room duty. It is her responsibility to monitor the lunch room while students are eating. This is a noisy and somewhat stressful duty. In today's lunch room, two boys become unruly and nearly get into a fight. She sends them to the office for discipline, but the situation is quite upsetting.

The second half of fourth period is Ms. Bell's lunch time. She usually has 25 minutes to eat lunch and relax before fifth period begins. Today, however, she must use part of that time to drop by the office for a follow-up discussion with the assistant principal concerning the incident with the two boys in the lunch room.

In fifth period, Ms. Bell teaches eighth-grade health. Today is a test day. While the students are taking their test, Ms. Bell works at her computer to update the online Web page that lists student assignments for the week.

Sixth period is Ms. Bell's planning period. Today she tries to make a phone call to the parents of one of her students who is having problems in health class, but no one is home. She then grades the test papers from her previous class and records the grades. She averages the grades and starts to develop interim reports for the fifth-period class, but she runs out of time. Seventh and eighth periods are also eighth-grade health classes. While students take their tests, Ms. Bell grades papers from the previous classes and writes her interim reports.

School ends for the students at 2:57 P.M. After monitoring the hall while students leave the building, Ms. Bell hurries to the cafeteria for the monthly teachers' meeting. General information and announcements are presented by the principal. The meeting ends at 4:00 P.M.

In addition to her teaching responsibilities, Ms. Bell coaches the junior high girls' volleyball team. Practice usually goes from 3:15 P.M. to 5:00 P.M. Today's practice will go from 4:00 P.M. to 5:30 P.M. because of the teachers' meeting. After practice, Ms. Bell waits until the last girl leaves the locker room, then returns to her classroom to prepare for the next day's classes. She leaves the school at around 6:00 P.M.

After dinner and her family responsibilities, Ms. Bell spends 20 minutes on the phone with the student's parents who were not at home earlier in the day. She then finishes grading the tests she gave in class and continues working on interim reports. It will take her at least one more evening to finish the interims. At 11:00 P.M. she turns off the light and goes to bed.

Additional Responsibilities

In addition to the lesson planning, grading, parent meetings, disciplining, coaching, and the various administrative duties, teachers may have still more responsibilities. They may be involved in curriculum development, the review of materials for classroom use, the chaperoning of dances or other after-school activities, fund-raising, and the advising of student groups such as yearbook, debate, or student council. Many teachers now keep active Web pages that can be accessed by students and parents. These Web pages may contain announcements, assignments, and grades or progress reports. Teachers need to be responsive to their e-mail accounts because parent, student, and school district communication is often conducted in this manner. School health education specialists should also be active members of their professional organizations. This allows them to network with other health education specialists and to stay up to date in the field. Finally, school health education specialists should be strong advocates for health and health education/promotion (see **Box 7.1**). They must make certain that fellow faculty, administrators, school boards, and the community as a whole are aware of the unique contributions of a school health program. (See **Table 7.3**.)

SCHOOL HEALTH EDUCATION/PROMOTION Carolyn Conley

CURRENT POSITION: Teacher, Health and Physical Education

EMPLOYER: South Carolina Public Schools

DEGREE/INSTITUTION: B.S., University of Toledo, 2010, Health Education and Physical Education

Describe your past and current professional positions and how you came to hold the job you now hold (How did you obtain the position?): After graduating from the Health Education Program at the University of Toledo in the winter of 2010, I decided to take a little vacation and lived with my sister for a few months in California as I searched and applied for Health and Physical Education jobs through the Internet. I had never been a fan of Ohio winters so besides looking through a few Ohio teacher job search sites, I was also looking in North and South Carolina, Florida, Georgia, and California. I spent no less than 3 hours each day searching and applying for positions without much luck. I moved back to Ohio in April after being contacted by a public charter school that immediately needed a part-time PE teacher. When I arrived home, I also was accepted to three local school districts to substitute teach. For the remainder of the 2011 school year, I worked as many hours as I could in all four positions.

After many disappointing leads and a few job offers in places I was not interested in working, I was contacted by the administrators from a Title I high school in rural South Carolina. It was the first week of August and they needed to quickly fill a health and physical education position. After receiving an employment offer, I took a quick drive down to South Carolina to make sure that the school was a fit for me. The town was very small without much to offer a girl in her 20s, but the weather was great, the people seemed friendly, and the teaching position was full-time. At this point in the search it was hard to pass up a job. I have now finished my second year in this position.

Describe the duties of your current position: In my current position, I have a lot

of different and eclectic duties. In addition to teaching two health education classes, three Freshmen Focus classes, and one physical education class I have normal responsibilities like every teacher has such as: parent/teacher conferences, lunch duty, faculty meetings, graduation assignments, etc. I also coach two varsity sports, volleyball and softball; am a site coordinator for implementation of a sexual health curriculum; run a "Safer Choices" peer group as part of the sexual health program; and am the high school liaison for the American Cancer Society's Relay for Life program.

Describe what you like most about this position: The thing I like most about this position is that I have a lot of freedom to do what I want with the classes I teach and the groups I lead. I have to stick to basic standards but can mold my lessons around them in creative ways and have fun with my students. I also like the relationships I have been able to make with the students. Since I was the outsider in their community, it was initially difficult to gain the students' trust. Now after two years the students and community know me better. When my students see me in the grocery store and see me running through their neighborhoods, they know I am a real person just like everyone else. It is also really good for them and the community to see that I follow a healthy lifestyle, exercise regularly, and in general, practice what I teach in class.

Describe what you like least about this position: The thing I like least about this position is the lack of organization, collaboration, and standards within the school building. The expectations for teachers and students are low and that is the level at which everyone performs. While I enjoy the freedom to mold my curriculum, at the same time there needs to be oversight and evaluation to be sure standards are met. It is hard to stay passionate and motivated

BOX 7.1 *continued*

when no one cares what you're doing. There needs to be more accountability and higher expectations. Teachers and administrators also need to work together more and to be on the same page to do the best they can to better the students.

What health education responsibilities (assessing, planning, implementing, evaluating, resourcing, communicating, advocating) do you use in your position? As a health educator, it is my responsibility to plan my overall curriculum and outline for the school year. I assess what concepts need specific focus in the community where the school is located and plan health education units to meet those needs throughout the year. I do research before implementing each unit to make sure I have the most up-to-date information possible and carry out the lessons I have planned in the most creative and effective ways possible. I evaluate each student in relation to the objectives that I establish. To be the most effective teacher I can be, I communicate with other teachers, administrators, and parents through phone calls, e-mails, letters, and personal conversations.

What recommendations/ advice do you have for current health education students that would like to eventually be school health educators? My advice to health education students would be to find one or more passionate health education faculty/professional mentors, learn all you can from them, and maintain contact with them after graduation. You will need these people to keep you motivated, write letters of recommendation and give you advice. I initially found teaching to be very challenging, especially in a position that is not fully supported and where there are no other health educators. I constantly have to advocate for health and health education to make sure it remains a priority for the school and community. I feel like my job is the most important one in the school and the field of health education is crucial for human happiness and success. You have to keep your passion even when you have terrible days at school. Force yourself to be positive, relax, and look at the big picture. Remember that you are making a huge difference. Challenge yourself everyday to be better than you were yesterday.

TABLE 7.3 Advantages and disadvantages of working in school health education/promotion

Advantages

- Health education specialists have the ability to work with young people during their developmental years.
- Health education specialists have the potential to prevent harmful health behaviors from forming instead of working with older people after such behaviors have been formed.
- Health education specialists have the opportunity to impact all students because health education/promotion is usually a required course.
- A graduate degree is not needed for entry-level employment.
- There is good job security.
- Summer months are free and there are nice vacation periods in December and in spring.
- Benefits are good.
- There is a multifaceted career ladder.
- There are typically good health and retirement benefit programs.

continued

TABLE 7.3 *continued*

Disadvantages

- Good health education specialists usually spend many long hours at their job, including weekends and evenings that may compensate for the long vacation periods.
- Health education specialists may have relatively low status in a school district when compared with teachers of more traditional subjects such as math, science, and English.
- Pay is low when compared with professionals in other fields but comparable with that of other health education specialists.
- Student discipline problems are often seen as a major disadvantage.
- Summer "free time" may be consumed with summer employment or returning to college for additional required coursework.
- It is difficult dealing with conservative school boards, parents, and community groups when teaching controversial issues such as sex education and drug education.
- Resources may be limited to support the program.

▷ Public or Community Health Education/Promotion

Within the health education/promotion profession, there has been much discussion concerning the terms community health education/promotion and public health education/promotion. Some believe these two terms are synonymous whereas others feel there are unique differences between them. It is the opinion of the authors that the terms are more alike than different and that the field is gradually evolving to accept the term public health education/promotion. Both community health education/promotion and public health education/promotion students have similar skill sets, meet the competencies of the National Commission for Health Education Credentialing, and compete for similar jobs in departments of public health and community health agencies. A survey of professional preparation programs (Miller, Birch, & Cottrell, 2010) found that 72.3 percent of respondents reported making modifications to their existing undergraduate health education/promotion program or concentration within the past three years to take on a more public health focus. Sixty-three percent of the programs surveyed indicated they would seek accreditation as a public health education/promotion program when available whereas only 19 percent indicated they would not seek accreditation as a public health education/promotion program. For that reason the authors use the term *public health education/promotion* to include both community health education/promotion and public health education/promotion programs.

According to the Association of Schools of Public Health (2010),

> [t]he work of public health educators (PHEs) is to change policies and environments as well as attitudes and behavior that affect health, and to operate in close association with community groups. PHEs plan and direct programs, design workshops and forums, work with community groups, and serve a broad public health agenda. They may conduct studies of public health education needs, evaluate the materials and methods used in programs, determine program effectiveness, and try to improve the general health in communities. They might do this by working with people and organizations addressing health-related issues such as pollution, drug abuse, nutrition, safety, and stress management. These professionals also write health education materials such as fact sheets, pamphlets, and brochures—a special and critical skill, as materials must often match the needs, preferences, and skills of underserved populations. (p. 82)

Public health programs target individuals, local communities, states, and the nation. There is a reciprocal relationship between these various targets. Over the years, it has become clear that the health of a community is closely linked to the individual health of community members. Likewise, the collective behaviors, attitudes, and beliefs of everyone who lives in the community profoundly affect the community's health. Indeed, the underlying premise of *Healthy People 2020* was that the health of the individual is almost inseparable from the health of the larger community, and that the health of every community in every state and territory determines the overall health status of the nation. This explains why the vision for *Healthy People 2020* was "A society in which all people live long, healthy lives" (U.S. Department of Health and Human Services, 2013).

The most likely sources of employment for public/community health education specialists are voluntary health agencies and public health agencies. **Voluntary health agencies** are created by concerned citizens to deal with health needs not met by governmental agencies (McKenzie, et al., 2012). "Their missions can be public education, professional education, patient education, research, direct services and support to or for people directly affected by a specific health or medical problem. They may also serve families, friends, or loved ones of those affected" (Daitz, 2007, p. 4). As their name implies, they rely heavily on volunteer help and donations. There are usually paid staff members who are responsible for administration, volunteer recruitment and coordination, program development, and fund-raising. Health education specialists are hired to plan, implement, and evaluate the education component of the agency's programs. They often, however, are involved in other aspects of the agency as well. Voluntary health agencies are usually nonprofits and are funded by such means as private donations, grants, fundraisers, and possibly United Way contributions. Examples of voluntary health agencies include the American Cancer Society (see **Figure 7.2**), American Heart Association, and American Lung Association. Most of these large, well-known voluntary agencies have national, state, and local divisions.

▶ **Figure 7.2** The American Cancer Society is a nationwide voluntary health organization dedicated to eliminating cancer as a major health problem by preventing cancer, saving lives from cancer, and diminishing suffering from cancer through research, education, advocacy, and service. Health education specialists often work for voluntary agencies such as the American Cancer Society.

In addition to the large national voluntary associations, there are many other nonprofit health-related organizations that provide a variety of services to the public. One such organization is Smile North Carolina, which is a part of the Smiles Program mobile dentists. See **Box 7.2** for more information about working in such a program.

BOX

7.2

Practitioner's Perspective

COMMUNITY AGENCY Jennifer C O'Donnell, CHES

CURRENT POSITION: Oral Health Educator
EMPLOYER: Smile NC
DEGREE/INSTITUTION/MAJOR: B.S., University of North Carolina Wilmington, 2012, Community Health Education

Describe your past and current professional positions and how you came to hold the job you now hold (How did you obtain the position?): Working as an Oral Health Educator has been my first health-related job since graduation. During college, I worked on two internships, both dealing with different aspects of community health. Each internship provided me with important experience that helped prepare me for my current role. I worked with Project Tobacco Free UNC, which was trying to change the state constitution to allow state universities to create their own tobacco use policies, including the decision to be a tobacco-free campus. While with this project, I worked on many initiatives, including letter writing campaigns to the Board of Governors, speaking with state legislators, creating and implementing a smoking prevention workshop for middle-schoolers, and joining advocacy initiatives to help turn a local beach into a smoke-free beach. For my second internship, I worked as a campus representative for NARAL Pro-choice North Carolina, the state subsidiary of a national reproductive rights organization. I was a founding member of NARAL Pro-Choice NC at the University of North Carolina Wilmington and drafted the constitution to become a school-sponsored organization.

After graduation, I took a month off to help transition from the role of full-time student back into the role of mother to two elementary-school-aged children. While searching for health-related jobs on Indeed.com, I found this job listed and realized that it would be a perfect fit with my desire to help people and be involved in raising my children. This position was the first and only position I applied for post-graduation. I was contacted for an initial telephone interview and was hired during a follow-up Skype interview a few days after I applied for the job.

Job responsibilities in your current position: As an Oral Health Educator for Smile NC, my main priority is to increase the number of children who are able to receive preventative and restorative dental services. I do this in three ways. Firstly, I encourage administrators, directors, and other key people to allow us to offer our services to the children in their communities. I also work to remain in communities by strengthening relationships between my organization and the stakeholders to be able to continue to educate and provide care to the children already in our care. Lastly, I spend time with these children educating them about how to have a healthy mouth, and getting them excited about healthy teeth to open conversations with their parents. I spend a lot of time on the road, traveling to various communities, daycares, schools, and administrative offices across the eastern part of North Carolina.

Describe what you like most about this position: I feel so fortunate to have the ability to work for an organization that provides direct and indirect help to children across the state, especially those from disadvantaged backgrounds. North Carolina has a large number of children with limited access or that have no access to dental

BOX 7.2 *continued*

services. There are many communities with a large part of their population that live in extreme poverty. Poor oral health can lead to reduced academic achievement, as 58 hours per 100 elementary students and 80 hours per 100 high school students are missed due to dental problems each year. (Seirawan, Faust, & Mulligan, 2012). I feel that I am helping these children have a chance at a better future. I love that we find a way to help every child that has parental consent. No child is turned away because they can't afford to pay.

I love talking with the children about their teeth. To me, so many things about dental health are obvious, but they are not obvious to many of students I work with. I now understand better than ever how misinformation, fear, and a lack of resources contribute to poor health outcomes. In a short period of time, I can teach proper brushing techniques, help alleviate fears about going to the dentist, improve the self-esteem of those with dental restorations, and give hope to those who've never been to the dentist. I love seeing the pride in the faces of students when they answer tricky anatomy questions correctly. I love feeling the joy and gratitude of the students when they receive a new toothbrush. It breaks my heart to hear that some of these kids didn't even have a toothbrush of their own. I also love talking with the parents and teachers of the students. They play such an influential role in the health of students

Describe what you like least about this position: In all honesty, I love every aspect of my job. Every workday is different, every school I visit has a different way for me to get the information to the students, and the long car rides provide me the opportunity to listen to audiobooks! The hardest part of my job is that the main office is in Michigan, while I operate out of my home office in North Carolina. Even though there are regular e-mail, telephone, and teleconferencing communications with the main office and Oral Health Educators across the country, I don't always feel as if I am part of a larger team.

What health education responsibilities (assessing, planning, implementing, evaluating, resourcing, communicating, advocating) do you use in your position? There are many health education responsibilities that I use in my job. I have had to plan and implement school assemblies, create and teach lesson plans for various age groups, and constantly update and improve ways to disperse as much age-appropriate retainable information as possible in a short amount of time. Currently, I do not assess the needs of each community, but other employees use data collected from the census to target schools with a large percentage of students living in poverty or have students receiving free or reduced school lunches. At the end of the school year, the State Manager compiles a report for each specific community. These reports detail the schools serviced, the number of students seen, the number of cleanings, sealants, and cavities corrected, and the estimated number of classroom hours saved by having these services performed. I present this information to community stakeholders, including school system administrators and nurses. During these meetings, I also try to strengthen the relationship between the communities and my program by addressing any concerns and offering suggestions on how to increase student participation.

Communication is the most important part of my job. I have to speak to people of all ages in ways that enable them to learn and retain information. While it is easy to speak with a classroom filled with eager kindergarteners while entertaining them with a puppet with gigantic teeth, it becomes challenging to find ways to engage apathetic middle schoolers (showing and explaining real x-rays works wonders!).

My job includes the opportunity for a lot of advocacy. I need to develop ways to explain to community officials why our mobile dental unit will help their community

BOX

7.2

continued

and I teach children how to advocate for themselves while talking with their parents about the possibility of receiving dental care at their school.

What recommendations/advice do you have for current health education students that would like to eventually be working in a community agency? I actually have two things I'd recommend to a current health education student who would like to work in a community agency. The first and most important would be to discover your passion and find a way to incorporate it into your career. Participate in relevant experiences, internships, and volunteer opportunities that will help expand your resume. A résumé filled with pertinent experiences will help you land an interview. Demonstrate your passion when you speak to interviewers so they will want to bring that passion into their team. There is no greater feeling than having the ability to get paid while working on something you love. This will increase your life satisfaction and make you a more effective health educator.

The second thing I would recommend would be to become extremely proficient in health communications. This is such a diverse field, with diverse situations in which we need to convey information. Whether it is helping a senior citizen take their prescriptions correctly and consistently, encouraging local politicians to help provide funding for a safe driving program, or organizing a community to help prevent a cement plant from moving into town, we will need to find a way to convince people of the importance of our information. The ability to find a way to help any demographic in a manner which helps them understand, learn, and retain information is what health education is all about. Effective written and oral communication is the key to improving the health of an individual, community, state, or nation.

Public health agencies, or official governmental health agencies, are usually financed through public tax monies. Government has long been responsible for doing for the people as a whole what individuals cannot do for themselves. Thus, governments provide police protection, educational systems, clean air and water, and many other important services. Departments of public health, thus, are formed to coordinate and provide health services to a community. Health departments may be organized by the city, county, state, or federal government. They operate primarily with paid staff and typically provide health education/promotion services as part of their total program. They may also seek grants and hire health education specialists on grant funds. Public health agencies are known for their bureaucracies, protocols, policies, and procedures. It often takes considerable time to accomplish tasks, and work often needs to be reviewed and approved by higher-level administrators. On the positive side, public health agencies often work with the groups of people most in need of health services and offer good benefit packages for employees (Hall, 2007). **Table 7.4** contains a list of agencies that have programs for which public health education specialists may be employed.

More diversity in terms of job responsibilities exists in the public/community health education/promotion settings than in the other major settings in which health education specialists are employed. This is as a result of the large number of community and public health agencies that exist and the vast differences in their missions, goals, and objectives. In some agencies, health education specialists serve administrative functions such as coordinating volunteers, budgeting, fund-raising, program planning, and serving as liaisons to

TABLE 7.4 **Possible sources of employment in public/community health education/promotion**

State, local, city health departments
U.S. Public Health Service
U.S. Food & Drug Administration
U.S. or state departments of agriculture
U.S. or state departments of transportation
County extension services
U.S. Department of Health and Human Services
U.S. Centers for Disease Control and Prevention
National Institutes of Health
Environmental Protection Agency (EPA)
Health Resources and Services Administration (HRSA)
Substance Abuse and Mental Health Services Administration (SAMHSA)
Indian Health Service
U.S. or state penal institutions
Voluntary health agencies
Private health agencies/foundations

other agencies and groups. They often use population-based strategies such as advocating for laws, policies, rules, and regulations that impact health. In other public/community agencies, the health education specialist may be more involved in direct program delivery to the clientele of that agency and/or the community at large. Most frequently, however, health education specialists are involved in a little bit of everything.

A Day in the Career of a Community Health Education Specialist

Mr. Fischer is the health education specialist for a local division of the American Cancer Society (ACS). In that role, he has the responsibility of conducting health education/promotion programs in a five-county area of the state. Mr. Fischer usually arrives at the office between 8:30 and 9:00 A.M. Today, however, he had an 8:00 A.M. meeting with a local coalition that is working with local school districts to implement comprehensive school health education/promotion into their curricula. This is an important issue because the ACS has made comprehensive school health education/promotion one of its major priority areas at the national level. Mr. Fischer has been responsible for forming this coalition and was recently elected to serve as its chairperson. As such, he sets the agenda, runs the meetings, takes minutes, and always plans for juice and bagels to be served.

It is 9:30 A.M. when Mr. Fischer finally arrives at his office. He spends the next half-hour opening his mail, responding to e-mail, and returning telephone calls. From 10:00 A.M. to 11:00 A.M. is the biweekly staff meeting, which is run by Mr. Fischer's supervisor, who is director of the local ACS unit. In these meetings, staff members provide updates on projects for which they are responsible. Issues and problems facing the local unit are discussed, with the intent of involving the group in identifying potential solutions. Information from the state and national levels is also provided by the director.

From 11:00 A.M. to 12:00 P.M., Mr. Fischer has time to sit at his desk and work on planning for "Cancer Survivor Day." This is a special event open to all cancer survivors where they are encouraged to participate in cancer screenings, can obtain information on healthy lifestyles and staying cancer free, talk with fellow cancer survivors and various vendors of health-related products and services, and listen to free entertainment. Mr. Fischer is responsible for this event. He has to recruit local sponsors to donate money or prizes for the event, plan a variety of activities to promote the event, contact local media to cover the event, distribute materials to numerous participating groups, coordinate volunteers to assist with the event, develop letters of understanding with each group assisting with the event, and provide letters of thanks to all groups and individual volunteers who assist with the event after it is over. Twice during this hour, Mr. Fischer is interrupted by phone calls from individuals needing information on various cancers. Mr. Fischer writes down their request on a referral slip, along with their name and contact information. Twice a week he has a volunteer who comes in and mails or e-mails all of the information that has been requested. It is Mr. Fischer's responsibility to recruit, train, monitor, evaluate, and acknowledge all of the volunteers he uses in his program.

At 12:00 P.M. Mr. Fischer heads out for lunch. He usually eats lunch at his desk while working, but today he is speaking to the local Rotary Club about the Cars for a Cure program. This is a program that encourages people to donate old cars, truck, motorcycles, boats, and such to the ACS so that they can be auctioned and the money used to support ACS programs. Although Mr. Fischer enjoys public speaking, he does not have enough time to handle all of the requests and frequently coordinates volunteers to speak on behalf of the ACS.

Mr. Fischer returns to his office shortly before 2:00 P.M. He takes another hour to answer phone calls and e-mails that have come in since the morning and writes some correspondence related to the Cancer Survivor Day program. From 3:00 P.M. to 5:00 P.M., Mr. Fischer is on the phone, calling volunteers to participate in a fund-raiser called Relay for Life. At this event, teams of people camp out at a local high school, park, or fairground and take turns walking or running around a track or path. Each team is asked to have a representative on the track at all times during the 24-hour event. Donations are made to the teams by those wishing to support the event. This is a good fund-raiser and a lot of fun, but it takes considerable staff time to prepare for the event.

Mr. Fischer leaves the office at 5:00 P.M. to have dinner with his family. Tonight, however, he has to be back at the office at 7:30 P.M. for a meeting of the Skin Cancer Prevention Committee. As the name implies, this committee of volunteers is responsible for all local ACS programs dealing with skin cancer and reducing sun exposure. As the health education specialist, Mr. Fischer has to be present for all of their monthly meetings. In addition to the Skin Cancer Prevention Committee, there are also board meetings, volunteer recognition nights, support group meetings, and numerous other speaking engagements and responsibilities that require Mr. Fischer to work in the evenings. He usually spends one to three nights a week on the job. In addition, he occasionally has to work on weekends during special ACS events like Relay for Life.

Additional Responsibilities

As can be seen from the Mr. Fischer example, public/community health education specialists are involved in numerous and varied activities (see **Box 7.3**). Planning, implementing, and evaluating programs and events are major tasks, but, in conducting these tasks, health education specialists get involved in fund-raising, coalition building, committee work, budgeting, general administration, public speaking, volunteer recruitment, grant writing, media relations, and advocacy. (See **Table 7.5**.)

Practitioner's Perspective

BOX
7.3

COMMUNITY HEALTH EDUCATION SPECIALIST Patricia Stewart

CURRENT POSITION/TITLE: Director of Coordinated School Health Programs (CSHP)

EMPLOYER: Idaho State Department of Education (SDE)

DEGREE/INSTITUTION/YEAR: Bachelor's of Science, Dakota State University, Madison SD

MAJOR/MINOR: Physical Education and Health

How I obtained my job: My education and work experience prepared me well for my job. I have worked in the field of health education/promotion for over 30 years, starting my career teaching health and physical education at the secondary level. Teaching provided me with an opportunity to work with students from different cultural backgrounds, which broadened my perspective regarding health risks and protective factors influencing student behavior and educational outcomes. I worked as a consultant for a health education/promotion curriculum company training staff in school districts in several states, which increased my insight into the level of health education/promotion implementation occurring in the United States. My previous experience as director of CSHP in the South Dakota Department of Education is probably the best preparation for moving into my current position at the Idaho State Department of Education (SDE). Working in state government gave me the experience of writing grants, collecting data, informing policy, and evaluating the process and the outcomes of health-related projects/initiatives. Since CSHP is funded by the Centers for Disease Control and Prevention, Division of Adolescent School Health, I was exposed to the public health perspective. CDC bases funding and programming on data and research, so the importance of data collection and following research best practice to prioritize and focus programming became clearer to me. My involvement in professional organizations helped me build a broad network of health promotion partners across the country. This network has provided resources and funding support for various projects in programs and even opened doors for career opportunities. I am still a health educator, but now my opportunities to advocate for health education/promotion are expanded beyond the classroom to include community partners.

How I utilize health education/promotion in my job: As Director of CSHP, I collaborate with the Department of Health and Welfare and other organizations involved in health promotion to address health issues facing ID youth. Initially, I brought together lead health educators from pre-K to post-secondary, utilizing our partnership with the Idaho Association for Health, PE, Recreation and Dance to review and revise the ID Health Education Standards. I also worked closely with our physical education coordinator to follow the same process to revise the ID Physical Education Standards. I believe that these two content areas, although different, complement one another and are now closely aligned to the national standards. There has been a philosophical change in health education/promotion over the past ten years, resulting in a greater focus on skill building within each of the health education/promotion topics rather than focusing only on providing health information to students. Our program has provided significant professional development to health educators in schools focused on helping teachers align curriculum with standards and performance assessment to ensure that students have both the knowledge and the skills to practice healthy behavior for a lifetime. Our goal in providing this type of professional development is to help teachers change student health behaviors to reduce youth risk behaviors.

What I like about my job: My position provides a unique opportunity to work collaboratively with both government agencies and outside health-promoting organizations to gather data, garner resources, assist in policy change, and evaluate

BOX
7.3

continued

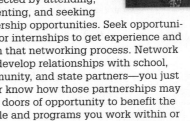

effectiveness of programs to promote the health of children and youth. Serving as a coordinated school health director allows me to work collaboratively with other areas to find the resources to address health needs. A CSHP Director has to look at the big picture and work collaboratively with health educators, physical educators, food service staff, school nurses, school counselors, the safe and drug-free school personnel, staff wellness, and parents and community partners. I enjoy providing professional development in health education/promotion and also helping school staff develop a coordinated approach to address health issues by utilizing their school and community partners.

What I like least about my job: Working in a state-level position in CSHP removes me from the direct contact I have with students, which is why I entered the education field initially. The CSHP staff are involved in so many initiatives and partnerships that sometimes one feels like it is difficult to follow a project from implementation to completion taking the time to fully evaluate both the process and the outcome. It is important to remain focused on key priority areas and recognize limitations in my time and resources. Funding from CDC for CSHP programs is highly competitive and very limited within states, so the need to continually write grants and seek funding to support programming through partnerships is an ongoing process. This challenge allowed me to grow in my skills to advocate for programs using data and collaborative partnerships to create an effective message of change.

Recommendations for those preparing to be health educators: To be effective you must remain committed to the hard work and passionate about what you do and why you do it. In order to remain dedicated to the profession, strive to be a lifelong learner with a commitment to seeking

professional development. Join your professional organization(s) even before leaving your undergraduate program and stay connected by attending, presenting, and seeking leadership opportunities. Seek opportunities for internships to get experience and begin that networking process. Network and develop relationships with school, community, and state partners—you just never know how those partnerships may open doors of opportunity to benefit the people and programs you work within or provide you with a new and challenging career opportunity.

The role of health educators/health promotion specialists in the future: Primary prevention should be the most important priority of health care reform in this country. We cannot continue to react to chronic health issues and health care costs in this country, but must strive to be more proactive. Health educators will continue to have an ever-increasing role to play in schools and communities as part of a comprehensive health care system. Using the coordinated school health approach, health educators will work in partnership with public health and health care providers to plan, implement, and promote programs to reduce risk behaviors and increase the practice of health-enhancing behaviors significantly, reducing morbidity and mortality in the United States. Health educators should bring to these partnerships a passion for working with youth, knowledge of current best practices in health education/promotion, and teaching skills to effectively facilitate student learning. I believe these unique traits will impact positive health behavior change in youth and, ultimately, reduce the burden of health care costs in this country.

TABLE 7.5 **Advantages and disadvantages of working in public/community health education/promotion**

Advantages

- Job responsibilities are highly varied and changing.
- There is a strong emphasis on prevention.
- There is usually a high community profile.
- Health education specialists work with multiple groups of people.
- There is a high degree of self-satisfaction.
- These positions typically offer good benefit packages.
- These positions typically allow flex time when working evenings or weekends.

Disadvantages

- Pay may be low, particularly in voluntary agencies.
- When hired directly by a community or public health agency, job security tends to be good. In such situations, the health education specialist is said to be employed on **hard money**. Sometimes, however, these agencies hire health education specialists on money secured through grants, which is known as **soft money**. In these situations, positions are terminated when grant funding is discontinued, so job security can be a concern.
- Relying heavily on volunteers can be frustrating. Although most volunteers are great, some do not demonstrate the same level of commitment as might a paid employee.
- There never seems to be enough money to run all the programs that need to be offered in the way they should be offered.
- These positions often require irregular hours that may include evenings and weekends.
- There is a lot of bureaucracy in public health agencies.

▷ Work-Site Health Education/Promotion

In describing Work-Site Health Promotion programs, the CDC notes, "The workplace and the health of the workers within it are inextricably linked. Ideally, workplaces should not only protect the safety and wellbeing of employees but also provide them opportunities for better long-term health and enhanced quality of life. Effective workplace programs, policies, and environments which are health-focused and worker-centered have the potential to significantly benefit employers, employees, their families, and communities" (CDC, 2013c). Since the mid-1970s, business and industry in the United States have been offering work-site health promotion programs for their employees. Why are work sites interested in offering these programs and why are health education specialists interested in working in these settings? Chapman (2006) offers an insightful and succinct response to these questions:

> Increasing employer-related health care costs continue to provide a serious threat to the economic life of virtually all American employers. Behavioral issues of employees and their family members continue to loom large as a major reason for increasing health costs. In addition more than 131 million individuals are in the U.S. work force and another 55–65 million are linked through family relationships or retirement relationships, putting employers in a key role related to health and wellness issues for approximately 80% of the U.S. population. This and several other characteristics of the worksite itself, such as the amount of time people spend at work each week and the economic role of employers in the health of employees, make it an excellent place to conduct wellness programs. (p. 6).

These work-site wellness programs offer an additional setting for health education specialists and allow them to reach segments of the population that are not easily reached through traditional community health programs.

In the United States, annual healthcare expenditures surpassed 2.6 trillion dollars in 2010 or an average of $8,402 for every man, women and child living in the Unite States. This is more than three times the $714 billion spent in 1990, and more than 10 times the $253 billion spent in 1980. Healthcare expenditures accounted for 17.9 percent of the gross domestic product (GDP) in 2010 and are projected to be nearly 20 percent or one-fifth of the GDP in 2020 (California Health Care Foundation, 2013). Approximately one-third of these healthcare costs are picked up by business and industry in the form of health insurance premiums (Chenoweth, 2011). Starbucks, for example, pays more for its U.S. employees' health insurance each year than it does for coffee (Rubleski, 2007). Can work-site health promotion programs reduce these costs? According to the Wellness Councils of America (2006), the advantages of work-site health promotion are no longer a matter of speculation. In 2006 there were more than 600 articles that provided both circumstantial and direct evidence of the value of work-site health promotion programs. The tangible benefits include reduced sick leave absenteeism, reduced use of health benefits, reduced workers' compensation costs, reduced injuries, and reduced presenteeism losses (losses resulting from poor productivity in those employees that are present). Beyond the tangible benefits there are also intangible benefits including improved employee morale, increased employee loyalty, less organizational conflict, a more productive workforce, and improved employee decision-making ability.

Goetzel and Pronk (2010) conducted a systematic review of 51 work-site health promotion studies. They found that certain health behaviors, biometric measures, and financial outcomes could be influenced through work-site health promotion programs although the effect sizes for these improvements were modest when compared to clinical trials. The impact, however, of modest changes when applied to large groups of people combined with the relatively low cost of work-site programs when compared to clinical interventions confirmed their value. They went on to say that, "Many of the programs considered in the work-site review fall under the broad umbrella of primary prevention (e.g., encouraging workers to be more physically active; providing them with education about and access to a healthy diet; teaching techniques for managing stress; helping employees stop smoking; and mandating seat belt use) and thus may achieve long-lasting population based health improvements at a low cost. Further, it was observed that health promotion interventions delivered at the work-site can be efficiently and cost-effectively provided, especially when company leadership, norms, culture, and policies are aligned to support adoption of healthy habits and prevention practices" (p. S224).

Health promotion programs at work sites differ greatly from site to site (U.S. Department of Health and Human Services, 2003; Chenoweth, 2011). Some are extensive, include elaborate facilities, and are conducted by full-time staff members hired by the company (see **Figure 7.3**); others are minimal programs that may include only a brown bag lunch speaker's program or a discount at the local YMCA or health club (Chenoweth, 2011). For a list of work-site health promotion activities, see **Table 7.6**.

The proportion of employers who provide work-site health promotion programs has increased over the years. It is reported that health improvement programs of some kind are now being offered by more than 80 percent of work sites with 50 or more employees and almost all large employers with more than 750 employees (U.S. Department of Health and

▶ **Figure 7.3** Health education specialists are employed by business and industry to provide programs to improve the health of employees.

TABLE 7.6 **Work-site health promotion activities**

Smoking cessation	Cancer risk awareness	Lending libraries
Stress management	Cardiovascular risk awareness	Physical examinations
Weight loss		Smoke-free policies
Exercise/physical fitness	Skin cancer screenings	Counseling hot lines
Nutrition	Flu shots	Hypertension screenings
Safety	Health fairs	HIV/AIDS prevention
First aid & CPR	Bulletin boards	Paycheck stuffers
Mammography screenings	Newsletters	Web site development

Human Services, 2003). Despite these impressive numbers for large employers, more needs to be done. Many of these large employers have only minimal health promotion offerings. The majority of U.S. employees work in small and medium-sized companies that are much less likely to offer any health promotion opportunities. Certain types of employers, such as retailers, seldom offer health promotion programs, and any employer with a high rate of workforce turnover has no motivation to offer health promotion programs. Further, only 28 percent of employees aged 18 years and older participate in employer-sponsored health promotion activities (U.S. Department of Health and Human Services, 2000).

Work-site health promotion received a significant boost from the passage of the Patient Protection and Affordable Care Act. As a result of the wellness and prevention provisions in this act, a national work-site health policies and programs survey will was done to more thoroughly assess what employers were doing in relation to worksite health promotion. In 2011, five-year grants to small employers (less than 100 employees) were made available to provide technical assistance and other resources to establish wellness programs for employees. In 2014, employers will be permitted to provide employee rewards in the form of insurance premium discounts, waivers of cost-sharing requirements, and so forth for employees participating in wellness programs and meeting certain health-related standards (Society for Public Health Education [SOPHE], 2013).

Though positions exist in the work-site health promotion setting that are strictly health education/promotion, more frequently expertise in exercise testing and prescription is also required. This is because many work-site health promotion programs are centered around a fitness center. It is often the fitness center that is the most visible aspect of a work-site health promotion program and attracts many employees to health promotion activities. Therefore, skills related to exercise are important, and these skills are not part of the competencies required by a health education specialist. As a result, health education specialists preparing for employment in work-site health promotion should strongly consider a minor or second major in exercise science (see **Box 7.4**). Peabody and Linnan (2007) recommend that those wanting careers in the work site setting consider getting two degrees: one a more generalist degree (health education, public health, health promotion), and the second a specialist degree (exercise physiology, nutrition science, nursing, athletic training). They indicate that it does not matter which degree is the undergraduate and which is the graduate, but that an individual with both a generalist and a specialist degree "will have many more options than someone with two degrees in either field" (Peabody & Linnan, 2007, p. 31). Beyond specialty expertise, a master's degree is also required for many entry-level health education/promotion positions in business and industry. In addition to the Certified Health Education Specialist (CHES) or Master Certified Health Education Specialist (MCHES) credential, certifications more specific to exercise are available from the American College of Sports Medicine and may be required at some work-site settings. Certifications for specific aspects of work-site health promotion, such as aerobic dance, first aid, and cardiopulmonary resuscitation (CPR), and for smoking cessation instructors are also available and encouraged. In general, the more degrees, certifications, and credentials one has, the better one will compete for worksite health promotion positions.

A Day in the Career of a Work-Site Health Education Specialist

The day begins early for Alisa. The fitness center opens promptly at 5:00 A.M. so that employees who start work at 6:00 A.M. have time to work out before beginning their shift. Alisa has to be there at 4:45 A.M. to open the doors, turn on the lights, and greet the first members. The first two hours of her day are spent working the floor. This means she greets members as they enter the facility; walks around the machines, providing instruction where needed; chats with the members; answers health-related questions; and basically makes everyone feel important and welcome. By 7:00 A.M., all of the shift workers have left the fitness facility and, by 9:00 A.M., the managerial employees have cleared out.

From 9:00 A.M. to 11:00 A.M. is a slow time in the center. A few retired employees and spouses use the machines, but this is basically the time for Alisa to get other tasks done. She begins by laundering the dirty towels and folding those that come out of the dryer. Next she provides the routine maintenance to the machines. This involves cleaning them with disinfectant and applying a lubricant to the moving parts. Once this is completed, Alisa has about an hour to work at her desk. Today she is writing an article on the different

WORKSITE HEALTH PROMOTION Nicole Gaudette

CURRENT POSITION: Manager, Health Education & Wellness
EMPLOYER: Geneia
DEGREES/INSTITUTION: MPH, Boston University
MAJOR: Social and Behavioral Science Concentration

Job history: After graduating from Boston University with my Master of Public Health degree and participating in multiple innovating internships in Boston I moved back to my hometown in Pennsylvania. I was offered employment at Global Secure Systems in a grant funded one-year position as a Public Health Training and Outreach Specialist. In this role I independently designed and delivered interactive presentations catered to the individual needs of Pennsylvania participants within an alert network system. I managed and administered the logistical components of this alert network, coupled with the creation of novel documents and protocols. While directing this system, I communicated and disseminated pertinent information regarding the significance of this network at the same time establishing effective working relationships with city, government and community agencies.

After completion of this one-year role, I moved to Capital BlueCross as a Health Education Consultant. In this role I delivered professional consultation and high-level wellness implementation to employer groups, individual members and the community for health management programming and employee lifestyle enhancement in the workplace. I also evaluated health prevention and promotion strategies, specific to diverse work environments, for application and execution of programs and synthesis of program validity and cost benefit to group customers. Another job responsibility was the generation of specific recommendations for customer-specific reference through research of employee population needs based on disease prevalence, utilization, associated costs and trends designed to impact positive health outcomes. After five years in the health education and wellness unit, I have advanced from Consultant to Team Lead to Manager of the unit.

My current job responsibilities: I am the Manager for a team of health education specialists. Within my scope of job duties I supervise seven individuals whose main function is to support employer groups for health management programming. As a team we have staff meetings once every two weeks, case reviews every quarter, intrinsic motivation skill building sessions once a month, and individual one-on-one meetings every two weeks all which I develop, coordinate and lead. Having a healthy work culture is vital in my view so I focus on staff members in various ways, such as creating consistent awards and recognition processes, clearly communicating new program development, assessing motivation of staff for change and development of novel implementation strategies for staff led programming. Being a compelling role model for change as the team leader is crucial with exemplification of a positive attitude and stance on changes. With changes and as part of a sound communication strategy, I conduct feedback loops to evaluate specific procedures within health and wellness to assess job duties and functions and analyze individual performance. As the manager, I also attend finalist presentations and answer request proposal summaries both for prospective and current group customers.

What I like most about my position: The best part of my position is working within a team of fun, passionate, energetic, knowledgeable and inspiring individuals. We genuinely have a healthy and happy work environment that makes everyday enjoyable and something I look forward to each day. We function in a high energy, fast-paced environment that generates different and exciting days. As a unit we steadfastly support one another and are true team members, just like a professional

BOX

7.4

continued

sports team, who have concern, care and perpetual encouragement for everyone.

What I like least about my position: One of the biggest challenges in my position is the variety of tasks and pace of schedule that I face. In many cases, we support a large and wide-ranging set of customers and maintain a large customer base with assorted set of needs and objectives. As our product offerings and success relies on tailoring of our products and services to meet the unique needs of a customer, it is not uncommon that week-to-week, there is a different set of tasks with fluctuating schedules to perform. To meet this challenge, I find that dedicating time each week to organizing and planning is essential. This strategy includes detailed preparation of near-term activities and high-level scoping of longer-term activities. Implementing this planning cycle allows me to be proactive in identifying and scheduling specific tasks to ensure that the output of my and unit work exceeds customer's expectations and is completed and conducted on schedule.

Recommendations for future students: There are so many opportunities within the realm of health education and wellness I would encourage students to follow their passion that will enhance their intrinsic motivation for traveling down their chosen path. It is important to inherently motivate yourself that can lead to heightened success in the area you have chosen. Doing something you like keeps you motivated because it is enjoyable. Through choosing to do something you have satisfaction in

doing, it is important to seek out and master optimal challenges. The reward for choosing a path such as this is that it will foster your sense of what you enjoy doing, it will allow for accomplishment of and provide an enhanced view of what you want to do thereby making you a positive contributor to society.

A day in the career of a health education and wellness manager: Every day is a bit different depending on the immediate needs of staff members and/or employer groups with whom we work. Being connected to staff members is essential as decisions and feedback is at times needed promptly. Meetings typically infiltrate into the day very quickly, making being adaptable essential and a strong skill set for this position. At times, employer group requests arise which need to be addressed in a time sensitive manner. These get boosted to the top of the list of the day for priority completion. There is always an open door guiding principle for staff members to discuss challenging group situations or anything that needs senior level support. There is also a lot of interaction within the Clinical Management department as a whole within a day. Many of the scheduled meetings involve various projects and/or initiatives in the department and interacting and dialoguing with these individuals is important to move forward in a productive, streamlined manner.

types of dietary fats, to be included in the Wellness Center newsletter she publishes each month. The newsletter is distributed to all active employees and retirees of the company. Alisa is always amazed at how important writing skills are to her position in work-site health promotion.

Between 11:00 A.M. and 12:15 P.M., Alisa teaches two aerobics classes for the employees. The first is a beginners' class for new members. The second is supposed to be a more advanced class. Unfortunately, many of the shift employees have no choice in their lunch time, so Alisa ends up with some very advanced members in the beginners' class and some beginners in the advanced class. This is frustrating and could be avoided if there were another fitness center employee. There are, however, only two employees in the center, and Rob, the other health education specialist, must work the floor with the lunch crowd while Alisa teaches. Alisa is going to pursue the possibility of hiring a part-time aerobics instructor just for the lunch hours. This would allow her to offer a beginning and an advanced class at each time slot.

From 12:15 P.M. to 1:00 P.M., Alisa runs an ongoing support group for employees trying to lose weight. All participants bring a brown bag lunch that is supposed to contain food appropriate for a weight-loss diet. They weigh in weekly, and Alisa provides each participant with a voluntary body composition (fat vs. lean) analysis every three months. At least twice a week, Alisa prepares a 20-minute lecture on a weight-loss topic or invites a guest speaker from the community.

At 1:00 P.M. the employees are back at their work stations, and there is again a quiet time in the health promotion center. Alisa spends the next hour eating lunch at her desk and working on a new incentive program for employees to join the health promotion center that will be offered next month. She has to develop all of the brochures, promotional material, and registration forms and arrange for the purchase of incentive items.

At 2:00 P.M. she has a meeting with upper management of the company. She has been advocating for the company to establish a no-smoking policy for the past five years. Two years ago, the company did restrict smoking to specified smoking areas, which was a major accomplishment. Today she will present a proposal to phase out all smoking over a one-year period. Alisa would be responsible for offering several smoking cessation classes over the 12-month period before the no-smoking policy takes effect. She has already decided that her next advocacy effort will be to have more healthy alternatives available in the vending machines, snack rooms, and cafeteria. She has begun a literature review to learn what other companies have done to improve the nutrition of their employees.

By 2:30 P.M. she is back in the health promotion center. The second shift employees are in the center now ahead of their shifts, so Alisa is again working the floor. Today she has to do initial fitness assessments on three new employees. This involves running the employees through a standardized series of tests. Based on the results of these tests and each employee's fitness objectives, she prescribes an individualized exercise program for each employee. She then takes the employees through the fitness center and teaches them how to use the equipment and maintain a record of their progress.

By 3:30 P.M. Alisa is finished with the assessments. Because she had the early shift, opening the facility, she is finished for the day. Rob, who came in later, will stay and close the facility at 8:00 P.M.

Additional Responsibilities

The responsibilities involved in working in a corporate health promotion center are many and varied. In some facilities, maintaining records such as who is using the center, which programs are most popular, fitness assessment results, and health profiles is a major task. Fortunately there are software programs available to assist with this. There are always many little things that need to be done, such as the creation and updating of bulletin boards, equipment maintenance, and towel distribution and laundering. Many times, annual health fairs, company-wide health screenings, and flu shot programs are

TABLE 7.7 **Advantages and disadvantages of working in work-site health promotion**

Advantages

- It affords excellent opportunities for prevention.
- It provides access to individuals who may not participate in community programs.
- Health education specialists work with multiple and diverse groups of people, including everyone from upper management to shift workers.
- Most health education specialists in the corporate setting enjoy their positions and report a high degree of job satisfaction.
- Pay is usually higher than in other health education settings. Benefits are usually good, but they vary considerably from employer to employer.
- Health education specialists have access to fitness facilities for personal use.

Disadvantages

- Hours are long and irregular. To cover employees on all shifts in a company may necessitate health education specialists' working hours early in the morning or late in the evening. It is not unusual to work more than eight hours a day.
- Upward mobility may be a problem. Typically, there are only one or two managerial positions in health promotion at any given work site. This makes it difficult for health education specialists to move up. In addition, those holding managerial positions as directors of health and fitness have nowhere to move up in a company unless they are willing to get out of the health promotion field.
- Health promotion programs and fitness centers often seem to be low on a company's priority list. Such programs are often the first to receive budget cuts in difficult times and often seem to be short of the staff necessary to run optimal programs.
- Some companies subcontract their health promotion and fitness programs to outside vendors. Some of these outside vendors hire part-time health education specialists, pay lower wages, and provide few or no benefits.
- Health education specialists have strong pressure to be extremely fit and be healthy role models for other employees.

the responsibility of the health promotion staff. In addition, advocating for population-based, corporate-wide policies, rules, and regulations to enhance the health of employees is important. These policies, rules, or regulations may relate to tobacco use, food service, safety, violence, stress, and so forth.

Being a health education specialist in a work-site setting is not easy. It is imperative that work-site health education professionals stay up to date with health information and the operational processes of running a work-site program. As noted by the American College of Sports Medicine (2003), "the worksite health promotion professional needs to have a good handle on where to find the information, knowledge, resources and expertise that are needed to access the underlying foundations on which programs are built, the operational processes that allow programs to flourish, and the motivation to continually keep a heads-up attitude toward new and innovative strategies that allow well-established programs to maintain their cutting edge" (p. xi). See **Table 7.7** for a listing of the advantages and disadvantages of employment in worksite health education/promotion.

Those who combine health education/promotion with a fitness background may find employment in settings beyond the business world. See **Table 7.8** for a partial listing of employment opportunities for those with both health education/promotion and exercise training.

TABLE 7.8 **Employment opportunities in health education/promotion with an emphasis in exercise and fitness**

Corporations, business, and industry	Outside commercial vendors that provide programs to work sites
Corporate/industrial parks	
YMCAs/YWCAs	Entrepreneurial enterprises (aerobics studios, consulting, club owner, personal training)
Private health and fitness clubs	
Special-population clubs (women, elderly, etc.)	Fitness product/service companies (sales and marketing)
Community parks & recreation programs	
Colleges/universities	Condos and apartment complexes
Hospitals	Hotels
Sports medicine centers	Spas
Insurance companies that offer health education/ promotion programs to their corporate clients	Resorts and cruise lines

▷ Health Education/Promotion in Healthcare Settings

Positions are available for health education specialists in a variety of **healthcare settings**, including clinics, hospitals, and managed care organizations (McKenzie, Neiger, & Thackeray, 2013). "Typically in the medical care field, health education specialists serve as administrators, directors, managers, and coordinators, supporting and consulting on health education programs and services" (Totzkay-Sitar & Cornett, 2007, p. 8). Health education specialists have also been used in healthcare settings to provide patient education (Byrd, Hoke, & Gottlieb, 2007). For example, a patient is diagnosed with heart disease. That patient is then referred to the health education specialist for information about exercise, nutrition, weight control, stress management, smoking cessation, and so on. This could involve one-on-one education or counseling sessions with the patient, or it might involve group programs in which multiple patients receive the same program at the same time.

In hospitals and other healthcare settings, health education specialists have also been hired to direct health and fitness programs for company employees, much the same as in other worksite settings (Breckon, et al., 1998) (see **Figure 7.4**). Sometimes these programs

▶ **Figure 7.4** Hospitals employ health education specialists to provide programs for employees, patients, or the community at large.

HOSPITAL MAIN ENTRANCE

are also open as an outreach service to community members. Other times, health education specialists are responsible for developing and conducting health and fitness programs specifically designed for community members through fitness facilities that are affiliated with the hospital (see **Box 7.5**).

HEALTH CARE EDUCATOR Carrie Wilcox, RN, M.S.

CURRENT POSITION/TITLE: Community Health Educator

EMPLOYER: Jay County Hospital

DEGREE/INSTITUTION/YEAR: B.S./M.S. Ball State University, 2001–2002; A.S.N. Ivy Tech 2007

MAJOR(S): Health Science and Nursing

Job responsibilities: I have a number of job responsibilities in my role as Community Health Educator for Jay County Hospital. I am responsible for teaching diabetes education, congestive heart failure education, and smoking cessation classes to members of our community. I also provide this type of education to patients admitted to the hospital during their stay. I created a wellness program that was implemented in our local high school to teach students the importance of making healthy lifestyle choices. I also serve as the facilitator for a childhood weight management program entitled *Stop Taking On Pounds*. Lastly, I coordinate community health awareness events for the hospital.

How I got my job: The position was posted in my local newspaper. The requirements for the job included being a registered nurse, experience in community health, and interest in diabetes. I possessed all three qualities. As part of my health science education, I interned with the Diabetes Prevention Program on the Tohono O'odham Indian Reservation in Sells, Arizona. This experience made me a prime candidate for this position to deliver diabetes education to a population in a rural community.

What I like most about my job: I love the variety of my work. Every day is different and there is a great deal of opportunity for creativity. Program development allows me to assess a population, determine their needs, and plan a program to meet such needs. I have freedom in this planning process and am able to make connections with other community members as a result of such programs.

What I like least about my job: Working at a small, rural hospital limits the resources available for programs. Funding is always an issue that has to be considered before starting a project. In addition to funding, personnel resources are limited, so I carry the entire responsibility for my work. I am expected to provide education both inside and outside of the hospital, which can be challenging at times.

How my work relates to the responsibilities and competencies of a health education specialist: My job as Community Health Educator requires me to constantly assess the needs of the community. From this assessment, I plan, implement, and evaluate health education/promotion programs. When working with patients admitted to the hospital, I must assess their learning levels and readiness to change to provide the most effective health education/promotion resources. I serve as a resource for health education/promotion to our community and hospital as a whole. I also coordinate health education/promotion services between Jay County Hospital and the community.

Recommendations for those preparing to be health education specialists: I would strongly suggest choosing internships that allow you some valuable hands-on experience with program planning. Developing health education/promotion programs is

BOX 7.5 *continued*

the heart of your responsibility as a health education specialist. Gaining experience and becoming comfortable with assessing patient/population needs, developing a program to meet these needs, and evaluating the outcomes is vital in preparing you for future employment. Also, create a portfolio of the projects you complete both in the classroom and in your internship experiences to share with potential employers in an interview. Proof of your ability to provide effective health education/promotion and develop needs-appropriate programs will speak volumes to a potential employer. Finally, get involved. Eta Sigma Gamma was a wonderful experience for me as a health science student and allowed me to take leadership within my field of study. There are many opportunities on campus to participate in health education/promotion-related activities. Be proactive and get involved in a club or organization you believe in.

Unfortunately, patient education has not emerged as a major source of employment for health education specialists. Although it seems like an ideal activity for health education specialists, third-party reimbursement is not provided by health insurance companies to cover a health education specialist. Third-party reimbursement refers to the system whereby healthcare providers can submit their bills to the patient's insurance company for reimbursement (McKenzie, et al., 2012). Thus, patient education does not happen or it may be done by nurses who can also serve other functions in the healthcare setting that are reimbursable. Although health insurance companies are certainly concerned about reducing healthcare costs, their strategies to date have been more short term. The impact of health promotion and education programs may not be seen for years, and cause-and-effect relationships are difficult to establish. Therefore, without the availability of third-party payment, there is a major disincentive for hospitals, clinics, and private practice physicians to offer health promotion and education services to their patients. In response to this problem, SOPHE has made third-party reimbursement one of its major advocacy issues.

Of all healthcare settings, health maintenance organizations (HMOs) have been most receptive to hiring health education specialists. The first HMOs were established in the 1970s as a result of federal money that was made available to help with start-up costs and to study the effectiveness of this healthcare delivery mechanism. In essence, patients belonging to an HMO pay one set fee for all their medical services in a given year. It therefore benefits the HMO to provide preventive health services and health education/promotion programs to keep their patients healthy. The fewer services a patient uses, the greater the cost benefit to the HMO. In the initial HMO legislation, one of the criteria for establishing an HMO was providing health education/promotion. Unfortunately, there were no stipulations on the professional preparation of the health education/promotion provider. Often, nurses or other individuals with little or no health education/promotion preparation or experience were given the responsibility of providing health education/promotion programs. As a result, some HMOs have developed outstanding health education/promotion programs with health education specialists, whereas others do very little.

There is, however, reason to be optimistic about future employment opportunities in healthcare settings for health education specialists. The Health Promoting Hospitals

Network (HPH) is working with partners such as the World Health Organization (WHO) to incorporate more health promotion and education programs in hospitals worldwide (WHO, 2013). With changes in the U.S. medical care system rapidly occurring, the increased emphasis on cost-cutting measures, and movement toward more managed care, it is likely that prevention will take a higher profile in the future. As these changes occur, health education specialists will be the best prepared professionals to assume responsibility for helping individuals adopt healthy lifestyles.

A Day in the Career of a Healthcare Setting Health Education Specialist

Mary's day begins at 8:30 A.M., when she arrives at the hospital, picks up her mail, and proceeds to her office. She is the only health education specialist employed by this large metropolitan hospital, but she does have a secretary/assistant who works closely with her to carry out the duties of the position.

At 9:00 A.M. Mary has to attend the weekly staff meeting. This is a meeting with all department heads at the hospital. Much of the agenda does not concern Mary directly, but it is important for her to know what is going on in all departments. At today's meeting, it was decided to have an open house for the public to see the newly renovated obstetrics wing of the hospital. Mary is given the responsibility of planning and advertising this event.

At 10:00 A.M. Mary has an appointment with the administrative head of the Cardiac Rehabilitation Program at the hospital. The purpose of the meeting is to begin planning the development of two brochures that will eventually be distributed to all cardiac rehabilitation patients and will be posted on the hospital education Web site that Mary maintains. One brochure will be on stress-management strategies, and the other on different types of dietary fat. They brainstorm ideas, and Mary agrees to develop a rough draft of the content of the brochures for the administrative head to review prior to their next meeting. They will also discuss graphics, layout, and production at the next meeting.

At 11:00 A.M. Mary leaves the hospital to drive to one of the local malls. The mall has decided to conduct a three-day health fair, and the hospital has agreed to be a co-sponsor of the event. Today is a planning meeting for all of the agencies and businesses that will participate. In addition to serving on the planning committee, Mary is responsible for setting up the hospital's display and coordinating nurses and physicians to work in several screening stations. During the health fair, Mary will be at the hospital's booth all day, handing out materials, answering questions, and promoting the hospital's community outreach health promotion programs.

After lunch, Mary returns to the hospital around 1:00 P.M. and spends the next two hours working on the hospital's health and wellness newsletter. As a public service and to promote the hospital, Mary is responsible for developing a newsletter every other month that is mailed to all households in the hospital's immediate service area. Each edition of the newsletter features one department in the hospital and contains several additional articles about health and wellness. Mary writes much of each newsletter, using information she obtains from the Internet and from a variety of health journals and newsletters to which she subscribes. She designs and formats the newsletter with a desktop publishing program she has on her computer. She marvels at how important good writing skills are to her position.

At 3:00 P.M. Mary leads a weight-loss support group for hospital employees. Most of the participants are nurses and housekeeping staff from either the first or second shift. At each session, participants weigh in, share their experiences over the previous week, and listen to a 20-minute presentation designed to enhance their weight-loss program. Mary is responsible for each week's presentation. In addition, she provides participants with healthy recipes, exercise tips, motivational incentives, and recognition awards. The weight loss support group also has a Web site that Mary maintains where additional recipes and information on weight loss is posted. In the future Mary plans to expand the Web site and develop an online hospital based weight loss program that will be made available to the entire community.

After class, Mary returns phone calls, answers e-mails, and ties up loose ends until it is time for her to go home at 5:00 P.M. It is not unusual for Mary to take some work home in the evenings or on weekends. Tonight, however, Mary must return to the hospital at 7:30 P.M. to teach a stress-management class for the community. The stress class is part of the hospital's ongoing community outreach program. Each month a different health topic is taught, and Mary is responsible for either teaching the class or lining up the instructor for the class.

Additional Responsibilities

Health education specialists working in healthcare settings are involved in numerous and varied activities. The actual responsibilities can differ greatly from one healthcare setting to another. Planning, implementing, and evaluating programs and events are certainly major tasks. Health education specialists may also be involved in grant writing, one-on-one or group patient education services, publicity, public relations, employee wellness activities, and various collaborative efforts with other hospital staff, community agencies, or departments of public health.

Administration is a major responsibility of many health education specialists working in hospitals. They are often hired as managers, directors, or coordinators of programs. Hospitals often adopt a "team" approach to health education/promotion, in which doctors, nurses, physical therapists, and other health specialists are all part of the team. Health education specialists plan and coordinate the programs and serve as resources for the other team members, who actually present the programs. In this type of position, the health education specialist provides little direct client service (Breckon, et al., 1998). (See **Table 7.9.**)

▷ Health Education/Promotion in Colleges and Universities

Colleges and universities are another source of employment for health education specialists. Within the college setting, there are typically two types of positions that health education specialists hold. The first is an academic, or faculty, position, and the second is as a health education specialist in a student health service or wellness center.

As a faculty member, the health education specialist typically has three major responsibilities: teaching, community and professional service, and scholarly research (Preparing Future Faculty, 2013). The amount of emphasis on each of these major responsibilities is dependent on the institution. In large research institutions, faculty may spend most of their time writing grants and conducting research. In smaller four-year colleges, teaching may be the major responsibility. In addition to the major responsibilities, faculty may be asked to

TABLE 7.9 **Advantages and disadvantages of working in a healthcare setting**

Advantages

- Job responsibilities are highly varied and changing.
- There is increased credibility due to the healthcare connection.
- There is usually a high community profile.
- Health education specialists work with multiple groups of people.
- Wages and benefits are good.
- There is a high degree of self-satisfaction.

Disadvantages

- Health education/promotion may have low status and low priority within health care settings.
- Health education specialists must continually justify the program's value.
- Jobs are difficult to obtain.
- Turf issues over educational responsibilities can develop.
- Hours may be long and irregular.
- Some medical doctors may be difficult to work with.

advise students, serve on committees, coordinate or lead student groups, attend professional conferences, and accept administrative duties.

The minimum qualification for working as a faculty member in the college/university setting is usually a doctoral degree in health education/promotion. Though some junior colleges and small four-year schools may hire faculty with only a master's degree, most tenure-track positions require a doctorate. In addition, depending on the position for which one is applying, it may be necessary to have had prior experience or academic training in school health, public/community health, or work-site health promotion. Holding or being eligible for a CHES or MCHES credential is often listed as a preference or requirement for faculty positions.

For a health education specialist in a university health service or wellness center, the major responsibility is to plan, implement, and evaluate health education/promotion programs for program participants (see **Box 7.6**). In some universities, the program participants are students, whereas in others it is the faculty and staff. Often both groups are included as program participants. In addition to program planning, the health education specialist may be responsible for maintaining a resource library; maintaining a Web site, one-on-one advising with students; developing and coordinating a peer education program; speaking to residence hall, fraternity, and sorority groups; conducting incentive programs; and planning special events.

The minimum qualifications for working in a university health service or wellness center typically include a bachelor's or master's degree in health education/promotion. A master's degree is usually preferred. Students interested in working in this setting are advised to work as volunteers or consider completing a practicum or internship in the campus wellness center while an undergraduate. Many universities have peer education programs in which undergraduate students are trained by the professional health education specialist to conduct programs for their peers. This type of experience is invaluable, whether or not a student is subsequently employed in a university health service or wellness center. It is also important to obtain the CHES or MCHES credential for work in this area.

UNIVERSITY WELLNESS CENTER Jodi Brawley, M.S., CHES

CURRENT POSITION/TITLE: Health Educator

EMPLOYER: Boise State University

DEGREE/INSTITUTION/YEAR: Master's of Science, California Polytechnic State University, San Luis Obispo, 1999

MAJOR: Kinesiology, Exercise Science and Health Promotion

How I obtained my job: After seven years working in a variety of health promotion positions, I decided I wanted a job in higher education. Having lived in California all my life, I was open for a change. I found the position on a national job recruiting Web site. After being offered the position, I relocated to Boise, Idaho. Four years later, I am very pleased with my choice to move.

How I utilize health education/promotion in my job: The health education/promotion tools that are intrinsic to my daily work are planning, designing, and evaluating health promotion outreach programs that meet the needs of our students and staff. I also use learning outcomes for all programs and outreach as a way to keep focused on the educational purpose for all events.

What I like most about my job: I thoroughly enjoy supervising the Wellness Works Peer Education internship program. I have the opportunity to mentor students as Peer Educators, watching them develop as young professionals while coordinating health promotion events and educational campaigns. The Peer Educators program deals with a variety of health topics including fitness and nutrition, body image and eating disorders, stress, sleep, sexual health, back health, and depression and anxiety. It is a great experience watching these student leaders grow and make a lasting impact on our campus and in the lives of our students.

What I like least about my job: Every job has its downside. My least favorite aspect of my current job is not having enough resources to provide the services needed on our campus. Staff and funding are often limited, although there is additional need for services, and only so much can be done with the resources available. In an ideal world there would be adequate professional staff and a sufficient budget to help all the students and staff meet their health and wellness goals.

Recommendations for those preparing to be health education specialists: I highly encourage students to participate in an internship program. Internships are a great opportunity to experience various work environments and apply classroom knowledge to real-life settings. Health education/promotion can vary diversely from work place to work place, so the more internships or practica you can do, the greater likelihood you will find a setting that you enjoy and can flourish in.

The role of health educators/health promotion specialists in the future: The future is ours to create. Health care continues to be a hot topic, and as the population ages, the role of the health education specialist will continue to grow. Health education specialists are going to be called upon to work with individuals for behavior modification programs, develop and support public policy, and influence changes that create healthy environments for people to live, work, and play.

▷ International Opportunities

Health education/promotion specialists may wish to consider working in foreign countries for all or a portion of their careers. There is great need for professionals with health education/promotion skills in many developing countries. These positions often require special dedication because the living and working conditions may be more challenging than those experienced in the United States. For those so inclined, however, the rewards in terms of personal satisfaction and accomplishment can be tremendous. Further, the experience gained by planning, implementing, and evaluating health promotion and education programs in foreign countries can be invaluable to one's professional development (see **Box 7.7**).

Working in developing countries often requires the health education specialist to examine different health problems and to try different approaches. For example, instead of helping people reduce high-fat, high-cholesterol diets, as in the United States, the health education specialist may be helping people deal with problems of starvation, malnutrition, and parasitic and bacterial infections. Instead of dealing with heart disease and lung cancer, the health education specialist in a developing country may be facing schistosomiasis, diarrhea, and ascaris and tapeworm infections.

Consider the case of Sofia. Sofia was working as a community health education specialist for the health department in a rural community of about two thousand people in a developing country. The water source for this community consisted of several large ponds. These ponds were the only source of drinking water and were also used for bathing, clothes washing, and care of animals. Many people were getting sick with severe diarrhea, and there had been several deaths among the elderly and very young. To alleviate this problem, it was decided to develop an educational campaign to get people to boil their water before consumption. Sofia was given the responsibility for developing this campaign. There were no local newspapers or radio stations and no billboards, and many of the people could not read. After consulting with local leaders, it was decided that the best way to spread the information would be to use a "mobile communication system." This was accomplished by hooking up an old stereo system to a car battery and driving around the community, broadcasting information about the importance of boiling water. In addition, Sofia set up several demonstrations around the community about how to boil water effectively. These sessions were also advertised via the "mobile communication system."

As can be seen from Sofia's experience, health education specialists working in foreign countries must be able to develop creative, innovative programs to solve identified health problems. Most often, these programs must be low-cost, easily developed and implemented, acceptable to the social and cultural norms of the community, and available to all aspects of the public. It is imperative that these programs be developed in conjunction with the local people being served. It is also helpful when programs are sponsored by organizations seen as credible by the priority population.

One of the best ways to begin a career in international health is to volunteer with the Peace Corps. Health education/promotion professionals are in demand by the Peace Corps, and students should begin the application process early in their senior year. Many colleges and universities are visited by Peace Corps recruiters every year, and talking to one of these Peace Corps volunteers is a good place to start. Faculty members on your campus may have been former Peace Corps volunteers and talking to these individuals can provide valuable insight into the Peace Corps experience.

There are many advantages to volunteering with the Peace Corps. The Peace Corps provides volunteers with some of the best language and technical training in the world. Each Peace Corps volunteer is granted a monthly allowance for housing, food, clothing, and miscellaneous expenses. Free dental and medical care are provided, as well as free transportation to the placement setting and 24 vacation days per year. Deferment of federal student loans

TABLE 7.10 **International health organizations**

National Council for International Health
American Association for World Health
World Health Organization (WHO)
Joint United Nations Program on HIV and AIDS (UNAIDS)
Pan American Health Organization
U.S. Agency for International Development (U.S.A.I.D.)
Foundations such as the Bill and Melinda Gates Foundation
Nongovernmental organizations such as Save the Children
CDC Coordinating Office for Global Health

is also possible while serving in the Peace Corps. After completing the two-year experience, volunteers are given a post-service readjustment allowance of $7,425. They are also given preference for federal jobs and have enhanced scholarship and assistantship opportunities at many major colleges and universities (Peace Corps, 2013). In addition, a successful Peace Corps experience may serve as a stepping stone to paid positions in other international health organizations (see **Table 7.10**).

The CDC is expanding its presence overseas. This may create future opportunities for health education specialists. "CDC is committed to ensuring that people around the world will live safer, healthier, and longer lives through the achievement of its Global Health Goals: Global Health Promotion, Global Health Protection, and Global Health Diplomacy" (CDC, 2013a.).

BOX 7.7

Practitioner's Perspective

GLOBAL HEALTH Emily Miller, B.S.

CURRENT POSITION/TITLE: International Medical Programs Coordinator; Tena, Ecuador
EMPLOYER: Timmy Global Health
DEGREE/INSTITUTION/YEAR: Bachelor of Science, Ball State University, 2013
MAJOR/MINOR: Health Science/Spanish

My global health experience: Global health is an all-encompassing term that refers to health equity and prosperity both locally and globally. During my freshman year of college, I became actively involved in global health. In 2009, I participated in an international medical brigade hosted by the Ball State University Timmy Global Health chapter (BSU Timmy). Our team of students and doctors visited five rural communities surrounding Quito, Ecuador, and treated over 500 patients in the span of one week. Throughout the week, I was given the opportunity to collect patient history, record patient vitals, shadow medical professionals of various specialties, administer fluoride for all the children, as well as manage a mobile pharmacy.

Along with this clinical experience, I was also given the opportunity to further expand upon several health education initiatives. Water sanitation, dental hygiene, malnutrition, and prenatal care are the four main health disparities within these communities. Waterborne parasites are extremely common within these communities, so it is important to teach community members how to properly boil and treat their water source in order to lessen and/or eliminate this illness.

BOX 7.7 *continued*

Dental hygiene is another major health concern, particularly among the children. Many children will arrive to the clinic with a mouthful of cavities, so teaching proper brushing and flossing techniques is very important in promoting good oral hygiene. All pregnant mothers are also given prenatal vitamins for which I explained the importance of prenatal care and encouraged the mothers to receive periodic check-ups prior to their delivery. Although medical treatment is important, primary and secondary prevention are imperative. Health education plays a major role in the prevention of communicable diseases and the overall offset of chronic diseases.

To say it was an enriching experience is an understatement—this first trip to Ecuador revolutionized my view of health. The various determinants of health (i.e., social, political, environmental, biological, etc.) play a significant role in the health outcome of poor, rural communities. For example, the majority of patients we treat during brigades do not have regular access to a health clinic. Furthermore, several patients must walk over five hours to reach a mobile clinic, while others must wait several months before the next mobile clinic is in their area. The field of global health attempts to minimize these determinants through various interventions and programs. This initial experience granted me the opportunity to intern with the organization and eventually obtain my current position.

How I obtained this experience: I obtained this experience through the Timmy Global Health chapter at Ball State University (BSU Timmy). The organization has nearly 30 university chapters across the U.S., and I was fortunate enough to have a chapter at my school. Being originally from Texas, I had never heard of the organization, so this was a great opportunity to learn more about the organization and get involved in global health. Stemming from my experience with the BSU Timmy chapter, I was able to work my way up and intern at the organization headquarters in Indianapolis. Consequently, I worked closely with the organization staff and was fortunate enough to receive my current position as an international medical programs coordinator. In this position, my responsibilities include organizing medical brigades, coordinating meetings among the community health workers, developing and implementing health education programs, and conducting research; all of which tie in nicely with the seven areas of health education responsibilities.

Why I have chosen to work in global health: Health is a fundamental human right, and everyone deserves the opportunity to a happy and fruitful life. Unlike the majority of the world's population, I was born into a privileged, healthy life. I believe it is my responsibility to give back to those less fortunate to ensure that the communities with whom I work are given the same opportunities and health resources that I received throughout my numerous stages in life.

What I like most about working in global health: Working in global health allows me to combine my three passions in life: health, servitude, and travel. After my first medical brigade in Quito, Ecuador, I was immediately hooked. The demand for health education in poor, rural communities is undeniable and the broad scope of this field allows me to address an endless list of health disparities. My particular position as a medical programs coordinator gives me the ability to provide health services and resources to individuals who otherwise lack such amenities. Simply teaching an individual how to properly wash their hands or treat their water drastically impacts their health. These seemingly small accomplishments play a much larger role in these communities, which make this occupation all the more enjoyable and rewarding.

BOX
7.7

continued

What I like least about working in global health: Working in global health is a never-ending endeavor. Unfortunately, there are millions of individuals and families living in abject poverty with little opportunity to improve their circumstances. As a health education specialist, I am limited in the amount of work I can do in these communities, and unfortunately, several circumstances (e.g., social, environmental, biological, etc.) are out of my control. For example, the poverty level and isolated location of these communities limits the amount of health resources and services they are able to receive. Additionally, the patriarchal or '*machismo*' culture within these communities greatly hinders the health status of women and children. Furthermore, shifting community health behaviors is not a short-term process. After investing a lot of time and energy and waiting patiently for my work's impact to unfold, I am continually learning the full impact of my job.

Health education responsibilities I use in my global health work: My work in global health allows me to encompass all seven areas of health education responsibilities. Alongside my responsibilities as a medical programs coordinator, I also received a grant through Timmy Global Health to design and implement a women's health program in Tena, Ecuador. Through these combined duties, I am able to address each area of health education responsibilities. Specifically, in order to understand my international communities, it is imperative that I assess the needs, assets, and capacity for health education within my adopted community (Area I). Once I determine the level of health intervention needed, I am able to plan, implement, and evaluate my health education program(s) (Areas II-IV). Research is another important component of the health education process, which allows one to understand, evaluate, and improve existing and future health programs within their community (Area IV). Within my occupation, I am also able to administer and manage health education within my community health programs (Area V), serving as a health education resource person and advocate for health and health education (Area VI-VII). Needless to say, my work in global health has given me the opportunity to exercise all seven areas of health education responsibilities.

Recommendations for other health education specialists who would like to work in global health: One advantage of working in global health is the ability to work anywhere in the world. Begin your exploration in the classroom and enroll in global health courses. If your school does not offer courses in global health, MIT offers free international health courses (https://www.edx.org/ and http://ocw.mit.edu/index.htm). For those interested in tackling modern global health issues, consider volunteering for both local and international health organizations (e.g., health clinics that serve impoverished communities, homeless shelters, health education facilities, etc.). It is important to note that it is not absolutely necessary to travel to another country to experience poverty and disease; there are countless communities here in the U.S. that desperately need help, as well. However, to fully understand the complexities of health disparities around the globe, considering studying abroad in an impoverished country and make sure to study the language beforehand. Last, but not least, remain curious; make a point to explore and cultivate your interests.

▷ Nontraditional Health Education/Promotion Positions

In addition to the traditional settings for health education/promotion that have been described in this chapter, there are a variety of nontraditional jobs that health education specialists may wish to consider. These positions may or may not carry the title of health education specialist. In some cases, they require the health education specialist to use the skills and competencies in different or unique ways. Further, it is often necessary for health education specialists to sell themselves to get these positions, as the persons doing the hiring may be unfamiliar with the skills and training of a health education specialist.

Given health education specialists' knowledge of health and fitness, sales positions related to health and fitness products are a real possibility. Pharmacy sales, fitness equipment sales, and the sales of health-related textbooks are all areas in which health education specialists have found employment. Life and health insurance are two additional options to consider in the area of sales.

By emphasizing the communication competencies that are part of the professional training in health education/promotion, the health education specialist may seek employment in journalism, TV, or radio. Many television stations have a regular health or medical reporter who does feature stories on health-related issues. Newspapers may have a health column that could and should be written by a health education specialist. Writing articles for health-related Web sites or actually developing Web sites for health-related organizations are other possibilities (see **Box 7.8**). Again, it is necessary for health education specialists to sell themselves to obtain these positions. Taking elective classes or minors in media, communications, and journalism and doing one's internship in these settings also may assist those interested in this career field.

Health education specialists should always be alert to unique job opportunities, many of which may not even carry the title of health education specialist. One health education specialist, for example, was hired by a state mental hospital as a "Teacher II." His job was to provide drug education to patients who had a history of drug problems and sex education to patients who had a history of sex problems. The remainder of his work schedule involved tutoring patients in math and science who were studying to obtain their high school general equivalency diploma.

▷ Landing That First Job

At first, it may seem unusual to discuss landing one's first job while still in an introductory course, but this is the best time to consider the issue of future employment. There are several actions students can take during their college years to enhance their chances of obtaining employment. By following the suggestions made in this section, a student will be far ahead of those who wait until the end of their degree program to address these issues.

No matter what the setting in which a health education specialist hopes to eventually work, landing the first job can be a frustrating experience. Students often find themselves in a dilemma. Employers want their new employees to have had "experience," but where

BOX
7.8

NONTRADITIONAL HEALTH EDUCATION/PROMOTION POSITIONS
Nicole Nichols

CURRENT POSITION: Content & Editorial Director; Resident Fitness Expert

EMPLOYER: SparkPeople, Inc. (SparkPeople.com and BabyFit.com)

DEGREE, INSTITUTION, MAJOR: B.S.Ed., University of Cincinnati, 2005, Health Promotion & Education with Exercise & Fitness Emphasis

Current job responsibilities: As the primary content developer and editor for SparkPeople.com and BabyFit.com, it's my responsibility to create and manage all of the content on our Web sites. SparkPeople.com is the fastest growing health site on the Web and covers a wide variety of health, nutrition, fitness, and weight loss topics, while BabyFit.com helps women have healthier pregnancies and babies by focusing on good nutrition and prenatal exercise.

"Content" can mean a wide range of things for both sites. It's my job to either create the content by writing it myself, or by hiring and managing freelancers or health experts for certain projects. I write and edit articles, create interactive quizzes and assessments, conduct polls, review products and books, write instructions for our exercise demos, create online workout videos, summarize current research studies that apply to our members, and write and manage our 13 different daily and weekly e-newsletters. While this type of content focuses on general health, fitness, and nutrition, it's also my responsibility to proof, edit, and sometimes write other pieces of content on the sites—like instructions for using the site, member surveys, announcements, technical FAQs, company press releases, and promotional pieces for other magazines and newspapers.

While content creation and management makes up the bulk of my job, I'm also involved with our Community Message Boards as a Resident Fitness Expert. When members ask questions about weight loss, exercise, nutrition, and more, I can answer their questions and point them to other helpful resources. Lastly, I create and manage our unique employee wellness program, which we call the SparkPeople Adventure. It entails daily, weekly, and monthly nutrition and fitness goals that everyone must meet in order to earn a year-end bonus.

Health education/promotion responsibilities I use most in my job: Although my job is nontraditional, I use a lot of the core responsibilities of a health education specialist on a daily basis:

- Assess Needs: I have to assess the needs of the members of our site in order to create content that is appealing and helpful to them. After all, we want them to return to the site and reach their goals. I can assess these needs by conducting polls or surveys, and by skimming the message boards to see the types of questions that are asked most often.

- Plan and Implement Effective Programs: When I find the needs of our members, I brainstorm topics to meet those needs and come up with the most effective way of educating members on a topic, whether it be an article, a quiz, or an in-depth guide. I'll either write the content myself, or assign it to one of our in-house experts or freelancers as a way of "implementing" the program.

- Evaluate Program: Because members can easily contact us via e-mail or message boards, they are able to ask additional questions, point out errors, or give feedback about the content on the site. This lets me know whether the content is doing well, or if I might need to revisit it.

- Act as a Resource: This is probably what I do most. By writing and generating content, I'm taking the steps to find accurate, reliable, and helpful information that members can use. All of our content is backed by research and is medically accurate. If and when generally accepted guidelines on fitness, nutrition, and health change, then I also need to

continued

BOX 7.8

react and update our resources on the site. Regarding message boards, I have to know when I'm qualified to answer questions on certain topics, or when another expert (or resource) is needed, and be able to point people in the right direction.

How I got my job: In college, I knew that I wanted to be a health and fitness writer, so I took additional courses in journalism and copyediting. I obtained a part-time job at the college newspaper, writing health articles. That led me directly to SparkPeople, because one of their employees saw my work and asked me if I'd want to write for them as a freelancer. After I wrote my first article, they contacted me for an interview, and hired me on the spot. I worked as the assistant editor part-time while in school and got a full-time job offer upon graduation.

What I like most about my job: I love knowing that each day my efforts are directly helping and educating people. Since we're a small company, I can work independently and make decisions without waiting for the approval of others. This way, I'm much more efficient and able to get a lot accomplished. I feel fortunate that staying on top of current health trends and news is part of my job, and that I help people interpret that information and apply it to their own lives to become healthier. Making the workout videos is one of my favorite tasks—and getting free products and books from other companies who hope we'll mention or use their stuff is a fun perk. My co-workers and our company culture are also pluses. Everyone is passionate about doing their job well so SparkPeople and BabyFit can help millions of people around the world.

What I like least about my job: I'd say the only downside to my job is the lack of face-to-face contact with the people I am educating. Although my work is online and can potentially help more people than most health professionals can expect to reach with traditional health programs, I do it all from behind a desk, without any real interactions with these people.

Recommendations for students preparing to be health education specialists: I have what many people would consider to be a fun job with an excellent company. And the reason I am here today, especially so early in my career, is directly related to my undergraduate work and experience. Whether you hope to write for a magazine or Web site, or just want to get the best job possible, I believe these points are keys to success:

- Take your classes seriously and really learn the material. I have to apply things that I learned in college on a daily basis—I'm expected to know certain things so that every piece of content on our site is accurate, safe, and easily understood. No matter where you work, you'll need to be an "expert" on something. A high GPA is a highlight on a résumé that might help you land that first job.

- Get work experience in the field. This will help you narrow down what you want to do as a career, and help you stand out against the competition. Try a variety of part-time jobs and volunteer opportunities while in college.

- Work to improve your writing and communication skills. No matter what health education/promotion job you get, you'll have to write and speak well to be taken seriously and increase your credibility.

- Network. Get to know your professors, your boss, and other professionals in the field. Attend events that will expand your network and join professional associations. After all, you never know who might recommend you or tell you about a job opportunity.

- Find your passion. Whether it's a type of work (like writing, in my case), or a particular area in the health field, it's important to care about the nature of your work. That makes you more effective in your job, and makes your job more rewarding.

are students supposed to get experience if they can't get hired? There are several possible answers to this question. One way to gain experience is to obtain part-time or summer employment in one's preferred health education/promotion setting. Typically, there are many more students looking for this type of employment than there are employment situations. Should such an opportunity be available, however, it is an excellent way to gain experience before graduation. Another way to obtain experience is to volunteer time in the chosen health education/promotion setting. Most professional health education specialists working in the field are more than willing to accept and use the volunteer time of health education/promotion students. In addition to experience, volunteering also begins the important process of **networking**. Networking involves establishing and maintaining a wide range of contacts in the field that may be of help when looking for a job and in carrying out one's job responsibilities once hired.

Some health education/promotion programs now offer **service learning** opportunities to their students (Cleary, Kaiser-Drobney, Ubbes, Stuhldreher, & Birch, 1998). Organized service learning opportunities provide course credit for students to work with a community agency to meet an identified community need. For example, health education students develop a service learning project with the local health department to collect trash out of an urban streambed (National Service Learning Clearinghouse, 2013). Collecting the trash is a valuable community service, but they go further and analyze the content of the trash to determine possible sources of pollution. They then share their results with residents of the neighborhood where the stream is located and develop a plan to address the problem. This service learning experience provided hands-on, practical, real-world experience that students could not obtain from the classroom. Service learning can also be beneficial in broadening one's professional network, which is so important in the health education/promotion field. Take advantage of as many service learning opportunities as possible. The experience and networking gained through service learning can give new health education/promotion professionals a tremendous advantage in the job market.

Carefully planning internships and practicums can help students obtain their first professional position (see **Box 7.9**). Required field experiences are often the best way to obtain practical experience in one's chosen setting. Students should consider what they would like to be doing five years after graduation and select an experience that closely matches that goal. Frequently students are hired by the agency after completing their practicum or internship experience.

In addition to obtaining experience, students should strive to obtain an excellent academic record. When there is heavy competition for an open position, one of the first strategies in making hiring decisions is to examine grade point average. This is not to say that the person with the highest grade point average is always the best person or will always get the job. But, when there are 50 applications for one job, grade point average is an easy way to begin limiting the field.

Develop a well-organized, professional-looking portfolio. A **portfolio** is a collection of evidence that enables students to demonstrate mastery of desired course or program outcomes. In health education/promotion, the responsibilities, competencies, and sub-competencies should be emphasized. Many health education/promotion programs now require portfolios as part of their professional preparation programs. Even if the portfolio is not required, students should develop a portfolio on their own. Thompson and Bybee

Practitioner's Perspective

BOX 7.9

STUDENT INTERNSHIP Melinda Hershey

INTERNSHIP LOCATION: Kampala, Uganda, and Bwindi, Uganda

INTERNSHIP ORGANIZATION: Conservation Through Public Health (CTPH)

DEGREE/INSTITUTION, AND GRADUATION DATE: B.S. from The University of Cincinnati, Health Promotion and Education, Public/Community Health Concentration; September 2010

Internship placement: I was interested in pursuing a career in international health and decided that I wanted to explore health promotion issues in Africa. I did an online search for organizations in Africa that dealt with health and came across CTPH. The organization studies the relationships between human and animal diseases in Uganda.

Internship description: My major responsibility during this internship was to conduct health interviews within two separate parishes in the Bwindi community. I explored the hygiene and sanitation standards within the community and advised community members on how to better their health by improving their hygiene and sanitation practices. I also asked questions about family planning awareness and explained to community members the connection between smaller families and better overall health. In addition, I spoke with key community members such as hospital administrators and school principals to learn about the pressing health issues in their communities. I also created brochures and flyers to create awareness about health issues, including an Anthrax epidemic in nearby Queen Elizabeth National Park.

Pros and cons of my internship: I really enjoyed the fact that I was able to experience my internship in Uganda. It was truly a learning experience and allowed me

to compare and contrast the health issues of the United States with the health issues of Africa. It was also an extremely culturally rich experience for me and I learned so much about an entirely different group of people. However, working in Africa is much different than working in the United States. Sometimes you have to really fend for yourself and work independently on your own projects with very little guidance, which was a lesson in perseverance for me. Overall, I am glad that I chose to do my internship in Uganda because it opened my eyes to what it's like to work in a different country.

Internship importance: Participating in this internship was extremely important in helping me determine my future career. I came to Uganda thinking that I wanted to do international development work for the rest of my life. However, working there made me realize that I have so many other interests, like environmental health and women's empowerment. I came out of this experience with a whole new perspective on what I want my life's work to be, which turns out to be much different than I had initially imagined.

Recommendations for health education/ promotion students: When you're looking for an internship, do your research. What do you want to get out of the experience? Is it really going to help you determine your future career? Don't just pick an internship because it's easy, close by, and convenient. Pick one that you think is going to help you both professionally and personally; this is your chance to explore the field before you jump into a real job, so make it count!

(2004) note that a portfolio is a "living document that is ever-changing with the increasing depth of knowledge and experience of the individual" (p. 52). They go on to identify five basic elements that should be included in any portfolio: (1) table of contents, (2) résumé, (3) education and credentials, (4) samples of work, and (5) references. The samples of work could include such exhibits as student papers or course projects, audio- or video-tapes of students giving a presentation, analyses of student work by professors or outside reviewers, student goal statements, reflections, and summaries (Cleary & Birch, 1996, 1997). Another way to design the portfolio is to structure it around the NCHEC health education specialist competencies. Essentially exhibits are included in the portfolio for each competency. Students may also want to consider developing the portfolio in an electronic format instead of the more traditional notebook or binder. In addition to providing more flexibility in the way exhibits are presented and displayed, an electronic format also provides the opportunity to showcase one's creativity and to demonstrate technology skills to potential employers (McKenzie, Cleary, McKenzie, & Stephen, 2002). Imagine the impact on a prospective employer when a new health education specialist provides a well-developed, attractive portfolio that clearly demonstrates health education responsibilities and competencies.

Your résumé is extremely important in obtaining your first job. The résumé is your advertisement for yourself. It is the first item of yours that most prospective employers will see. It will create a first and lasting impression of you. What you include in the résumé and how you present the information may make a difference in whether or not you are hired. You should start now to involve yourself in experiences that will look good on your resume. As you develop your résumé make sure that there are no spelling or grammar errors. One former student actually lost a job opportunity because of three spelling errors on her résumé. The more specific you can be in describing your accomplishments on the résumé, the better. Jeff Brizzolara, a health education specialist and Chief Clinical Officer for Viverae Health Care, has some suggestions on how to be more specific; these can be seen in **Table 7.11**.

Beyond the portfolio and resume, consider what certifications are going to be important in landing your first job and carefully plan to make sure they are awarded either before graduation or as soon after graduation as possible. All professional health education specialists should pursue the CHES and MCHES credential. In the future, this may be a prerequisite for many health promotion and education positions. Other certifications should be obtained depending on work setting and need.

Get to know your faculty. They are a great source of information about jobs and how to compete for them successfully. Often employers contact faculty directly, asking for the

TABLE 7.11 **Résumé—Words of wisdom**

Out-of-Date Résumé (Overused Clichés)	More Effective Résumé (Be Specific—Provide Examples)
Results Oriented	Describe a problem that you solved
Team Player	Describe a team project you were part of and the results
Excellent Communication Skills	Demonstrate how your communication skills produced meaningful results
Strong Work Ethic	Provide an example of how you went "above and beyond" to produce results
Meets or Exceeds Expectations	Explain how you were recognized for your effort/work

Source: Jeff Brizzolara, PhD, MPH, MBA. Chief Clinical Officer, Viverae Health Care, Inc. Used by permission.

names of students who might be interested in a particular position. But unless a faculty member knows a student by name and knows that the student is in the job market, there is little the faculty member can do.

Most colleges and universities have placement centers that provide a variety of services to students, including help in developing an effective resume. They may also assist by maintaining a list of job openings, providing workshops or handouts on interviewing skills, and establishing reference files for students. The placement center at the University of North Carolina Wilmington provides in depth trainings for students on how to use LinkedIn to help land a job. It would be a good idea to contact the placement center well before graduation to determine when and how to access its services.

A final suggestion is to join one or more of the health education professional associations (see Chapter 8). Employers are typically impressed when they see that a young professional has been a member of a professional association and perhaps has attended one or more professional meetings. "Professional meetings and conferences are filled with opportunities.... Where else can you find hundreds, even thousands, of education professionals from all over the world coming together to share cutting-edge knowledge through presentations, sessions, workshops, socials, and other events, than at professional meetings and conferences?" (Dixon-Terry, 2004, p. 16). If your campus has a chapter of Eta Sigma Gamma, the professional health education/promotion honorary, try to get involved. Eta Sigma Gamma recognizes high academic achievement, provides opportunities to obtain valuable leadership experience, and allows students to plan, implement, and evaluate various service projects and social activities.

In addition to the aforementioned suggestions, one caution is in order. Be careful what you place on social networking websites such as Facebook and Twitter. Prospective employers are savvy and often will look online to see what additional information they can find about you. "Susan Masterson, a recruiter with TeamHealth in Knoxville, TN, said, using social networking sites is a strategy that anyone in recruiting, whether it be physicians or otherwise, needs to incorporate in their plan. It's here. It's here to stay" (Dolan 2009). Health education/promotion internship site supervisors have even looked online before accepting a student for internship. One author of this text actually received a letter from a prospective employer indicating that he had not hired a particular student because of offensive content he found online. Further, he admonished the program to caution students about what they include online. Students' posting questionable information online seems to be a somewhat common practice. According to an *AMNews* article, in one study 60 percent of U.S. medical schools surveyed reported incidents of students posting unprofessional content on line (Dolan, 2009). What is questionable content is difficult to define. Certainly pictures involving sex, alcohol, or drugs are not appropriate, but anything that causes doubt should be removed. Students should also restrict who can be friends and can access their information as much as possible.

Students who follow the aforementioned suggestions will be better positioned to obtain initial employment in the health promotion and education profession. This is a good time to be a health education specialist, and the future looks even brighter than the present. According to the U.S. Department of Labor Bureau of Labor Statistics (2013), the number of health education specialists will need to grow from the 63,400 jobs in 2010 to a projected 86,800 by the year 2020 for a growth rate of 37 percent, which places health education in the growth category of "much faster than average." Floyd and Allen

(2004) noted, "As the field of health education continues to expand, the number and type of careers will continue to expand. Health education professionals must be willing to implement innovative and quality school and non-school programs for an increasingly diverse population in increasingly diverse settings. The future of health education is here" (p. 36).

Excelling in Your Health Education/Promotion Career

Landing a job is merely the first step in becoming a successful health education specialist. Once you have the job, it is critical that you excel in the job. This is important for two reasons. First you must excel to demonstrate that you are an important and contributing member of the organization that hired you and to enhance your career potential. Second, you need to excel to help further the health education/promotion profession. Your work reflects on all health education specialists and may determine whether your organization or other organizations will hire more health education specialists in the future.

What does it take to excel in health education/promotion? Obviously, one must demonstrate the ability to meet the competencies and sub-competencies of a health education specialist, but one must also meet the standards of a good employee. Numerous authors writing about careers in health education/promotion have elaborated on what is needed to excel as an employee in a health education/promotion position. In talking about how to excel in a voluntary health agency position, one author wrote, "Completing your tasks and projects on time, under budget, and with minimum problems is your most obvious goal, but do not underestimate the value of attitude, spirit, and the ability to work under pressure and with difficult people. A positive, can-do attitude, a willingness to learn new and different skills on the job, and the ability to work in an environment that values teamwork is a 'must'" (Daitz, 2007, pp. 5–6). Other authors writing about working in health and medical care note, "Being successful means meeting and exceeding the expectations of the job and showing initiative in achieving organizational goals" (Totzkay-Sitar & Cornett, 2007, pp. 9–10). In discussing federal health education/promotion positions, Howze (2007) said, "With any job, success requires continually showing how you add value to the organization. For example, many federal agencies are struggling to find workers with language skills, so consider becoming fluent in a second language" (p. 13). And finally, if you are trying to excel in a public health department position (see **Box 7.10**), "Become known as a high achiever/performer and a good team player. Make a positive and lasting impression on your supervisor as well as upper level managers with whom you may have contact through your assignments. Anticipate what needs to be done" (Hall, 2007, p. 17).

The aforementioned quotes clearly indicate that, regardless of the setting, you must go beyond simply meeting the minimum expectations of the job to being a good employee and a good health education specialist. To excel you must go the extra mile and do the unexpected as well as the expected. You need to be a good "people person," demonstrate a positive attitude, and be willing to learn and take on new tasks. These are the things that will separate you from other employees and establish you as a truly outstanding health education specialist.

BOX
7.10

EMPLOYER OF HEALTH EDUCATION SPECIALISTS Louise Villejo, MPH, MCHES

CURRENT POSITION: Executive Director, Patient Education Office
EMPLOYER: University of Texas MD Anderson Cancer Center
DEGREE/INSTITUTION: University of Houston, BS; University of Texas School of Public Health, MPH
MAJOR: Health Administration

My employment history: I have been privileged to serve MD Anderson Cancer Center patients and their family members for the last 31 years. I began as a health education coordinator in the Patient Education Office and was promoted to director in 1984. Before I came to MD Anderson I did an internship at the National Cancer Institute as a health communications intern and felt that this opportunity had a major impact on my career. I was able to experience health education/promotion program planning from a national public health perspective. After college, I worked for an organization that provided administrative support to migrant health care centers across the southwest and saw how important these organizations were in addressing the disparities of access to basic health care.

My current job responsibilities: In my current position I am responsible for developing and directing a system-wide infrastructure so that patients/family members and clinical staff have access to the wide array of health education programs and resources developed by our team and interdisciplinary health care providers.

I work with staff to assure our strategic initiatives to develop or improve cancer patient education programs are in line with the institutional goals, and assist the organization to meet regulatory compliance standards. We engage patients/family members using patient- and family-centered methodologies to inform our efforts. I believe that it is my responsibility to make sure we are developing cutting edge educational resources while also assuring that we address health literacy and the educational needs of diverse populations.

An essential skill when working in a health care environment is collaborating with the health care team. I work with every multidisciplinary disease-site center in the institution and our patient education programs address cancer across the continuum of care from prevention, screening, treatment, recovery, surveillance, relapse and survivorship or hospice.

My goal is to continually educate leadership and staff of the importance of using best and evidence-based practice and engaging patients/family members in their care. The bottom line is helping the patients/family members participate in their care, develop the skills they need and improve their health outcomes.

To do this work it is critical to recruit, train and retain a cadre of highly trained health educators. I have eight health educators on staff and they must confidently lead the clinical team in patient education program and resource development.

People management and planning, directing and monitoring a program budget are also my key responsibilities.

How I develop a job description: The organization has a framework for developing job descriptions that I follow which includes overall function and scope, essential job functions, supervision given and received, physical requirements, certifications, education and experience. I use the seven areas of responsibilities of a health education specialist as the framework for the essential job functions. I start by outlining what we need done and list the specific responsibilities competencies, skills and abilities that are needed. It is always helpful to have other managers, staff and someone from Human Resources review the draft to make sure it is clear and is in the appropriate format.

What I look for in reviewing applications: When I am reviewing applications for a position, I develop a spreadsheet and include column headings of the most important aspects of the position, for

BOX 7.10

continued

example, education and experience in: management, health education program development, budget, strategic planning, personnel management, etc. This helps me prioritize at a glance characteristics of preferred candidates to interview.

What I look for in an interview: As when reviewing applications, I develop an interview guide and interviewee spreadsheet. The guide makes sure that I am asking each applicant similar questions. I use it strictly as a guide and not a rigid interview script. The interviewee spreadsheet does provide at a glance an accurate comparison of applicants. Beyond the interview guide, however, I delve deeper into their work experience and try to understand why they are interested in the position. I try to determine their leadership style and experience working with diverse groups.

I am thrilled if they are able to frame their experiences in the health education specialist's seven areas of responsibility. Even a newly graduated student with little work experience can use their class projects and volunteer activities. Bringing a well-prepared portfolio of work products is a plus.

Recommendations for health education specialists looking for employment: Health educators looking for employment should work their networks, join one or more professional organizations, attend meetings, and contact leadership. Sites liked LinkedIn and a growing number of mobile job search apps can assist in networking and provide job opportunities. The networking is not only critical for your job search but is key for a public health professional. Public health work relies strongly on collaborations to leverage limited assets and build capacity.

Volunteering with nonprofits is another way to build your portfolio. If you want to develop or sharpen your skills volunteer to participate or co-lead a project.

Network with everyone you know and discuss what type of position you are looking for and your experience and background. Even if they are not in the field they might know someone you can contact. Call all of your professional contacts and don't forget your professors. Ask each person you talk to if they would recommend someone else that you can contact. Don't just ask them if they have a job opening, ask broader questions to assist you to understand all the field has to offer. Ask them about what they do and how they got in to the field. Most people are very willing to help and connect you with others if they do not have a job opening. Don't stop looking even if you get an interview, keep reaching out and applying for positions. You don't want to lose momentum if you don't get that job.

Read everything you can regarding advice on job-hunting and interviewing. Looking for employment is a full-time job. Organize and keep track of your efforts. If you get an interview be prepared, follow-up with a thank you letter and ask when they expect to fill the position. Have your elevator speech prepared regarding why it is important to hire an academically trained health education specialist. Let them know how interested you are and what a great fit you would be and why. Don't hesitate to follow-up several times if necessary. Be upbeat and ask specific questions.

From my perspective as someone who hires health educators, I recommend that health education specialists looking for employment submit high quality, well written letters of application and résumés, focus on the responsibilities and competencies required in a position and tie those to your training as a certified health education specialist, be well prepared for any interview opportunities, be well versed on the organization to which one is applying, have questions ready for interviewers about the job duties and responsibilities, dress professionally, and demonstrate a sense of self assurance and confidence.

Summary

There are many settings in which a health education specialist can seek employment. In this chapter, we have discussed in detail health education/promotion positions in schools, public/community health agencies, work sites, healthcare facilities, colleges and universities, and international settings. In addition, we have examined the potential for employment in nontraditional settings and have considered what introductory-level undergraduate students can do to help themselves obtain their first job. Finally, we discussed what it takes to be successful in a health education/promotion position.

Review Questions

1. Identify four major settings and two nontraditional settings in which health education specialists are employed.

2. Compare and contrast the roles and responsibilities of health education specialists working in schools, public and community health agencies, work sites, and healthcare facilities. How are all of these settings similar? How are they different?

3. What is the difference between a position funded with hard money and a position funded with soft money? Which position is preferable and why?

4. Explain why it might be said that health education/promotion has never reached its real potential in the healthcare setting. What factors have kept health education/promotion positions at a minimal level in this setting?

5. What is networking and why is it important in health education/promotion?

6. What can introductory-level health education/promotion students do now that might help them land their first job after graduation?

Case Study

Marla has a B.S. degree in health education/promotion and is CHES certified. For the past five years, since graduating from college, she has been working as a health education specialist for a private vendor who then contracts with companies to offer health education/promotion and fitness services to their employees. During this time the vendor has placed her at three different corporations. All three corporations have been extremely satisfied with her services and the vendor/employer has also given her positive evaluations.

Recently Marla has become dissatisfied with her position. She feels that her $29,000 annual salary is too low, and she gets no retirement, dental, vision, or pharmacy benefits. With her current employer, there is no opportunity for promotion, and raises are small and infrequent. She has two specific goals for the future. One, she wants to continue working in health education/promotion, but she is open to working in any setting. Two, she wants to earn a higher salary and have better benefits. If you were advising Marla, identify options you could suggest. What things could she do to make herself more marketable? What additional education or professional development does she need? What does she need to do in terms of networking? What types of positions and settings should she be considering? Outline a plan for Marla in the next 12 months that will help her to realize the two goals she has established.

Critical Thinking Questions

1. Select any health education/promotion setting and give specific examples of how a health education specialist working in that setting would need to use all seven responsibilities of a health education specialist (i.e., when thinking about assessment at the work-site setting, a health education specialist might have to assess the health needs of employees, assess the current health behaviors of employees, assess how responsive employees would be to a given health promotion program, assess upper management support for a given program, etc.).

2. If you were in a position to hire a new health education specialist, what qualities, traits, and experiences would you look for in making your hiring decision? Compare this with the qualities, traits, and experiences you currently possess. Make a list of things you could do to enhance your marketability prior to graduation.

 Activities

1. Select the one setting you think you would most like to work in. Develop a short essay describing why you prefer this setting to other health education/promotion settings and what you think you will need to do to land a job in that setting.

2. Visit a health education/promotion professional who works in the setting in which you would most like to be employed. Develop a job description for this person's position that explains the qualifications and responsibilities needed for the job.

3. Examine the online classified ads of a major-city Sunday newspaper. Identify those jobs you find that specifically ask for a health education specialist. Next, look through the same classified ads and identify those that do not ask for a health education specialist but require competencies and skills similar to those of a health education specialist. Compare your results with others in the class.

4. Interview someone who is responsible for hiring health education specialists. Find out what that person looks for in a letter of application, a vita, and a personal interview.

5. Contact the placement office at your institution. Determine what services it offers and when these services should be accessed.

 Weblinks

1. **http://www.bls.gov**

   U.S. Bureau of Labor Statistics

   Go to this Web site and run a search for "health education specialists." Review the various documents you find to determine workforce size, average salaries, states with most health education specialists employed, states with highest average salaries, metropolitan areas with highest average salaries, and other important information about health education specialists.

2. http://www.peacecorps.gov

   Peace Corps

   This Web site provides information about the Peace Corps, what volunteers do, where the Peace Corps is active, benefits of Peace Corps service, how to become a Peace Corps volunteer, and much more.

3. http://www.welcoa.org

   Wellness Council of America

   The Free Resources section of this site indexes a number of free worksite health promotion resources that can be easily downloaded in PDF format.

4. http://www.cdc.gov/nccdphp/dnpao/hwi

   Centers for Disease Control and Prevention's Healthier Worksite Initiative

   This page provides access to a number of resources to help one plan, implement, and evaluate work-site wellness programs.

5. http://www.cjhp.org

   Californian Journal of Health Promotion

   Use the Past Issues section to access Volume 5, Issue 2 of the *Californian Journal of Health Promotion* and specifically an article written by Byrd, Hoke, and Gottlieb titled "Integrating Health Education into Clinical Settings." This is an excellent article that describes a successful use of health education specialists in a clinical setting.

6. http://www.cjhp.org

   Californian Journal of Health Promotion

   Use the Past Issues section to access Volume 2, Issue 1 of the *Californian Journal of Health Promotion* and specifically an article by Eleanor Dixon Terry titled "Attending Professional Health Education Meetings: What's In It for the Student and New Professional." This is an excellent article with good advice for students or new professionals attending their first professional health education/promotion meeting.

7. http://www.acha.org

   American College Health Association

   In the Publications section of the Web site, go to the Guidelines, Recommendations, and White Papers area. There you can download a document titled "Guidelines for Hiring Health Promotion Professionals in Higher Education." Compare yourself against the guidelines and recommendations presented in this document. While this document was designed specifically for health education specialists working in college or university wellness programs, many of these guidelines and recommendations would be appropriate for employers in other settings.

 # References

Allensworth, D., & Kolbe, L. (1987). The comprehensive school health program: Exploring an expanded concept. *Journal of School Health, 57,* 409–412.

American College of Sports Medicine (ACSM). (2003). *ACSM's worksite health promotion manual.* Champaign, IL: Human Kinetics.

American School Health Association (ASHA). (2013). What is school health? Retrieved May 29, 2013, from http://www.ashaweb.org/i4a/pages/index.cfm?pageid=3278.

Association of Schools of Public Health (ASPH). (2010). Careers in public health. Retrieved September 6, 2007, from http://www.whatispublichealth.org/careers/index.html.

Breckon, J., Harvey, J. R., & Lancaster, R. B. (1998). *Community health education: Settings, roles, and skills for the 21st century.* Gaithersburg, MD: Aspen Publishers, Inc.

Byrd, T. L., Hoke, M. M., & Gottlieb, N. H. (2007). Integrating health education into clinical settings. *California Journal of Health Promotion, 5* (2): 18–28.

California Health Care Foundation. (2013). *California Health Care Almanac.* Retrieved June 3, 2013, from http://www.chcf.org/~/media/MEDIA%20LIBRARY%20Files/PDF/H/PDF%20HealthCareCosts12.pdf.

Centers for Disease Control and Prevention (CDC). (2013a.). CDC jobs overseas. Retrieved June 3, 2013, from http://www.cdc.gov/globalhealth/employment/.

Centers for Disease Control and Prevention (CDC). (2013b). Components of Coordinated School Health. Retrieved June 1, 2013, from http://www.cdc.gov/healthyyouth/cshp/components.htm.

Centers for Disease Control and Prevention (CDC). (2013c). Workplace Health Promotion. Retrieved June 3, 2013, from http://www.cdc.gov/workplacehealthpromotion/.

Chapman, L. S. (2006). Fundamentals of worksite wellness. *Absolute Advantage, 5* (4), 3–23.

Chenoweth, D. H. (2011). *Worksite health promotion.* 3rd ed. Champaign, IL: Human Kinetics.

Cleary, M. J., & Birch, D. A. (1996). Using portfolios for assessment in the college personal health course. *Journal of Health Education, 27* (2), 92–96.

Cleary, M. J., & Birch, D. A. (1997). How prospective school health education specialists can build a portfolio to communicate professional expertise. *Journal of School Health, 67* (6), 228–231.

Cleary, M. J., Kaiser-Drobney, A. E., Ubbes, V. E., Stuhldreher, W. L., & Birch, D. A. (1998). Service learning in the "third sector": Implications for professional preparation. *Journal of Health Education, 29* (5), 304–311.

Daitz, S. J. (2007). Health education careers at nonprofit voluntary health agencies. *Health Education Monograph, 24* (1), 4–6.

Dixon-Terry, E. (2004). Attending professional health education meetings: What's in it for the student and new professional? *California Journal of Health Promotion, 2* (1), 16–21.

Dolan, P. L. (2009). Social media behavior could threaten your reputation, job prospects. AMNews. Retrieved October 13, 2009, from http://www.ama-assn.org/amednews/2009/10/12/bil21012.htm.

English, G. M., & Videto, D. M. (1997). The future of health education: The knowledge to practice paradox. *Journal of Health Education, 28* (1), 4–7.

Fisher, C., Hunt, P., Kann, L., Kolbe, L., Patterson, B., & Wechsler, H. (2003). Building a healthier future through school health programs. In *Promising practices in chronic disease prevention and control: A public health framework for action.* Atlanta: Department of Health and Human Services. 2-25.

Floyd, P. A., & Allen, B. J. (2004). *Careers in health, physical education and sport.* Belmont, CA: Wadsworth-Thompson Learning, Inc.

Goetzel, R. Z., & Pronk, N. P. (2010). Worksite Health Promotion: How much do we really know about what works. *American Journal of Preventive Medicine 38* (2) Supplement 2, S223–S225.

Hall, J. Y. (2007). Entering and navigating a health education career in the local public sector. *The Health Education Monograph, 24* (1), 15–17.

Howze, E. H. (2007). Health education jobs in the federal government. *The Health Education Monograph, 24* (1), 11–14.

Jalloh, M. G. (2007). Health education careers in schools. *The Health Education Monograph, 24* (1), 18–22.

Joint Committee on National Health Education Standards (JCNHES). (2007). *National Health Education Standards: Achieving Excellence.* 2nd ed. Atlanta: American Cancer Society.

McKenzie, J. F., Cleary, M. J., McKenzie, B. L., & Stephen, C. E. (2002). E-portfolios: Their creation and use by pre-service health education specialists. *International Electronic Journal of Health Education, 55,* 79–83.

McKenzie, J. F., Neiger, B. L., & Thackeray, R. (2013). *Planning, implementing, & evaluating health promotion programs.* 6th ed. Boston, MA: Pearson Education, Inc.

McKenzie, J. F., Pinger, R. R., & Kotecki, J. E. (2012). *An introduction to community health.* 7th ed. Sudbury, MA: Jones & Bartlett Learning.

Miller, B., Birch, D., & Cottrell, R. R. (2010). Current status and future plans for undergraduate public/community health education program accreditation. *American Journal of Health Education, 41* (5), 301–307.

Naidoo, J., & Wills, J. (2000). *Health promotion: Foundations for practice.* 2nd ed. Edinburgh, Scotland: Bailliere Tindall.

National Center for Educational Statistics (NCES). (2013). Back to School Statistics. Retrieved June 1, 2013, from: http://nces.ed.gov/fastfacts/display.asp?id=372.

National Commission for Health Education Credentialing (NCHEC). (2013). Health education credentialing. Retrieved May 29, 2013, from http://www.nchec.org/credentialing/healthedfaqs/.

National Service Learning Clearinghouse (NSLC). (2013). What is service learning? Retrieved June 3, 2013, from http://www.servicelearning.org/what-is-service-learning.

Peabody, K. L., & Linnan, L. A. (2007). Careers in worksite health promotion. *The Health Education Monograph, 24* (1), 29–32.

Peace Corps. (2013). Peace Corps: What are the benefits? Retrieved June 3, 2013, from http://www.peacecorps.gov/index.cfm?shell=learn.whyvol.finben.

Preparing Future Faculty. (2013). Faculty roles and responsibilities. Retrieved June 3, 2013, from http://www.preparing-faculty.org/PFFWeb.Roles.htm.

Rubleski, J. (2007). Embracing workplace wellness. *Absolute Advantage, 6* (5), 30–33.

Society for Public Health Education (SOPHE). (2013). Wellness & prevention provisions in the Patient Protection and Affordable Care Act (H.R. 3590). Retrieved June 3, 2013, from http://www.sophe.org/Sophe/PDF/Health%20Care%20Reform.pdf.

Seirawan, H., Faust, S., & Mulligan, R. (2012). The impact of oral health on the academic performance of disadvantaged children. American Journal of Public Health, 102 (9), 1729–1734.

Thompson, S. E., & Bybee, R. F. (2004). Professional portfolios for health education specialists and other allied health professionals. *California Journal of Health Promotion, 2* (1), 52–55.

Totzkay-Sitar, C., & Cornett, S. (2007). Health education options in health and medical care. *The Health Education Monograph, 24* (1), 7–10.

U.S. Department of Health and Human Services. (2000). *Healthy People 2010* (Conference Edition, in Two Volumes). Washington, DC.

U.S. Department of Health and Human Services. (September 2003). Prevention makes common "cents." Retrieved June 3, 2013, from http://aspe.hhs.gov/health/prevention/.

U.S. Department of Health and Human Services. (2013). About Healthy People 2020: Introduction. Retrieved June 1, 2013, from http://healthypeople.gov/2020/about/default.aspx.

U.S. Department of Labor Bureau of Labor Statistics. (2013). Occupational Outlook Handbook, 2012–13 Edition. Health Education, Retrieved June 5, 2013, from http://www.bls.gov/oco/ocos063.htm#projections_data.

Wellness Council of America. (2006). Planning wellness: Getting off to a good start—part 1. *Absolute Advantage, 5* (4). Retrieved June 3, 2013, from http://www.welcoa.org/freeresources/index.php?category=8.

World Health Organization (WHO). (2013). Health Promoting Hospitals Network. Retrieved June 3, 2013, from http://www.euro.who.int/en/what-we-do/health-topics/Health-systems/public-health-services/activities/health-promoting-hospitals-network-hph.

Agencies, Associations, and Organizations Associated with Health Education/Promotion

Chapter Objectives

After reading this chapter and answering the questions at the end, you should be able to:

- Define each of the following terms and give several examples of each: *governmental health agency, quasi-governmental health agency,* and *nongovernmental health agency.*

- Briefly describe the levels of governmental agencies and provide several examples of each.

- List and explain the four primary activities of most voluntary health agencies.

- Explain the purpose of a professional association/organization.

- Identify the benefits derived from membership in a professional organization.

- Identify the primary professional associations/organizations and coalitions associated with health education/promotion.

- Describe the process by which a person can become a member of a professional association/organization.

- Describe what the National Commission for Health Education Credentialing, Inc., is and its mission and purpose.

There are many health agencies, associations, and organizations with which health education specialists interact. Most of these agencies/associations/organizations were created to help promote, protect, and maintain the health of individuals, families, and communities. For many health education specialists, these agencies/associations/organizations will be places of employment. These groups regularly hire health education specialists to plan, implement, evaluate, and coordinate their educational efforts. Health education specialists not employed by these groups will find them to be valuable sources of up-to-date information and materials. This chapter classifies the agencies/associations/organizations into three major categories: governmental, quasi-governmental, and nongovernmental. Because information on most of these agencies/associations/organizations that support the efforts of health education/promotion is available elsewhere (e.g., McKenzie, Pinger, & Kotecki, 2012) and because this text was written primarily as an introduction to the profession, the primary emphasis of this chapter is on the professional health education associations/organizations.

▷ Governmental Health Agencies

Governmental health agencies are health agencies that have authority for certain duties or tasks outlined by the governmental bodies that oversee them. For example, a **local health department (LHD)** has the authority to protect, promote, and enhance the health of people living in a specific geographical area. Authority is given by the county, city, or township government that oversees the local health department. Governmental agencies, which are primarily funded by tax dollars (they may also charge fees for services rendered) and managed by government employees, exist at four governmental levels: international, national, state, and local (city and county). **Table 8.1** provides examples of governmental agencies and their governing bodies.

▷ Quasi-Governmental Health Agencies

Quasi-governmental health agencies (see **Figure 8.1**) are so named because they possess characteristics of both governmental health agencies and of nongovernmental agencies. They obtain their funding from a variety of sources, including community fund-raising efforts such as the United Way, special allocations from government bodies, fees for services rendered, and donations. They carry out tasks that are often thought of as services of governmental agencies, yet they operate independently of governmental supervision.

Probably the best known quasi-governmental health agency is the **American Red Cross (ARC)**. Clara Barton founded it in 1881 as an outgrowth of her work during the Civil War.

TABLE 8.1 **Governmental agencies and their governing bodies**

Level/Agency	Governing Body
International Level	
World Health Organization (WHO)	United Nations (UN)
Pan American Health Organization (PAHO)	An independent agency
National Level	
Centers for Disease Control and Prevention (CDC)	U.S. government, Department of Health and Human Services (HHS)
Food and Drug Administration (FDA)	U.S. government, Department of Health and Human Services (HHS)
State Level	
State health department	Individual state governments
State environmental protection agency	Individual state governments
Local Level	
Local health department (LHD)	City, county, or township governments
Local school district	Local school boards

▶ **Figure 8.1** The American Red Cross is one of the best examples of a quasi-governmental agency.

Today, the ARC has several "official" responsibilities given to it by the federal government, such as providing relief to victims of natural disasters (Disaster Services) and serving as the liaison between members of the active armed forces and their families during family emergencies (Services to the Armed Forces and Veterans). The ARC also provides many nongovernmental services such as its blood drives and safety services classes such as water safety, first aid, and CPR.

▷ Nongovernmental Health Agencies

Nongovernmental health agencies operate, for the most part, free from governmental interference as long as they comply with the Internal Revenue Service's guidelines for their tax status (McKenzie et al., 2012). They are primarily funded by private donations, or, as is the case with professional and service groups, membership fees. The nongovernmental agencies can be categorized into the following subgroups: voluntary, philanthropic, service, religious, and professional.

Voluntary Health Agencies

Voluntary health agencies (see **Figure 8.2**) are some of the most visible health agencies in a community. Voluntary health agencies are a U.S. creation and grew out of unmet needs in communities. When governmental or quasi-governmental agencies were not in place to meet the needs of communities, interested citizens came together to form voluntary agencies. Such was the case with the American Cancer Society, the American Heart Association, the American Lung Association, the Alzheimer's Association, and the First Candle (formerly SIDS Alliance). The number of voluntary agencies seems endless, with agencies for about

▲ **Figure 8.2** Two of the largest voluntary health agencies are the American Cancer Society and the American Lung Association.
Sources: The American Cancer Society logo is reprinted by permission of the American Cancer Society. Logo of the American Lung Association, courtesy of the American Lung Association.

every disease and part of the body impacted by a disease or an illness. Most voluntary agencies have four primary purposes: (1) raise money to fund research and their programs, (2) provide education to both professionals and the public, (3) provide service to individuals and families affected by the disease or health problem, and (4) to advocate for beneficial policies, laws, and regulations that impact the work of the agency and in turn the people it is trying to help. Some of these organizations obtain their money from community fund-raising efforts like the United Way, but most raise their money through writing successful grant proposals, carrying out specific special events (i.e., dance-athons, golf outings), conducting door-to-door solicitation or direct-mail campaigns, and other means of receiving donations.

Philanthropic Foundations

Philanthropic foundations play an important role by funding programs and research on the prevention, control, and treatment of diseases and other health problems. *Philanthropy* means "altruistic concern for human welfare and advancement, usually manifested by donations of money, property, or work to needy persons, by endowment of institutions of learning and hospitals, and by generosity to other socially useful purposes" (Random House, 2010, ¶ 1). Although many philanthropic foundations accept charitable contributions, they differ from voluntary health agencies in two primary ways. First, they were created with an endowment and, thus, do not have to raise money. Second, they are able to finance long-term projects that may be too expensive or risky to be funded by other agencies. Examples of some philanthropic foundations that have supported work by health education specialists are the Ford Foundation, the Robert Wood Johnson Foundation, and the Rockefeller Foundation.

Service, Fraternal, and Religious Groups

Many different service, fraternal, and religious groups have also been important to health education specialists. Even though none of these groups has the primary purpose of enhancing the health of a community, they often get involved in health-related projects. Health education specialists commonly interact with these groups as part of community coalitions or when they are seeking resources to fund or enhance their programs. Examples of service and fraternal groups (and their health-related projects) include Rotary International (worldwide polio eradication), Lions (Lions Quest and preservation of sight), Shriners (children's hospitals), and American Legion (community recreation programs).

Religious groups also have contributed to the work of health education specialists' projects, both on a global level (e.g., the Protestants' One Great Hour of Sharing, the Catholics' Relief Fund, and the United Jewish Appeal) and on a local level (e.g., food pantries, sleeping rooms, soup kitchens).

Professional Health Associations/Organizations

As noted at the beginning of this chapter, the primary focus of this chapter is the professional health associations/organizations. The mission of **professional health associations/organizations** is to promote the high standards of professional practice for their respective profession, thereby improving the health of society by improving the people in the profession (McKenzie et al., 2012). The mission is carried out by advocating for the profession; keeping the members up to date via the publication of professional journals, books, and newsletters and providing the members with an avenue to come together at professional meetings. At these meetings, members have the opportunity to share and hear the new research findings, network with fellow professionals, and find out more about the latest equipment and published materials in the field. In addition, professional associations/organizations provide their members with benefits such as reduced rates on various types of insurance, participation in tax-deferred annuity programs, discounts (annual national conventions, car rental, eye wear, long-distance telephone calls, publications, travel), job placement, and a variety of other associated items (see **Box 8.1**).

BOX 8.1

Benefits of Joining a Professional Association/Organization as a Student Member

- Opportunity to interact, collaborate, and network with other professionals in the profession
- Opportunity to meet and interact with health education/promotion students and faculty from other colleges and universities
- Develop professional colleagues
- Have a professional identity
- Professional guidance and mentoring
- Leadership development
- Learn more about how the profession and the association/organization operate
- Keep up to date on happenings in the profession and new health information
- Opportunity to participate in the association's/organization's electronic listserv, e-newsletters, Web chats, Webinars, and e-learning communities
- Advocacy alerts and updates
- Opportunity to grow professionally and personally while being supported and encouraged by others

- Be exposed to current research and pedagogy of the profession through meeting attendance and reading the publications of the association/organization
- Make professional contacts for future practicums, internships, or jobs
- Get connected to job banks and internship opportunities
- Opportunity to make a presentation at a professional meeting
- Opportunity to serve the profession through an association/organization
- Discounted registration fees for professional meetings and publications
- If certified, opportunity to earn continuing education contact hours (CECHs) for recertification of the Certified Health Education Specialist and Master Health Education Specialist credentials and other licensures

Source: Adapted from Society for Public Health Education, Inc. and from Young & Boling (2004).

Professional associations/organizations are member driven and composed, for the most part, of professionals who have completed specialized education and training and who are eligible for certification/licensure in their respective professions. These associations/organizations are funded primarily by membership dues, but it is becoming more common for them to seek grant funds (*soft money*) to help promote their missions. Most of these associations/organizations hire staff for day-to-day operations, but the officers are usually elected professionals.

In the remaining portions of this chapter, we present information on the national professional associations/organizations that help promote the health education/promotion profession. The reader should also be aware that many of these national associations/organizations have affiliates and other related groups at the regional and/or state level. For example, the American Public Health Association is a national organization, but there are also state associations such as the Ohio Public Health Association or the Indiana Public Health Association. In addition, there are also some state-only organizations that are not affiliated with any national organization. (Ask your instructor if there are any such organizations in your state.) Often it is these regional or state affiliates/organizations that health education/promotion students become members of first because of their proximity to campus, opportunities to get involved in the professional organization, less expensive membership dues, and local networking benefits. **Table 8.2** contains information about the following organizations.

THE AMERICAN ALLIANCE FOR HEALTH, PHYSICAL EDUCATION, RECREATION AND DANCE

The **American Alliance for Health, Physical Education, Recreation and Dance (AAHPERD)** functioned for many years as an alliance of five national associations (American Association for Physical Activity and Recreation [AAPAR], American Association for Health Education [AAHE], National Association for Girls and Women in Sport [NAGWS], National Association for Sport and Physical Education [NASPE], National Dance Association [NDA]), six district associations (Central, Eastern, Midwest, Northwest, Southern, and Southwest), and a research consortium. (Note that the district associations comprised AAHPERD members located in the states represented by these parts of the country. Also, states have an affiliate organization of AAHPERD—for example, the Ohio Association of Health, Physical Education, Recreation and Dance.) AAHPERD is several generations of professional organizations removed from its beginning in 1885, when Dr. William G. Anderson gathered a group of individuals with interest in physical training. The association, at that time, focused on disseminating knowledge and connecting those with similar interests (Anderson, 1985). The association continued to grow and turned into the American Physical Education Association (APEA) in 1937. In that year, the APEA merged with the National Education Association's (NEA) School Health and Physical Education Department to become an NEA Department with divisions of health, physical education, and recreation (Anderson, 1985). The merger resulted in the formation of the American Association for Health and Physical Education. The word *recreation* was added to the title in 1938, creating AAHPER. In the mid-1960s, the NEA began to feel pressure, because of a challenge from the American Federation of Teachers, to become more active in the welfare movement for teachers. This challenge made the NEA look more closely at its focus. It was supporting 30 departments that had members of their own, most of which were not

TABLE 8.2 **Information about key professional associations/organizations**

The American Academy of Health Behavior
Address:
17 Indian Creek Drive
Rudolph, OH 43462
Telephone and Fax: 419/760-6020
Internet: http://aahb.wildapricot.org/

American Alliance for Health, Physical Education, Recreation and Dance (AAHPERD)
Address:
1900 Association Drive
Reston, VA 20191-1598
Telephone: 800/213-7193; 703/476-3400
Fax: 703/476-9527
Internet: http://www.aahperd.org

American Association for Health Education (AAHE)
Address:
1900 Association Drive
Reston, VA 20191
Telephone: 800/213-7193; 703/476-3400 *Fax*: 703/476-9527
Internet: http://www.aahperd.org/aahe

American College Health Association (ACHA)
Address:
1362 Mellon Road, Suite 180 Hanover, MD 21076
Telephone: 410/859-1500
Fax: 410/859-1510
Internet: http://www.acha.org

American Public Health Association (APHA)
Address:
800 I Street, NW
Washington, DC 20001
Telephone: 202/777-APHA (2742); 202/777-2500 (TTY)
Fax: 202/777-2534
Internet: http://www.apha.org

American School Health Association (ASHA)
Address:
4340 East West Highway, Suite 403
Bethesda, MD 20814
Telephone: 301/652-8072
Fax: 301/652-8077
Internet: http://www.ashaweb.org

continued

TABLE 8.2 *continued*

Eta Sigma Gamma (ESG)

Address:

2000 University Avenue

Muncie, IN 47306

Telephone: 800/715-2559; 765/285-2258

Fax: 765/285-3210

Internet: http://www.etasigmagamma.org

International Union for Health Promotion and Education (IUHPE)

Address:

42 Boulevard de la Libération

93203 Saint-Denis Cedex, France

Telephone: 33 1 48 13 71 20

Fax: 33 1 48 09 17 67

Internet: http://www.iuhpe.org

Society for Public Health Education, Inc. (SOPHE)

Address:

10 G Street, NE, Suite 605

Washington, DC 20002

Telephone: 202/408-9804

Fax: 202/408-9815

Internet: http://www.sophe.org

National Wellness Institute, Inc. (NWI)

Address:

1300 College Court

PO Box 827

Stevens Point, WI 54481

Telephone: 715/342-2969

Fax: 715/342-2979

Internet: http://www.nationalwellness.org

---

members of the NEA (Anderson, 1985). In 1968, the NEA changed its bylaws regarding their departments. As a result an autonomous associated organization was formed. In 1975, AAHPER became completely disassociated from NEA. AAHPER added *dance* to its title in 1979 (Anderson, 1985).

In April 2013, after two years of discussion, the Alliance approved unification of AAHPERD's five national associations, six district associations, and its Research Consortium into one unified organization (AAHPERD, 2013a). AAHPERD has changed its name to SHAPE America (Society of Health and Physical Educators) and now describes itself as "the largest organization of professionals involved in physical education, physical activity, dance, school health, and sport" (AAHPERD, 2013b, ¶1), with a mission to "advance professional practice and promote research related to health and physical education, physical activity, dance, and sport" (AAHPERD, 2013b, ¶2). As a result of the unification process, AAHE, the association most directly related to the discipline of health education, formally separated from AAHPERD and is collaborating with the Society of Public Health Education (SOPHE) to form one organization with a stronger voice for the health education profession (SOPHE, 2013e). (See SOPHE for more information.)

As the collaboration of SOPHE and AAHE and the separation from AAHPERD is only a few months old, many aspects of the impact and outcomes of these new arrangements are yet to be known. But because of AAHE's long history, it is important to have a sense of the contributions this organization made to the profession to this point. The **American Association for Health Education (AAHE)** formally, the Association for the Advancement of Health Education evolved from the School Health Division of AAHPER when the AAHPER was reorganized in 1973 (Nolte, 1985). Its acronym is pronounced as "Aah-hee." Membership in AAHE included current, retired, and student (preparing for careers as) health education specialists and health promotion specialists regardless of their work setting. Before the collaboration with SOPHE, membership was approximately 6,500 members. The mission of AAHE, when associated with AAHPERD, was to advance "the profession by serving health educators and other professionals who strive to promote the health of all people through education and other systematic changes" (AAHE, 2010, slide 3). As of May 1, 2013, the AAHE formally retired (SOPHE-AAHE, 2012).

AAHE has produced several publications that health education specialists find useful. AAHE has had three peer-reviewed journals (a journal in which other professionals in the field decide what is published and what is not). The *American Journal of Health Education* (*AJHE*) has been a bimonthly publication that was available in both print and online versions. Most of the articles published in the *AJHE* have been research articles, but the journal also publishes commentaries, and has a special column for community, care setting, and work-site initiatives. Specific articles are designated as continuing education articles, so Certified Health Education Specialists (CHES) and Master Certified Health Education Specialists (MCHES) can earn Category I credits toward recertification by reading and answering questions about the articles. AAHPERD is responsible for publishing this journal.

Two additional journals that were previously published by AAHE have recently been transferred to the Foundation for Advancement of Health Education as a result of the recent AAHPERD/AAHE changes. The *Journal of Health Education Teaching Techniques* (JHETT) was formerly the electronic *Health Education Teaching Technique Journal*. This journal was originally launched in 2011 and focused on publishing new teaching ideas, techniques, and strategies for K–12 health educators (AAHE, 2013a). The *JHETT* will be available in both print and online editions and will focus on publishing health education teaching techniques (Foundation for Advancement of Health Education, 2013). The *Global Journal of Health Education and Promotion* (GJHEP) has recently been established to replace the *International Electronic Journal of Health Education* (*IEJHE*). The *IEJHE* was first available in 1997 and was the first Web-based peer-reviewed journal for health education, promotion, and behavior. The *IEJHE* provided a complete text of articles ranging from research to theory-based manuscripts. The *GJHEP* will feature international programs and initiatives in health education and promotion. In recent years, AAHE was involved in several activities of note:

- The AAHE offered four networking communities that focused on communicating and creating relationships with individuals in the health education/promotion profession (AAHE, 2013b). The networking sites included AAHE4ME (for university students majoring in health education), the Health & Wellness Teaching Community (for instructors of college-level personal health classes), AAHE on Ning (for all professional members of AAHE), and AAHE on Twitter (for all who want to follow AAHE).

- AAHE was recognized as a multiple event provider of health education continuing education contact hours (CECHs) by the National Commission for Health Education Credentialing (NCHEC). This designation allowed AAHE to offer CECHs for CHES and MCHES through the *American Journal of Health Education* and other special publications, and for participation in the annual AAHPERD/AAHE National Convention.

- The SOPHE/AAHE Baccalaureate Program Approval Committee (SABPAC) was a joint committee of SOPHE and AAHE responsible for directing the SAPBAC Program Approval process, which is a voluntary credential for undergraduate professional programs in community health education.

- AAHE was an active partner with three other professional associations and the American Cancer Society (ACS) in the creation of the *National Health Education Standards* (ACS, 2007). The standards were developed to assist in the creation of health-enhancing behaviors in children in all grades—pre-K through grade 12. Now in their second edition, the standards are used to guide school health curriculum development.

- The National Council for Accreditation of Teacher Education (NCATE) allowed AAHE to be the professional health education association/organization responsible for reviewing folios submitted to NCATE by colleges and universities when they were seeking NCATE accreditation for their teacher education programs.

AMERICAN PUBLIC HEALTH ASSOCIATION

The **American Public Health Association (APHA)** "is the oldest and most diverse organization of public health professionals in the world" (APHA, 2013a, ¶ 1). The APHA was founded in 1872 "as a result of the public health movement to combat yellow fever and other diseases in the 1870s" (APHA, n.d., p. 3). The mission of APHA is to "improve the health of the public and achieve equity in health status" (APHA, 2013a, ¶ 7). The association works toward this mission by providing public health leadership and collaborating "with partners to convene constituencies; champion prevention; promote evidence-based policy and practice, and advocate for healthy people and communities" (APHA, 2013a, ¶ 7).

Membership in the APHA is open to professional, student, and retired health professionals, as well as non-profit organizations interested in supporting the mission of the association. APHA currently has about 25,000 members. In addition, the organization represents another 25,000 individuals who are members of their affiliated state and regional health associations who are committed to creating a healthy global society (Winslow, N., personal communication, June 11, 2013). Once individuals become members, they have the opportunity to select one or more of the subgroups of the organization—called Sections and Special Primary Interest Groups (SPIGs). The basic organization unit of the APHA is the Sections. The 29 Sections "represent major public health disciplines or public health programs. These sections are designed to allow members with shared interests to come together to develop scientific program content, policy papers in their areas of interest or fields of practice, provide for professional and social networking, career development and mentoring" (APHA, 2013b, ¶ 1). SPIGs are open groups "of self-selected APHA members sharing a common occupational discipline or program area interest and electing no primary Section affiliation" (APHA, 2013b, ¶ 2). More specifically, these subgroups propose policy statements, advise on publications, provide testimony and reports, help develop the content and structure of annual meetings, and assist in APHA governance (APHA, n.d.). The sections most closely related to health education are (1) Public Health Education Section, which formed in 1922 and in 1991 changed its name to Public Health Education and Health Promotion Section, and (2) School Health Education Section, which formed in 1942 and in 1980 changed its name to School Health Education and Services Section. The Public Health Education and Health Promotion section "promotes the advancement of the health promotion and education profession and provides a forum for public health educators and those involved in health promotion activities to discuss ideas, research, and training; promotes activities related to training public health professionals" (APHA, 2013b, ¶ 1), whereas the School Health Education and Services section "focuses on development and improvement of health services, health education programs, and environmental conditions in schools, colleges, and early childhood care settings; advances public health in all school settings" (APHA, 2013b, ¶ 1).

The primary publication of APHA is the *American Journal of Public Health* (*AJPH*). This peer-reviewed journal is published monthly. A typical issue of the *AJPH* includes editorials, commentaries, book reviews, job announcements, notification of upcoming meetings, and authoritative articles in both general and specialized areas of research, policy analysis, and program evaluation of public health. Areas covered in the articles include the environment, maternal and child health, health promotion, epidemiology, administration, occupational health, education, international health, statistics, and more. The association also publishes *The Nation's Health* 10 times per year. This newspaper includes reporting on current and proposed legislation, policy issues, news of actions within the federal agencies and Congress, and special features. The publication also includes association news, job openings, and information on upcoming conferences. In addition to the *AJPH* and *The Nation's Health*, the APHA also publishes books and other media on a variety of public health topics. Examples include the best-selling title *Control of Communicable Disease Manual* (Heymann, 2009) and recent publication *Designing Healthy Communities* (Jackson, 2011). The most recent addition to the APHA's publications is its online newsletter called *Inside Public Health*. This "e-newsletter communicates important activities and announcements to Association members" (APHA, 2013c, ¶ 8).

There are other professional health associations that have a more focused mission. Some of those include the American College Health Association (ACHA), the American School Health Association (ASHA) (see **Figure 8.3**), the National Wellness Institute, Inc. (NWI), the SOPHE, and the American Academy of Health Behavior.

AMERICAN COLLEGE HEALTH ASSOCIATION

The **American College Health Association (ACHA)** was founded originally as the American Student Health Association in 1920. In 1948, the name of the association was changed to its current name. ACHA's mission is to "provide advocacy, education, communications, products, and services, as well as promote research and culturally competent practices to enhance its members' ability to advance the health of all students and the campus community" (ACHA, 2013a, ¶ 1). The association has three distinct types of memberships. One is for institutions of higher education. Currently, there are more than 800 such members. ACHA also serves more than 2,800 individual members who are interested in college health—that is, the health of college students. Included in the members are administrators, physicians

▶ **Figure 8.3** David Satcher, MD, PhD, who was a former Surgeon General, Director for the Centers for Disease Control and Prevention, and Administrator of the Agency for Toxic Substances and Disease Registry, addressed the membership of the ASHA in 2010. Annual professional conventions are an important benefit of membership in a professional organization.

and physicians' assistants, nurses and nurse practitioners, health education specialists, pharmacists, dentists, support staff who care for this special group of young adults, and students who are dedicated to health promotion on their campus. Most of these individual members are associated with the health service facilities on their respective campuses. The third type of membership is called sustaining members. This group is made up of nonprofit organizations and corporations interested in being more connected with the college health field (ACHA, 2013b).

Like some of the other associations/organizations, the ACHA also has affiliates across the United States. ACHA is divided into 11 affiliate organizations, each providing regional leadership and annual meeting opportunities. ACHA members receive concurrent membership in the affiliate organization at no additional cost (ACHA, 2013b). In addition, ACHA has nine membership sections, which are defined by the disciplines of college health. The Health Education Section, now called the Health Promotion Section, was formed in 1958.

ACHA publishes several newsletters, numerous health information brochures, and other special publications. The members-only newsletter, *College Health in Action*, is available online at the Association's Web site. The professional journal of the ACHA is the *Journal of American College Health*, which is published bimonthly and is the only journal devoted entirely to the health of college students. The journal publishes articles encompassing many areas of college health, "including clinical and preventive medicine, health promotion, environmental health and safety, nursing assessment, interventions, and management, pharmacy, and sports medicine. The journal regularly publishes major articles on student behaviors, mental health and health care policies, and includes a section for discussion of controversial issues" (ACHA, 2013c, ¶ 4).

AMERICAN SCHOOL HEALTH ASSOCIATION

The **American School Health Association (ASHA)** began on October 27, 1927, as the American Association of School Physicians (see **Figure 8.4**). The organization began to use its current name in 1936 (ASHA, 1976). The mission of the ASHA "is to build the capacity of its members to plan, develop, coordinate, implement, evaluate, and advocate for effective school health strategies that contribute to optimal health and academic outcomes for all children and youth" (ASHA, 2013a, ¶ 1).

Membership in the association is comprised of individuals and institutions with an interest in the health and well-being of school-aged children and youth. The ASHA is a multidisciplinary organization with nearly 650 members. Included in its membership are administrators, counselors, dentists, health education specialists, physical educators, school nurses, school health coordinators, and school physicians who advocate for high-quality coordinated school health programs. With membership in the ASHA comes the opportunity to join subgroups of the association called sections and councils. These subgroups allow members to interact with others who have the same school health interests. Examples of a few of the councils are health behaviors, international health, school health instruction and curriculum, food and nutrition, and sexuality education and reproductive health.

The *Journal of School Health*, which is published 12 times a year, is the primary publication of the ASHA. The journal is recognized widely and "is committed to communicating information regarding the role of schools and school personnel in facilitating the development and growth of healthy youth and healthy school environments. This focus on healthy youth Pre-K to Grade 12 and healthy school environments encompasses a variety of areas including health education; physical education; health services; nutrition services; counseling, psychological, and social services; healthy school environment; health promotion for staff; and family/community involvement" (ASHA, 2013b, ¶ 2). The readership of the

▶ **Figure 8.4** The American School Health Association focuses on the health of the school-aged child.

journal includes administrators, educators, nurses, physicians, dentists, psychologists and counselors, social workers, nutritionists, dietitians, and other health professionals. These individuals work cooperatively with parents and the community to achieve the common goal of providing youths with programs, services, and environment needed to promote health and to improve learning.

NATIONAL WELLNESS INSTITUTE, INC.

The **National Wellness Institute (NWI)**, founded in 1977, "was formed to realize the mission of providing health promotion and wellness professionals unparalleled resources and services that promote professional and personal growth" (NWI, 2013a). The mission of NWI "is to serve the professionals and organizations that promote optimal health and wellness in individuals and communities" (NWI, 2013a, ¶ 2). The mission is accomplished by:

- Identifying quality resources
- Providing quality continuing education and resources
- Promoting opportunities for lifelong learning
- Providing new and innovative professional development programs
- Developing effective educational lifestyle assessments
- Serving professionals and organizations that promote health and wellness (NWI, 2013a, ¶ 2).

There are three types of membership in NWI: individual, organizational, and student. The organizational membership allows five individuals at the same location to receive full NWI benefits. With each type of membership there is regular membership or a plus membership option, which includes a subscription to the *American Journal of Health Promotion*. With membership comes a number of publications including: *Wellness Management*, a newsletter that includes information about successful programs, programming tips, resources, research, events, career opportunities, professional development, and more; *Wellness News You Can Use*, a collection of downloadable, reproducible consumer-oriented short articles, quotes, and flyers for use in newsletters, payroll stuffers, and promotional pieces; *Health Promotion Practitioner*, a newsletter providing innovative and practical ideas in a concise, easy-to-apply style; and *International Wellness Connection*, which includes a series of monthly essays for wellness professionals across the world (NWI, 2013b).

One of the most visible components of the NWI is its National Wellness Conference, held each July in Stevens Point, Wisconsin. The conference is open to members and nonmembers alike and is a unique conference because it is a week of immersion into a wellness experience.

SOCIETY FOR PUBLIC HEALTH EDUCATION, INC.

The Society of Public Health Educators (SOPHE), founded in 1950, is the only professional organization devoted exclusively to public health education and health promotion. In 1969, the organization changed its name to the **Society for Public Health Education, Inc. (SOPHE)**. Its acronym is pronounced "sew-fee." The mission of SOPHE "is to provide global leadership to the profession of health education and health promotion and to promote the health of society" (SOPHE, 2013a, ¶ 2). At the national level, SOPHE's membership includes more than 4,000 professionals from throughout the United States and many foreign countries. Members work in a variety of places, including K–12 schools, universities, medical and managed care settings, corporations, voluntary health agencies, international organizations, and federal, state, and local government. There are currently 20 SOPHE chapters covering 29 states (SOPHE, 2013a) (see **Box 8.2**). Like several of the other associations or organizations, SOPHE members have the opportunity to associate with one or more smaller working groups. In SOPHE the smaller groups are called Communities of

BOX 8.2

Practitioner's Perspective

PROFESSIONAL ASSOCIATION (INDIANA SOCIETY FOR PUBLIC HEALTH EDUCATION) Leslie Gray, B.S., CHES

CURRENT POSITION/TITLE: Health Coach/Digital Strategist
EMPLOYER: Principal Wellness Company
DEGREE/INSTITUTION/YEAR: B.S., Ball State University, 2007
MAJOR: Health Science

Job responsibilities: I'm required to provide one-on-one telephonic health coaching to at-risk individuals. These individuals have completed a health screening provided by their employer. An individual would qualify for the health coaching program if one or more risks were "flagged," such as high blood pressure, blood sugar, high body mass index (BMI), or abnormal triglycerides or cholesterol levels. As a health coach, it's my responsibility to reach out to these individuals to educate, encourage, and support healthy behavior changes in the areas of exercise, nutrition, weight loss, smoking cessation, and stress management. A health coach is very similar to a sports coach, in the sense that the coach challenges, encourages, and guides the participants towards the goal of better health. During a coaching session, I will use various techniques to move a participant towards healthy changes. Some tools I use are: the Transtheoretical model, motivational interviewing techniques, up-to-date health information, and life experiences to relate and encourage healthy choices. My department also provides resources and information on various health topics we feel would be beneficial to use during coaching sessions. At the closing of a coaching session, which typically last 10–15 minutes, I schedule for a follow-up session to continue where we left off. We would continue this process until the participant has completed all of his/her coaching sessions.

How I obtained my job: I found this position through an online job posting using the Web site www.indeed.com. I applied for two positions within the company, a Health Coach and a Health Screening Specialist. After my interviews, it was decided I would fit best as a Health Coach because I had more experience with consultations and I held the Certified Health Education Specialist (CHES) credential.

What I like most about my job: I love hearing from my participants that I've helped them move towards living a healthier lifestyle, whether they've made large or small changes. It's an amazing feeling to know that I can help change people for the better. I find my motivation from each and every participant. It reminds me why I do what I do and it helps keep my passion alive.

What I like least about my job: The least enjoyable part of my position is the ever-growing workload. Because of lower than expected sales of our wellness products and the resulting layoffs, the health coaches are carrying more work than normal. Thus, I'm seeing a higher rate of burnout and frustration among my co-workers.

The impact of Indiana Society for Public Health Education (InSOPHE): Currently, I'm the Communications Director for InSOPHE. I obtained my position through the nomination process and membership vote. It has been an invaluable experience for me. When I first pursued this volunteer position I felt underqualified, because I only had a year and a half of professional experience and a bachelor's degree. However, the new and former

BOX 8.2

continued

board members have been extremely welcoming and it's been a pleasure growing and developing in this position. I would highly encourage involvement as a member within this or a similar organization for several reasons—networking, growth and development, and continuing education opportunities. InSOPHE also offers several workshops each year at a discounted rate for members, which helps me to maintain my CHES credential. The workshops have also provided networking opportunities where I've met other health education specialists who have become my mentors. If you have extra time on your hands, I strongly encourage you to take your membership with a professional organization a step further and serve on a committee or the board. Since joining the organization and serving on the board, I have found new interests and passions for health and it has shaped me into a well-rounded health education specialist.

Recommendations for those preparing to be health education specialists: My internship experience paved the way to finding my current job. I completed my internship for a small health clinic where our services were contracted out to a gas and electric company in Northwest Indiana. I gained invaluable experience developing incentivized wellness programs for the employees, conducting evaluations of existing and preexisting wellness programs, assessing and analyzing biometric results from a companywide health screening, developing and implementing individualized fitness programs, revamping all of the marketing material, helping plan and implementing a company health fair, and conducting bone density scans with one-on-one consultations about the importance of bone health.

I would also encourage you to become CHES certified. This certification opened several doors for me, professionally and personally. It has allowed me to differentiate myself from other health science graduates and confirm my ability to carry out the responsibilities of a health education specialist. It has provided me with several development and continuing education opportunities to maintain my certification as well as helped me develop my interests in the health field. I've attended workshops and training addressing sports nutrition, smoking cessation, stress management, urologic health, health literacy, health communications, and heart health.

Not only was I able to learn about specific health issues from the workshops, I also learned the importance of networking with other health education specialists with different preparation and work experiences.

Practice (CoP). CoP "promote continuing education, networking, information exchange and advocacy among SOPHE members interested in specific topics and/or work settings. Members share a similar role or a passion about a health topic or area of practice and a desire to exchange ideas, resources, research, or solutions to common problems. In addition to networking roundtables at SOPHE Annual Meetings, all CoPs maintain listservs throughout the year to encourage dialogue and exchange" (SOPHE, 2013b, ¶ 10).

SOPHE has four primary publications. They include two peer-reviewed journals, *Health Education and Behavior* and *Health Promotion Practice*, and two newsletters called "News & Views" and "News U Can Use." *Health Education and Behavior*, published bimonthly, is a well-respected journal that is aimed primarily at the dissemination of research findings, but a typical issue also includes perspective papers, practice notes, book reviews, and SOPHE-related information. *Health Promotion Practice* is published quarterly and is "devoted to the practical application of health promotion and education. The journal is unique in its focus on critical and strategic information for professionals engaged in the practice of developing, implementing, and evaluating health promotion and disease prevention programs" (SOPHE, 2013c, ¶ 4). "In an effort to 'go green,' this newsletter is posted in the Member Communities Section online six times a year. Along with its electronic posting, it is printed and delivered to National SOPHE members' homes twice a year" (SOPHE, 2013c, ¶ 2). "News U Can Use" is a weekly electronic newsletter that includes news items, new resources, funding opportunities, and job openings. SOPHE will publish a new peer-reviewed journal, *Pedagogy in Health Promotion: The Scholarship of Teaching and Learning*, beginning in spring 2015.

Over the years, SOPHE has had a good working relationship with the APHA. SOPHE regularly held its annual meeting the weekend prior to the APHA annual meeting in the same city as the APHA. More recently, the annual meeting has moved to spring. Like several of the other associations/organizations, the annual meeting of SOPHE provides opportunities to share and receive the most recent research findings, to earn continuing education contact hours, to participate in its job bank service, and to network with other professionals.

In addition to the aforementioned items, SOPHE has been involved in some other special projects. Some examples include:

- An annual health education advocacy summit at which health education specialists receive training in advocacy techniques and get to apply their new knowledge on a trip to Capitol Hill in Washington, D.C., to discuss health-related issues with staffers from key legislative subcommittees and representatives of their congressional districts

- An annual mid-year scientific conference in the spring, which focuses on a topic of special interest to those in the health education/promotion disciplines

- Partnership in the SOPHE/AAHE Baccalaureate Program Approval Committee (SABPAC) SOPHE also has taken the leadership for and partnered with a number of other organizations and agencies on several health promotion initiatives and professional development programs that are consistent with the mission and goals of SOPHE. At the time this book was written the SOPHE was involved in projects dealing with injury prevention, emergency preparedness and environmental health, school health, health disparities, and accreditation of academic health education programs (SOPHE, 2013d).

As mentioned in the AAHE section, SOPHE and AAHE leadership have entered into a collaborative relationship to create a stronger voice for the health education profession (SOPHE, 2013e). The combined membership will "focus on advocating for quality health education and promotion programs in all areas of society including schools, health care, government, community, and international arenas" (SOPHE-AAHE, 2012).

INTERNATIONAL UNION FOR HEALTH PROMOTION AND EDUCATION

Though all of the professional associations/organizations noted already in this chapter have members from countries other than the United States, there is one professional association that is truly worldwide: the **International Union for Health Promotion and Education (IUHPE)**. There are approximately 1,500 members worldwide. The IUHPE, founded in 1951 in Paris, is a global association with a mission "to promote global health and to contribute to the achievement of equity in health between and within countries of the world" (IUHPE, 2013a, ¶ 1). The IUHPE fulfills its mission by encouraging and facilitating the free exchange of ideas, knowledge, expertise, and experience and their dissemination, and by conducting collaborative projects, both at global and regional levels (Africa, Europe, Latin America,

North America, the Northern Part of the Western Pacific and the Southwest Pacific), with major intergovernmental institutions such as the United Nations and the European Commission, global, regional and local nongovernmental organizations, national agencies, foundations, academic institutions, and a broad range of practitioners. The IUHPE "core activity" in and for health promotion includes:

- Knowledge development, sharing, transferability (Building capacity, operating as a learning organization)
- Influence (advocate for and articulate health promotion positions of great importance)
- Representation and voice (as a professional organization)
- Engaging members in knowledge making, sharing, transferability, influence and representation.

The IUHPE defined priority action areas for 2011–2016 include the social determinants of health; health promotion in sustainable development; noncommunicable disease prevention and control; and health promotion systems. An obvious distinctiveness of the IUHPE is its global reach in every continent (Lamarre, M., personal communication, July 4, 2013).

Every three years the IUHPE holds a World Conference on Health Promotion as well as regional conferences, which have become important gatherings of health promotion experts and practitioners worldwide. The most recent one was held in Pattaya, Thailand, in August 2013. The IUHPE has a "family" of journals. The official membership journal, which is published quarterly, is *Global Health Promotion* (formerly called *Promotion & Education*). "It is a multilingual journal, which publishes authoritative peer-reviewed articles and practical information for a worldwide audience of professionals interested in health promotion and health education" (IUHPE, 2013b, ¶ 2). All IUHPE members receive a print copy of *Global Health Promotion* and have access to an electronic version as well. In addition, members can purchase, at a reduced rate, any of the other six journals (*Critical Public Health, Health Promotion International, Health Education Research, International Journal of Mental Health Promotion*, or the *International Journal of Public Health*) published in association through collaborative agreements with their respective publisher (IUHPE, 2013b).

AMERICAN ACADEMY OF HEALTH BEHAVIOR

The **American Academy of Health Behavior (AAHB)** is a professional organization unlike those presented so far in this chapter. Founded in 1997, the AAHB, or just The Academy, as it is referred to, is a society of researchers and scholars in the areas of health behavior, health education, and health promotion. The Academy "was created to improve the stature of health educators by supporting and promoting quality health behavior, health education, and health promotion research conducted by health educators" (Werch, 2000, p. 3). The mission of The Academy "is to serve as the 'research home' for health behavior scholars and researchers whose primary commitment is to excellence in research and the application of research to practice to improve the public's health" (AAHB, 2013a, ¶ 2). More specifically, The Academy's goals are:

"1. Establish financial solvency and security of The Academy to assure high quality and efficiency of The Academy.

2. Foster development and dissemination of knowledge through sponsorship of scientific meetings, symposia, and publications.

3. Increase member participation to improve The Academy.

4. Recognize outstanding achievements in the areas of health behavior, health education, and health promotion research.

5. Increase national/international influence of The Academy.

6. Encourage collaborative research efforts.

7. Influence health policy and allocation of resources within agencies, private foundations, and universities.

8. Foster the research career of young scholars" (AAHB, 2013a, ¶ 4).

Individuals must apply for membership in The Academy and acceptance is based on one's area of academic preparation and level of scholarly activity. The specific qualifications for membership are listed on The Academy's Web site (see Table 8.2). The official journal of The Academy is the *American Journal of Health Behavior*. In a typical issue of this bimonthly publication, readers will find a number of databased research articles along with articles on research techniques, uses of technology for research, biographical sketches of members of The Academy, and book reviews. In January 2010, the *American Journal of Health Behavior* changed from being published in a print format to an electronic (online) only format (AAHB, 2013b).

ETA SIGMA GAMMA

Founded in 1967, **Eta Sigma Gamma (ESG)** is the national health education honorary. The idea for the organization was born when three professors from Ball State University, Drs. William Bock, Warren E. Schaller, and Robert Synovitz, were on their way to a professional conference and were talking about the need for an honorary for the discipline. Their discussion led to the formation of the organization, which has had, from its beginning, the primary purpose of furthering the professional competence and dedication of individual members of the health education/promotion profession (ESG, 1991). The ideals of the honorary are symbolized in its seal. The seal (see **Figure 8.5**) "is divided into four equilateral triangles, each carrying a symbol. A lamp of learning is in the center triangle, surrounded by an open book representing teaching, a microscope signifying research, and an outstretched hand representing service. These three elements form the basic purposes of the organization and profession; teaching, research, and service. The unifying element of these purposes is symbolized by the lamp of learning, since it is through the learning process that each purpose is achieved" (ESG, 1991, p. 2).

▶ **Figure 8.5** Seal of Eta Sigma Gamma
Source: National Office of Eta Sigma Gamma, 2000 University Ave., Muncie, IN 47306. Used with permission.

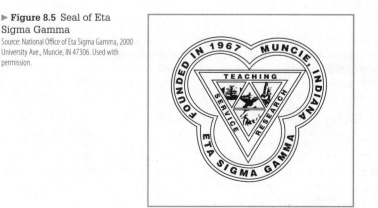

As noted in Table 8.2, the national office of Eta Sigma Gamma is located in Muncie, Indiana, on the campus of Ball State University in the Department of Physiology and Health Science. This is also where the Alpha Chapter (the first chapter of the honorary) is located. As of June 2013, there have been 129 chapters installed on university/college campuses throughout the United States. Chapters are awarded to colleges/universities based on a review and vote by the National Executive Committee of ESG on an application prepared by personnel at the petitioning college/university. From its beginnings, ESG has focused on the student members. Most individuals join the honorary when they are either undergraduate or graduate students. Membership is open to those who have a major or minor in health education and a grade point average equivalent to at least a *B–*. In fact, students can achieve membership only by affiliating through a collegiate chapter. Through their affiliation with the collegiate chapters they are eligible to apply for the awards and scholarships of the honorary. Professionals active in the discipline of health education/promotion and holding a degree can affiliate through the Chapter-At-Large (ESG, 1991) (see **Box 8.3**).

ESG regularly produces three publications: its journal, *The Health Educator*; *The Health Education Monograph Series*; and "The Vision," an online newsletter. Each of these

---

BOX 8.3

Practitioner's Perspective

PROFESSIONAL ASSOCIATION (ETA SIGMA GAMMA) Janet Kamiri

CURRENT POSITION/TITLE: Skills development specialist
EMPLOYER: Adult & Child Mental Health Center, Inc.
DEGREE/INSTITUTION/YEAR: B.A., Ball State University, 2010
MAJOR: School Health Education
MINOR: Oboe Performance

Becoming a health science major: When I started my undergraduate program, I was sure I was going to be a music teacher. I soon realized that even though I was passionate about music, it was not my professional calling. I began the search for a new major by taking career aptitude tests, talking to career counselors, and searching online for an answer. I finally asked myself, "What courses am I enrolled in that excite me? What courses have I taken that I have really enjoyed?" My favorite class in high school was health. I was currently enrolled in a personal health course at Ball State University and always found myself sharing what I learned in class with my friends. I set up an appointment to meet with a professor in the health science department to discuss options in health education. I enrolled in an introductory course for the next semester and was exposed to a variety of options in the field of health education. I decided health science would be my new major, with an emphasis on education in the school setting. I felt that this would be the ideal setting for me to help others.

Getting involved in health education: I wanted more from my education than just academics. I wanted to interact with people who had similar interests, develop professional relationships, make myself more marketable, and learn through real life, hands-on activities. I wanted to grow personally and professionally and make the most of my time at the university.

A few of my professors suggested that I look into joining Eta Sigma Gamma. In my first semester as a school health major, I attended meetings, interacted with the members, and participated in chapter events. I found that the students involved in Eta Sigma Gamma were serious and passionate about the field. They were actively applying their skills in a nonthreatening social environment. These students were creating a niche for themselves and a community to be a part of, which was especially beneficial at a large university where it is easy to get lost.

During my time as a student member of the Alpha Chapter of Eta Sigma Gamma,

BOX
8.3

continued

I was involved in many different projects and events on campus and in the community. On campus, we strengthened our program planning and implementation skills working on projects such as hosting an alcohol education program during *Spring Break Safety Week* and sponsoring activates during *Safer Sex Week* to educate students on safer sex practices and the importance of HIV awareness and testing. In the community, we cleaned our section of the highway through the Adopt-a-Highway organization, sponsored activities at the local Boys and Girls Club, and volunteered at a food bank. We also co-sponsored a "March for Babies" walk through the March of Dimes Foundation and hosted a breast cancer research fundraiser. These activities were not hypothetical. Rather, we were directly involved in improving peoples' health just as professional health education specialists are.

I served on the Executive Committee for the Alpha Chapter in the positions of Vice-President and President. Through these two positions, I gained valuable leadership skills, improved my organizational and planning skills, and learned how to balance details within the big picture.

Being a member of Eta Sigma Gamma also opened other doors for me. I attended a national student leadership conference, which helped improve my effectiveness not only as a leader on campus, but also as a teacher in the classroom. I also applied for a travel grant through Eta Sigma Gamma. This grant helped make it possible for me and another chapter member to attend the national meeting for Eta Sigma Gamma. At the meeting, we learned what other students were doing on their campuses and in their communities and gained valuable preprofessional advice from current health education specialists.

Completing an internship/student teaching: As a school health major, student teaching was required. I was fortunate, however, also to complete an internship with St. Vincent Health (a hospital system in the Indianapolis, IN area). These two experiences boosted my confidence in interacting within the professional world and broadened my skill set. I was able to integrate skills and educational approaches from two different health education settings. In both roles, I collaborated with other professionals, planned and implemented instruction, and evaluated and analyzed the effectiveness and the impact of my work.

Recommendations for those preparing to be health education specialists: First, get involved. Opportunities for personal and professional advancement are readily available for people who are willing to go beyond their academic course work. Being involved on campus and in professional associations such as Eta Sigma Gamma allows you to apply what you learn in the classroom to practical situations and provides you with more opportunities to interact with professors and students at your university as well as with professionals and students from all over the country. Preprofessional involvement in the field increases your marketability and better prepares you for a job as a health education specialist.

Second, develop relationships with leaders in the field. Find a professor with whom you connect with and create a mentor/mentee relationship with them. Professors have a wealth of knowledge about the field, a willingness to share advice that they want to share, and connections to opportunities that can benefit you both personally and professionally. Also, do not be afraid to approach professionals at conferences, especially if their work interests or inspires you. Taking the initiative to seek out information and opportunities and to build professional relationships will only benefit you in the future.

Third, do not be afraid to stand out. Working your hardest is not only personally rewarding, but also can open many doors. Dedication and passion increase your opportunities to effect positive change and improve the lives of the people you work with.

publications is distributed twice a year. Like the publications of the other associations/ organizations, these publications include the current works of the professionals in the field. However, unlike the others, only individuals who are current members of ESG can write articles for *The Health Educator* and *The Health Education Monograph Series.* Another unusual characteristic of the publications of ESG is that one entire issue of the *Monograph Series* each year is composed of articles written only by student members. This is another indication that the honorary is concerned about the preservice professional.

ASSOCIATIONS FOR DIRECTORS

There are two other professional groups that have ties to health education. They are the (1) Directors of Health Promotion and Education and (2) Society of State Directors of Health, Physical Education, and Recreation. Unlike all the other professional groups discussed, membership in these organizations is tied to one's employment. The individuals who belong to these organizations are employees of their respective state/territorial/Indian Health Service departments of health or education. There are two types of membership available in the Directors of Health Promotion and Education (DHPE)—regular/voting membership and associate membership. The number of DHPE regular/voting members is limited to the state or territorial level director of health promotion or public health education, Indian Health Services (IHS) director, or the equivalent. In states or territories where no such designation exists, the state, territorial, or IHS health official shall appoint an individual (DHPE, 2013a). Associate membership is open to individuals employed in the area of health education/promotion who support the purpose of the Association (DHPE, 2013a). The primary mission of the **Directors of Health Promotion and Education (DHPE)**, which was formed in 1946, is to strengthen "public health capacity in policy and in systems change to improve the health of all and achieve health equity (DHPE, 2013b, ¶1) .

This association is also an affiliate of the Association of State and Territorial Health Officials (ASTHO), which is the association for those who oversee state and territorial health departments. You can obtain more information about the DHPE by contacting any state or territorial department of health, or by logging on to the DHPE Web site (see the URL for this Web site in the Weblinks at the end of the chapter).

The Conference of State Directors of Health, Physical Education, and Recreation, which later changed its name to **Society of State Leaders of Health and Physical Education**, was founded in 1926 and is "a professional association whose members supervise and coordinate programs in health, physical education, and related fields within state departments of education. Associate members are those who are interested in the goals and programs of the Society who do not work within a state education agency" (The Society, 2013, ¶ 1). The mission of The Society is to use "advocacy, partnerships, professional development and resources to build capacity of school health leaders to implement effective health education and physical education policies and practices that support success in school, work and life" (The Society, 2013, ¶ 2)

You can obtain more information about The Society by contacting any state department of education or The Society Web site (see the Weblinks at the end of the chapter).

COALITIONS

Because of the large number of professional health education/promotion associations, there are times when there is a need to have a common voice for the profession. To help provide such a voice, coalitions of health associations/organizations have been created. The most prominent coalition is the Coalition of National Health Education Organizations, USA.

The **Coalition of National Health Education Organizations, USA (CNHEO)** is a non-profit federation of organizations dedicated to advancing the health education/promotion profession. The coalition is comprised of representatives (delegates and alternates) from six national associations/organizations with identifiable health education specialist memberships and ongoing health education/promotion programs. The associations/organizations included are the American College Health Association; the American Public Health Association, Public Health Education and Health Promotion Section; the American Public Health Association, School Health Education and Services Section; the American School Health Association; Directors of Health Promotion and Education; Eta Sigma Gamma; and the Society for Public Health Education, Inc.

The CNHEO was formed on March 1, 1972, after a series of three meetings in 1971 and 1972 to determine the feasibility of such an organization. The primary mission of the coalition is "the mobilization of the resources of the Health Education Profession in order to expand and improve health education, regardless of the setting" (CNHEO, 2013a, ¶ 2).

The work of the CNHEO is financed by funds obtained from coalition member organizations, public and private agencies, and contributions and gifts from individuals. Over the years, the working relationship of the member organizations has been outlined in the *Working Agreement of the CNHEO*. Also included in this document are the purposes of the coalition (CNHEO, 2006, ¶ 2).

1. To strengthen communications among the member organizations as well as between the health education profession and policy makers, other professions, and consumers

2. To develop, implement, and evaluate a shared vision and strategic plan for health education and the health education profession

3. To educate policy-makers on the need for federal and state public policies that support healthy behaviors and healthy communities

4. To collaborate on common issues, problems, and concerns related to health education

5. Increase the visibility of the health education profession and its member organizations

Unlike the other organizations and groups discussed in this chapter, the CNHEO functions with no paid staff members or permanent location. "The CNHEO carries on business by means of e-mail communication, monthly conference calls, and periodic face-to-face meetings during member organization conferences. Through these means it has made significant progress in addressing its purposes and priorities" (Capwell, 2004, p. 13). Since its inception, the CNHEO has operationalized its purposes in a number of ways, contributing to the growth of the profession. Below is a list of some of the recent activities and accomplishments in which the CNHEO has been involved. (Note: Some items in this list are discussed in greater detail in other chapters of this book when they apply to the content of that chapter.)

- Creation of position papers on topics of importance to the profession (e.g., preparation of elementary school teachers in the area of health education, and the strengthening of health education in the public health arena).

- Cosponsoring two invitational conferences in 1995 (NCHEC & CNHEO, 1996) and 2002 (CNHEO, 2003) to examine the status and future of the health education/promotion profession. These conferences led to the creation of goals and recommendations for the profession for the 21st century, and commitments by member organizations to lead or assist in addressing the recommendations (CNHEO, 2003). (See Chapter 10 for more on the future of health education/promotion.)

- Creation of a unified "Code of Ethics for the Health Education Profession" (see Chapter 5 and Appendix A).

- Cosponsoring the annual National Health Education Advocacy Summit that began in 1998. The purpose of the summit is to increase the capacity of health education specialists to engage in effective advocacy for a common health education/promotion agenda. At the summit attendees receive policy advocacy training and make legislative visits to educate congresspersons on priority issues in health education (CNHEO, 2013b).

- Support of the *Health Education Advocate* Web site. "The mission of the *Health Education Advocate* is to provide a central, timely source of advocacy information related to the field of health education and health promotion" (CNHEO, 2013b, ¶ 1). (See Weblinks at the end of this chapter for the URL of the Web site.)

More information about CNHEO can be obtained by contacting the office of any of the member organizations or by logging on to the CNHEO Web site. The URL for this site is presented in the Weblinks at the end of the chapter.

▷ Joining a Professional Health Association/Organization

Becoming a member of a professional organization is not difficult. With the exception of a few of the associations/organizations previously noted (CNHEO, AAHB, ESG, and DHPE and The Society), membership in a professional organization can be obtained by completing an application form (available from any of the organizations, included in many of the official publications, or found at the organization's Web site [see Table 8.2]) and sending the money with the desired length and category of membership (different rates apply to different types of membership—for example, student, professional, retired) to the association/organization of choice. Most individuals join a professional association/organization for a year at a time. Some associations, however, provide multiple-year memberships at a reduced rate or even a lifetime membership. In general, the cost of a membership in a state or regional association/organization is separate from and less than a membership in a national association/organization. If you are interested in joining a state or local association/organization, you can usually contact its national office to find out whom to contact locally.

▷ The Certification Body of the Health Education/Promotion Profession: National Commission for Health Education Credentialing, Inc.

The NCHEC (pronounced N-check) is unlike any other organization that has been discussed in this chapter. The NCHEC is not a professional organization that health education specialists join, but rather the organization responsible for the individual credentialing of health education specialists, thus it has no members. The history of the development of the NCHEC was presented in Chapter 6, while the information presented here is to give the reader an understanding of how the NCHEC operates.

"The mission of NCHEC is to enhance the professional practice of Health Education by promoting and sustaining a credentialed body of Health Education Specialists. To meet this mission, the NCHEC certifies health education specialists, promotes professional development, and strengthens professional preparation and practice" (NCHEC, 2013a, ¶ 1).

The charge of NCHEC "is to develop and administer national competency-based examinations; develop standards for professional preparation; and promote professional development through continuing education for health education professionals" (NCHEC, 2013a, ¶ 2). Four boards and the NCHEC staff carry out the work of the NCHEC. The boards include the Board of Commissioners [BOC], the Division Board for Certification of Health Education Specialists, the Division Board of Professional Development, and the Division Board for Professional Preparation and Practice. The four boards meet monthly via conference calls and have one or two face-to-face meetings each year.

The BOC, which is comprised of 11 commissioners, is the governing board and the board responsible for all the NCHEC activities (NCHEC, 2013a). The three division boards address the three activities noted in the NCHEC's mission statement: certification, professional development, and professional preparation. Those who hold either the CHES or the MCHES credential elect the directors and commissioners of the various boards, with the exception of one. The lone exception is the public member of the BOC, who is appointed by the BOC after a call for nominations. In addition, the elected directors and commissioners are volunteers and must hold an active CHES or MCHES credential (NCHEC, 2013a).

The primary responsibility of the Division Board for Certification of Health Education Specialists (DBCHES) is to create the two examinations of NCHEC—the CHES exam and the MCHES exam. More specifically, DBCHES, which is currently composed of 12 directors, along with the guidance of Professional Examination Services (PES) assures a periodic review and evaluation of certification and examination processes; recommends policies and procedures for administering the CHES and MCHES examinations; writes the examination questions; creates the exams; determines the pass point (i.e., minimum score on the examinations required to obtain the certification), and ensures that NCHEC's competency testing meets acceptable standards (NCHEC, 2013a).

The work of the Division Board for Professional Development (DBPD), which is composed of seven directors, is to oversee the recertification and annual renewal procedures for the two credentials (NCHEC, 2013a). "More specifically, the DBPD recommends policies and procedures related to the designation of continuing education providers, recertification and the annual renewal of CHES and MCHES; recommends fees for recertification, annual renewal and provider designation; and assures that the processes are monitored and periodically evaluated" (NCHEC, 2013b, ¶ 5).

The Division Board for Professional Preparation and Practice (DBPPP), which is also composed of seven directors, is responsible for promoting professional preparation (NCHEC, 2013c). "More specifically, the DBPPP works with colleges, universities and accrediting agencies to improve professional preparation programs and promote best practices in health education settings; and monitors and updates the certification application and eligibility review process" (NCHEC, 2013c, ¶ 5).

The CHES examination was given for the first time in 1990. The first MCHES examination was offered in 2011. Both examinations are offered twice a year—one in April and one in October—at approximately 120 locations throughout the United States. The examinations are each 165 questions long and candidates have three hours to complete the exam. The eligibility criteria to take the examinations are presented in **Box 8.4**.

NCHEC produces several different publications. The *NCHEC News* is NCHEC's newsletter for all CHES and MCHES (NCHEC, 2010a). The newsletter is published three times a year and is mailed to each current certification holder. Past issues of the newsletter are

Eligibility Criteria to Sit for the CHES and MCHES Examinations

CHES Examination

Eligibility to take the CHES examination is based exclusively on academic qualifications. An individual is eligible to take the examination if he or she has:

A bachelor's, master's, or doctoral degree from an accredited institution of higher education; AND one of the following:

- An official transcript (including course titles) that clearly shows a major in health education (e.g., Health Education, Community Health Education, Public Health Education, School Health Education, etc.). Degree/major must explicitly be in a discipline of "Health Education." OR
- An official transcript that reflects at least 25 semester hours or 37 quarter hours of course work (with a grade "c" or better) with specific preparation addressing the Seven Areas of Responsibility and Competency for Health Educators

http://www.nchec.org/exam/eligible/ches/

MCHES Exam Eligibility

The MCHES exam eligibility includes both academic and experience requirements.

Exam Eligibility
- For CHES: A minimum of the past five (5) continuous years in active status as a CHES.
- For Non-CHES or CHES with fewer than five years active status AND five years experience:
- A master's degree or higher in Health Education, Public Health Education, School Health Education, Community Health Education, etc.
- OR a Master's degree or higher with an academic transcript reflecting at least 25 semester hours (37 quarter hours) of course work in which the Seven Areas of Responsibility of Health Educators were addressed.
- Five (5) years of documented experience as a health education specialist

To verify applicants must submit:

1. Two verification forms from a current or past manager/supervisor, and/or a leader in a health education professional organization.
2. A current curriculum vitae/resume

In the verification form it must be indicated, and in the curriculum vitae/resume it must clearly be shown, that the applicant has been engaged in the Areas of Responsibility for at least the past five years (experience may be prior to completion of graduate degree).

http://www.nchec.org/exam/eligible/mches/

Source: The National Commission for Health Education Credentialing, Inc. (NCHEC). By permission.

available online at the NCHEC Web site (NCHEC, 2013c). NCHEC also publishes documents that are useful for those working in professional preparation programs, those offering continuing education opportunities, and those individuals preparing to take either the CHES or the MCHES examination. Included in these publications are a companion guide for the examinations (NCHEC, 2010a) and the competency-based framework (NCHEC, SOPHE, & AAHE, 2010). As noted, this later publication is a joint publication of NCHEC and its publishing partners AAHE and SOPHE. This document was generated from the findings of the

Health Education Job Analysis—2010 (HEJA-2010) and has "implications for professional preparation, credentialing, and professional development of all health education specialists regardless of the setting in which they are employed" (NCHEC, 2010b ¶ 1).

More information about NCHEC can be obtained by contacting the NCHEC office, 1541 Alta Drive, Suite 303, Whitehall, PA 18052-5642, Phone: (484) 223-0770, Toll-Free: (888) 624-3248, Facsimile: (800) 813-0727) or by logging on to the NCHEC Web site. The URL for this site is presented in the Weblinks at the end of the chapter.

Summary

This chapter discussed the various health agencies, associations, and organizations with which the profession of health education/promotion interacts. The agencies/associations/organizations were presented within three major categories: governmental, quasi-governmental, and nongovernmental. The primary emphasis of the chapter was to present information about a subcategory of the nongovernmental associations/organizations, the professional associations/organizations. Those discussed included the American Academy of Health Behavior; the American Alliance for Health, Physical Education, Recreation and Dance; the American Association for Health Education; the American Public Health Association; the American College Health Association; the American School Health Association; the National Wellness Institute, Inc.; the Society for Public Health Education, Inc.; the International Union for Health Promotion and Education; Eta Sigma Gamma; and associations for directors (Directors of Health Promotion and Education, and the Society of State Leaders of Health and Physical Education). Also, information about a coalition—the Coalition of National Health Education Organizations, USA—and information on how to become a member of a professional association/organization was presented. The chapter concluded with an overview of the National Commission for Health Education Credentialing, Inc., and the eligibility criteria for taking the CHES or MCHES examination.

Review Questions

1. Define and explain the differences among the following types of agencies: *governmental health agency, quasi-governmental health agency,* and *nongovernmental health agency.*

2. At what levels do governmental agencies exist? Provide an example of an agency at each level.

3. What are the four primary activities of most voluntary health agencies? Give an example of each.

4. What are the purposes of a professional association/organization?

5. What are the benefits derived from membership in a professional association/organization? Why should students become members?

6. What is the oldest and largest professional health association in the United States?

7. Name two professional health associations/organizations that focus their efforts on work settings for health education specialists. Name two other professional health associations/organizations that are not as focused on a work setting.

8. What is the name of the health education honorary? Where was it founded and where is the national office located? In general, where are the chapters of the honorary found?

9. What makes the AAHB different from the other professional organizations/associations presented in this chapter?

10. What is a coalition? Name one health education coalition. What is the primary purpose of this coalition? What are some of the recent activities of the coalition?

11. How does a person become a member of a professional organization?

12. What is the NCHEC? How is it different from the other organizations presented in the chapter?

▷ Case Study

Hilary has been employed by the XYZ voluntary health organization for almost a year now. The job has really gone well. She enjoys the work, likes her coworkers, and has been able to use much of what she learned during her health education/promotion professional preparation program. Just recently the organization received word that it had been awarded a $15,000 grant to conduct a health education/promotion program for a local senior citizens group on living a healthier life. Her supervisor, Ms. Denison, has given Hilary the responsibility to take the leadership for the project. One restriction on the use of the money is that the program must be planned by a representative group from local voluntary and governmental health education/promotion organizations. Therefore, Hilary's first task is to invite local groups to send a representative to the initial planning meeting. Hilary has set the goal of having seven different health voluntary and governmental agencies involved. If you were Hilary, which organizations would you invite to the initial meeting? Justify why you would select these seven.

▷ Critical Thinking Questions

1. For a number of years, many practicing health education specialists have pushed for a single professional health education/promotion association that would bring together many of the existing associations (i.e., ACHA, ASHA, SOPHE) so that health education/promotion would have a single professional association voice. Would you be in favor of or against combining all the health education/promotion professional associations into a single association? Defend your response. As part of your response, indicate what you think are the strengths and weaknesses of your position.

2. In this chapter you have read about a number of different professional health education/promotion associations. On graduating from college few new professionals have enough money to join several different professional groups. Assuming that you have enough money to join one national professional group on graduation, what association/organization would it be? Explain the reasoning you would use to select the one organization to join.

3. One of the major issues facing many professional health education/promotion associations is retaining members from year to year. Some members do not renew their membership because of cost. Others do not renew because they do not feel that they receive enough benefits. After conducting a membership survey, a professional health association

has decided to revamp the benefits provided to members. Assume that you have been appointed as a student member to the executive committee of the professional association and that the president of the association has charged the committee with revamping the membership benefits package. Each member of the executive committee has been asked to create a list of benefits. What would be on your list? Explain why you selected each item.

4. Throughout this book you have been introduced to the work of health education specialists. This chapter focused on the different professional organizations of our profession. We also presented information on the NCHEC. We stated that being a member of a professional organization is different than becoming certified as a health education specialist. Compare and contrast what you see to be the benefits of membership in a professional organization and becoming a CHES or MCHES. Aside from the financial costs, do you see any drawbacks of membership and certification?

▷ Activities

1. Closely examine one professional health association/organization and prepare a Power-Point presentation, poster, or other visual presentation on the history of that association/organization.

2. Interview two health education/promotion faculty members at your school and ask them the following:
   - Do they belong to any professional health education associations/organizations?
   - If they belong, why?
   - What benefits do they see in belonging to them?
   - What association/organization would they recommend that you join?

3. Does your school have a chapter of ESG? If not, make an appointment with the department head/chairperson to inquire about the possibility of starting one on your campus.

4. Write a one-page paper using the following two sentences to start the paper: "If I could join one professional health association/organization, it would be _____. My reasons for choosing that association/organization are _____."

5. Visit the Web site of the Coalition of National Health Education Organizations (CNHEO) (http://www.cnheo.org). Once at the site, read the "21st Century" reports: (1) *The Health Education Profession in the Twenty-First Century Progress Report 1995–2001*, and (2) *Coalition of National Health Education Organization's 2nd Invitational Conference: Improving the Nation's Health Through Health Education—A Vision for the 21st Century*. After reading the reports, create your own list of five activities that you feel the profession should engage in during the next 10 years to move the profession forward. Provide a brief (i.e., a couple of paragraphs) rationale for why you included each activity on your list.

▷ Weblinks

1. **http://www.astho.org**
   The Association for State and Territorial Health Officials (ASTHO)
   This is the Web site for the ASTHO, which is the national nonprofit organization representing the state and territorial public health agencies of the United States, the U.S.

territories, and the District of Columbia. Among other items, this site includes links to each of the state and territorial health departments.

2. **http://www.cancer.org/**

American Cancer Society (ACS)

This is the home page for ACS. The site presents the most up-to-date information on cancer, including treatment and prevention. The site also provides information about the ACS and the resources it can provide for cancer survivors and program planners.

3. **http://www.cnheo.org**

Coalition of National Health Education Organizations (CNHEO)

This is the home page for CNHEO. At the site, you will find information about all the member organizations, as well as the coalition's mission, goals, *Working Agreement*, the "Code of Ethics for the Health Education Profession," and the "21st Century" reports.

4. **http://www.americanheart.org**

American Heart Association (AHA)

This is the home page for the AHA. The AHA provides health education specialists with a wealth of information and materials about many of the cardiovascular diseases and stroke.

5. **http://www.lungusa.org**

American Lung Association (ALA)

This is the home page for the ALA. The ALA provides information about various lung diseases, including asthma, chronic obstructive pulmonary disease (COPD), and lung cancer; and stopping smoking resources.

6. **http://www.welcoa.org**

The Wellness Council of America (WELCOA)

This is the home page for the WELCOA. This site provides a variety of resources for those interested in worksite wellness programs.

7. **http://www.cdc.gov/**

Centers for Disease Control and Prevention (CDC)

This is the home page of the CDC. This Web site includes information for the lay public (i.e., traveler's health and emergency preparedness) as well as information to assist health education specialists (i.e., health topics A–Z, CDC recommendations, *MMWR*, and special funded initiatives).

8. **http://www.healtheducationadvocate.org/**

Health Education Advocate

This is the homepage of the Health Education Advocate that is sponsored by the CNHEO. This site provides up-to-date advocacy information for health education specialists, as well as links to other advocacy sites.

9. **http://www.nchec.org**

National Commission for Health Education Credentialing, Inc.

This is the homepage for NCHEC. At this site you can find out more about the CHES and MCHES examinations, order publications to help you prepare for the examinations, and get up-to-date on individual credentialing.

(Note: See Table 8.2 for the URLs of the various professional associations or organizations discussed in this chapter.)

References

American Academy for Health Behavior (AAHB). (2013a). *About AAHB.* Retrieved June 12, 2013, from http://aahb.wildapricot.org/About_AAHB.

American Academy for Health Behavior (AAHB). (2013b). *Publications.* Retrieved June 12, 2013, from http://www.ajhb.org/.

American Alliance for Health, Physical Education, Recreation and Dance (AAHPERD). (2013a). *Press Release: American Alliance for Health, Physical Education, Recreation and Dance Unifies As One.* Retrieved June 19, 2013, from http://www.aahperd.org/pressroom/aahperd-unification.cfm.

American Alliance for Health, Physical Education, Recreation and Dance (AAHPERD). (2013b). *Who we are.* Retrieved June 18, 2013, from http://www.aahperd.org/about/.

American Association for Health Education (AAHE). (2010). *About AAHE 2010.* Retrieved August 30, 2010, from http://www.aahperd.org/aahe/about/results.cfm.

American Association for Health Education (AAHE). (2013a). *AAHE publications.* Retrieved June 16, 2013, from http://www.aahperd.org/aahe/publications/.

American Association for Health Education (AAHE). (2013b). *Professional networking.* Retrieved June 16, 2013, from http://www.aahperd.org/aahe/proNetworking/.

American Cancer Society (ACS). (2007). *National Health Education Standards* (2nd ed.). Atlanta, GA: Author.

American College Health Association (ACHA). (2013a). *About ACHA.* Retrieved June 11, 2013, from http://www.acha.org/About_ACHA/Who_We_Are.cfm.

American College Health Association (ACHA). (2013b). *Membership.* Retrieved June 11, 2013, from http://www.acha.org/Membership/index.cfm.

American College Health Association (ACHA). (2013c). *Publications.* Retrieved June 11, 2013, from http://www.acha.org/Publications/JACH.cfm.

American Public Health Association (APHA). (2013a). *About us.* Retrieved on June 11, 2013, from: http://www.apha.org/about/.

American Public Health Association (APHA). (2013b). *Member groups and state affiliates.* Retrieved on June 11, 2013, from: http://www.apha.org/membergroups/sections/.

American Public Health Association (APHA). (2013c). *Publications & advertising.* Retrieved June 11, 2013, from http://www.apha.org/publications/.

American Public Health Association (APHA). (n.d). *The American Public Health Association: Keeping public health in the public eye for more than a century.* Washington, DC: Author.

American School Health Association (ASHA). (1976). *History of the American School Health Association, 1926–1976.* Kent, OH: Author.

American School Health Association (ASHA). (2013a). *ASHA & school health.* Retrieved June 11, 2013, from http://www.ashaweb.org/i4a/pages/index.cfm?pageid=3280.

American School Health Association (ASHA). (2013b). *Journal of School Health.* Retrieved June 11, 2013, from http://www.ashaweb.org/i4a/pages/index.cfm?pageid=3341.

Anderson, G. (1985). AAHPERD from the beginning. *Journal of Physical Education, Recreation and Dance, 56* (4), 94–96.

Capwell, E. M. (2004). Coalition of national health education organizations. *California Journal of Health Promotion, 2* (1), 12–15.

Coalition of National Health Education Organizations (CNHEO). (2003). *21st Century Report.* Retrieved September 1, 2010, from http://www.cnheo.org/index.html.

Coalition of National Health Education Organizations (CNHEO). (2006). *Working agreement.* Retrieved September 1, 2010, from http://www.cnheo.org/index.html.

Coalition of National Health Education Organizations (CNHEO). (2013a). *About us.* Retrieved June 13, 2013, from http://cnheo.org/aboutus.html.

Coalition of National Health Education Organizations (CNHEO). (2013b). *Health Education Advocate.* Retrieved June 13, 2013, from http://cnheo.org/hea.html.

Director of Health Promotion and Education (DHPE). (2013a). *DHPE membership.* Retrieved June 13, 2013, from https://dhpe.site-ym.com/?page=Membership_Main.

Director of Health Promotion and Education (DHPE). (2013b). About DHPE. Retrieved June 13, 2013, from https://dhpe.site-ym.com/?page=About_Main.

Eta Sigma Gamma (ESG). (1991, November). *Eta Sigma Gamma*. Muncie, IN: Author.

Foundation for Advancement of Health Education (2013). *Press release: JHETT call for reviewers.*

Heymann, D. L. (Ed.). (2009). *Control of communicable diseases manual* (19th ed.). Washington, DC: American Public Health Association.

International Union for Health Promotion and Education (IUHPE). (2013a). *About IUHPE.* Retrieved June 12, 2013, from http://www.iuhpe.org/index.html?page=5&lang=en.

International Union for Health Promotion and Education (IUHPE). (2013b). *The IUHPE journal family.* IUHPE. Retrieved June 12, 2013, from http://www.iuhpe.org/index.html?page=18&lang=en.

Jackson, R. J. (2011). *Designing Healthy Communities.* Hoboken, NJ: Wiley & Sons, Inc.

McKenzie, J. F., Pinger, R. R., & Kotecki, J. E. (2012). *An introduction to community health* (7th ed.). Sudbury, MA: Jones & Bartlett Publishers.

National Commission for Health Education Credentialing, Inc., & Coalition of National Health Education Organizations, USA (NCHEC & CNHEO). (1996). The health education profession in the 21st century: Setting the stage. *Journal of School Health, 66* (8), 291–298.

National Commission for Health Education Credentialing, Inc. (NCHEC). (2010a). *The Health Education Specialist: A companion guide for professional excellence* (6th ed.). Whitehall, PA: Author.

National Commission for Health Education Credentialing, Inc. (NCHEC). (2010b). *Health educator job analysis—2010: Press release.* Retrieved September 2, 2010, from http://www.nchec.org/news/what/#BM_NCH-MR-TAB2-169.

National Commission for Health Education Credentialing, Inc. (NCHEC). (2013a). *Mission and purpose.* Retrieved June 13, 2013, from http://www.nchec.org/aboutnchec/mission/.

National Commission for Health Education Credentialing, Inc. (NCHEC). (2013b). *What's new at NCHEC.* Retrieved June 13, 2013, from http://www.nchec.org/news/what/.

National Commission for Health Education Credentialing, Inc. (NCHEC). (2013c). *The NCHEC news bulletin.* Retrieved June 13, 2013, from http://www.nchec.org/news/bullet/.

National Commission for Health Education Credentialing, Inc. (NCHEC), Society for Public Health Education (SOPHE), & American Association for Health Education (AAHE). (2010). *A competency-based framework for health education specialists—2010.* Whitehall, PA: Author.

National Wellness Institute (NWI). (2013a). *History.* Retrieved June 11, 2013, from http://www.nationalwellness.org/?page=About_NWI.

National Wellness Institute (NWI). (2013b). *National Wellness Institute Member Benefits.* Retrieved June 11, 2013, from http://www.nationalwellness.org/?page=MemberBenefits.

Nolte, A. E. (1985). Health education: An alliance commitment. *Journal of Physical Education, Recreation and Dance, 56* (4), 107–108.

Random House, Inc. (2010). Philanthropy. In Dictionary.com *Unabridged.* Retrieved August 30, 2010, from http://dictionary.reference.com/browse/philanthropy.

Society for Public Health Education (SOPHE). (2013a). *About SOPHE.* Retrieved June 19, 2013, from http://www.sophe.org/mission.cfm.

Society for Public Health Education (SOPHE). (2013b). *Member communities.* Retrieved June 19, 2013, from http://www.sophe.org/community.cfm.

Society for Public Health Education (SOPHE). (2013c). *Programs & initiatives.* Retrieved June 19, 2013, from http://www.sophe.org/programs.cfm.

Society for Public Health Education (SOPHE). (2013d). *Publications & resources.* Retrieved June 19, 2013, from http://www.sophe.org/Publications_Resources.cfm.

Society for Public Health Education (SOPHE). (2013e). *Unification of the health education profession: SOPHE-AAHE updates.* Retrieved June 21, 2013, from http://www.sophe.org/SOPHE_AAHE.cfm.

Society for Public Health Education, Inc. (n.d.). *Health education professional organizations and you* (a handout). Washington, DC: Author.

SOPHE-AAHE. (2012). *SOPHE-AAHE joint statement, July 17, 2012.* Retrieved June 21, 2013, from http://www.sophe.org/Sophe/PDF/Statement_July17_final.pdf.

Society of State Leaders of Health and Physical Education (The Society). (2013). *About us.* Retrieved June 13, 2013, from http://www.thesociety.org/about.asp.

Werch, C. E. (2000). Editorial: What use, the American Academy of Health Behavior? *American Journal of Health Behavior, 24* (1), 3–5.

Young, K. J., & Boling, W. (2004). Improving the quality of professional life: Benefits of health education and promotion association membership. *California Journal of Health Promotion, 2* (1), 39–44.

The Literature of Health Education/ Promotion

Chapter Objectives

After reading this chapter and answering the questions at the end,
you should be able to:

- Describe the difference between a *primary*, a *secondary*, a *tertiary*, and a *popular press* literature source.

- Write an abstract or a summary of an article from a refereed journal.

- Critique a journal article using a logical sequence of questions.

- Become familiar with the most commonly used journals in the field of health education/promotion.

- Identify the most commonly used online computerized databases for finding health education/promotion information.

- Locate an article related to some aspect of health education/promotion using an online database.

- Conduct an Internet search for information about a health-related topic using one of the Web site URLs listed in the chapter.

- Critique the validity of the information obtained from searching a site on the Internet.

In her work as a health education specialist, Georgia administers a federally funded statewide center that distributes prevention information on alcohol, tobacco, and other drugs. Materials in the center include monographs containing the results of research studies on possible treatment protocols and prevention interventions; prevention and education materials from a variety of federal, state, and nonprofit agencies; information on evidence-based practice in both prevention and treatment; and an extensive video library. Almost daily, she and her staff receive requests for information from law enforcement agencies, legislators and organizational policy makers, community groups, school personnel, counselors, nonprofit organizations, treatment professionals, state agencies, churches, and individual patrons.

Over the past three or four years, more university health education/promotion students have been visiting to acquire materials for class projects, research studies, or potential thesis topics. These students often request Georgia or her staff to recommend the most up-to-date primary and secondary source materials and the most reputable Web sites related to substance abuse prevention.

After reading and digesting the information contained in this chapter, you should be able to address questions similar to those received by the staff of the center previously described. Serving as a resource for health information is a critical skill that must be acquired by those practicing as health education specialists.

The amount of information about any given topic is growing at almost an exponential rate. Terms such as *information overload* and *information burnout* are being heard more and more. Arguably, the area in which information is growing fastest and in which there is tremendous public interest is health. People today seem obsessed with gathering information about such health topics as diet, exercise, stress management, vitamins, drugs, sexuality, depression, safety, disease, violence prevention, healthcare policies, health insurance options, and the cost of medical procedures or prescription drugs.

The increasing demand for information, coupled with the fact that information is being produced at an ever greater rate, creates added need for health education specialists (see **Box 9.1**). Two of the major responsibilities of a health education specialist, as discussed in Chapter 6, involve being a resource person for health information (Responsibility 6) and communicating to others about health education needs, concerns, and resources (Responsibility 7) (see **Figure 9.1**). To perform these tasks, the health education specialist must have the skills to find information, evaluate the source of the information to determine its credibility, disseminate the information to consumers through the appropriate channels, and explain the meaning of the information in an understandable manner. This chapter introduces prospective health education students to the most common sources of health-related information used by health education specialists. It also describes how to access the information from these sources. When searching for information, it is always wise to seek the assistance of a reference librarian should questions arise.

▷ Types of Information Sources

When accessing information, it is important to note whether the source is primary, secondary, or tertiary. **Primary sources** of data or information are published studies or eyewitness accounts written by the people who actually conducted the experiments or observed the events in question. A journal that publishes original manuscripts only after they have been read by a panel of experts in the field (referees) and recommended for publication is termed a **refereed or peer-reviewed journal**. Examples of primary sources are research articles written by the researcher(s); personal records (autobiographies); podcasts or video/audio recordings of actual lectures (which may also be secondary sources depending on whether the information presented is the speakers' own work [primary] or a compilation of the works of self and others [secondary]); speeches, debates, or events; official records of legislative sessions or minutes of community meetings; newspaper eyewitness accounts; and annual reports.

Of note is the fact that some refereed/peer-reviewed journals now are published only in electronic format. These publications, known as **"open access" journals**, have articles that come in a variety of reader access levels. Some articles are immediately available to individual subscribers or subscribing institutions; others allow delayed access to articles for

USE OF HEALTH LITERATURE Stephanie Wheeler, B.S., CHES

DEGREE: B.S. in Health Promotion from Boise State University, 2004

CURRENT POSITION: Health and Wellness Center (HAWC) Health Educator

INSTITUTION: Minot Air Force Base, Minot, ND

EMPLOYER: Contract employee of the USAF

How I obtained my job: This position was obtained through sheer determination. At the time I applied, the company that held the central contract required a longer work history in the field than I possessed. After multiple contacts with the company (some may call it pestering) and going through extensive phone interviews, I was hired. Then the process of proving my abilities began.

How I utilize health education and the literature in health in my job: Perseverance is the key to health promotion. If one avenue does not lead the way to success, you must go back to the planning process and reevaluate. When a plan or program does not go as well as one would hope, there is no need to scrap the entire project. Take the pieces that worked well and build from them. Always go back to the original goal and make sure that it is a valid goal for both you and the population. One advantage to working for a military installation is that I have access to health data. At each chosen interval we can track changes to see if the desired outcome is surfacing. Additionally, we use surveys and sample groups to determine what was useful and what was not. Utilizing data from other studies can streamline efforts to what has worked for others and avoid their mistakes. While we all want our own ideas to be successful, it is ethically sound to research heavily before funding the plan. We have limited resources, which must be stretched maximally.

What I like most about my job: Seeing the joy of individuals and groups as they meet and exceed their goals is the best part of what I do. I love getting e-mails, phone calls, or visits from people telling me that they have learned from me and it has changed their life. Hearing newfound confidence in their voice and learning that they are sharing that information and enthusiasm with others are what health promotion is about.

What I like least about my job: Early in my career there was a particular point when I was contemplating whether or not I was making a difference. Often, we are planting the seeds without ever having the chance to see what the full harvest will yield. My mentor at the time asked me a question that seemed odd at the time. She asked me, "If your job was to make pigs fly and only one flew, would you have failed?" At the time, I recall thinking that it was a slightly silly question. Now I see her point. We cannot expect immediate results of our effort. We will not always see the return on investment (ROI). We must have faith that everything, every person, is worth our effort.

Recommendations for those preparing to be health education specialists: Anyone going into health education/promotion needs to have the ability to take criticism. Behavior change is difficult and sometimes painful. You may be the perceived source of pain! Criticism is opportunity for change for both me and my clients. Often, our greatest aggravation can become our stepping stone to the best success.

The role of health education specialists in the future: The future of HP means getting out into the community in a more assertive fashion. This does not mean that we will enter homes and exchange their cake for broccoli. However, the idea that providing information and hoping that people will show up to learn it is an old thought process. Rather than being entrenched in the medical community, health education specialists will be in more areas that the general population accesses such as grocery stores and shopping centers.

▶ **Figure 9.1** Health education specialists often make presentations to community groups.

anyone with an Internet connection; and some of the publishing sites have a mixture of the two availability types. The "open access" designation means that the article is copyrighted but generally can be used more liberally than articles with more traditional copyrights. Databases such as BioMed Central (biomedcentral.com) are repositories of these types of journals, many of which are new and most of which use scientists who have been editorial board members on highly prestigious paper-based journals for their editorial review boards. The increased cost of paper-based journals and publishing company charges will undoubtedly expand the number of open access primary sources of information in the future.

Secondary sources are usually written by someone who was not present at the event or did not participate as part of the study team. The value of these sources is that they often provide a summary of several related studies or chronicle a history or sequence of events. The writers of secondary sources may also provide editorial comments or alternative interpretations of the study or event. Secondary sources often provide a bibliography of primary sources. Examples of secondary sources are journal review articles, editorials, and non-eyewitness accounts of events occurring in the community, region, or nation.

Although refereed or peer-reviewed journals usually publish primary source articles, they occasionally contain secondary source articles. The types of secondary source articles most likely to be found in a refereed journal are articles summarizing the results of several studies, editorials, or positions deemed important enough (by a panel of expert reviewers) to be interesting and useful to those who read the journal.

Tertiary sources contain information that has been distilled and collected from primary and secondary sources. Examples include handbooks, informational pamphlets or brochures from governmental organizations (or hospitals, or national nongovernmental agencies such as the American Cancer Society or March of Dimes), newsletters such as the University of California's Berkeley Wellness Letter, almanacs, encyclopedias, fact books, dictionaries, abstracts, and other reference tools. At this stage, information from such sources is accepted as fact by the scientific community. The operative word in the preceding sentence is *fact*. Information that has no documentation and is laced with opinion or intended for marketing a service or product is not considered a tertiary source; publications of that type are classified as popular press sources.

A fourth source of health information, **popular press publications**, is probably the most difficult to check for credibility. Popular press publications range from weekly summary-type magazines (e.g., *Time, Newsweek, U.S. News & World Report*), regular articles in newspapers (e.g. Dr Oz's column), and newspaper supplements (e.g., *Parade*) to monthly magazines (e.g., *Reader's Digest, Better Homes and Gardens, Esquire*) and tabloids (e.g., *The Star*). At times, any of these may contain a primary source of information (as in an interview). Most often, however, they are secondary sources at best. Often, articles in the popular press include opinions or editorials that express the bias of the author or the editor of the publication. Popular press articles should be heavily scrutinized as to the source of the information before being cited as authentic and accurate.

Before concluding this discussion, it is important to note that, with the exception of open access journals, no Web site references were included in the literature types described. This is because Web sites are generally not refereed. Just about anyone can publish an article on the Web without an impartial reader or group of readers reviewing it beforehand. To be sure, Web pages are often wonderful sources of information, but they can just as often be replete with bad information. A discussion of methods to determine the accuracy of information on the Web is included later in this chapter. Sorting through the maze of health information can be a daunting task, even for the most skilled health education specialist. To equip the health education specialist for assuming the responsibilities of providing and disseminating information, several tasks need to be mastered. The next several sections of this chapter are designed to provide background for the student in: (1) identifying the components of a research article; (2) critically reading a research article; (3) ascertaining the accuracy of the information in articles that are non-research based or are from secondary or popular press sources; (4) writing an abstract or a summary of a journal article; (5) identifying and locating primary and secondary sources most commonly used by health education specialists using indexes, abstracts, and computerized databases; and (6) retrieving health-related information on the Internet.

▷ Identifying the Components of a Research Article

A research article usually begins with an abstract, which is a brief description of the study's results. The abstract describes the research questions that were tested, outlines the study design, and lists one or two major findings from the study. The abstract is meant to communicate essential information, so that readers will know whether the study has information related to the topic they are interested in. An example of an abstract (Hibbard and Greene, 2013) follows:

> Patient engagement is an increasingly important component of strategies to reform health care. In this article we review the available evidence of the contribution that patient activation—the skills and confidence that equip patients to become actively engaged in their health care—makes to health outcomes, costs, and patient experience. There is a growing body of evidence showing that patients who are more activated have better health outcomes and care experiences, but

there is limited evidence to date about the impact on costs. Emerging evidence indicates that interventions that tailor support to the individual's level of activation, and that build skills and confidence, are effective in increasing patient activation. Furthermore, patients who start at the lowest activation levels tend to increase the most. We conclude that policies and interventions aimed at strengthening patients' role in managing their health care can contribute to improved outcomes and that patient activation can—and should—be measured as an intermediate outcome of care that is linked to improved outcomes. (p. 207)

The introduction section, which sometimes is divided into subsections, follows the abstract. Its purpose is usually threefold: (1) to give readers a more detailed description of the research question(s) or hypotheses being tested; (2) to review related literature; and (3) to explain the need for or the significance of the study. This section communicates the rationale behind the researchers' decision to conduct the study.

The methodology section comes directly after the introductory material. In this section, there is usually a description of (1) the research design used, (2) the subjects who took part in the research, (3) the instruments used to gather the information necessary to answer the research questions, and (4) any administrative procedures involved in conducting the research, such as methods used to select the subject(s), gather the data, or protect the rights of the subject(s).

Following the methodology section are the results and discussion sections. The results section gives the research findings by describing the results of the statistical procedures used in analyzing the data (in the case of studies involving quantitative methods—methods involving the analyses of numerical data) and provides an overall answer to the research questions or hypotheses that were described in the introductory section. The discussion section provides a forum for the researcher to interpret the conclusions and meanings and to comment on the implications of the data analyses. In addition, the researcher often includes a narrative about the limitations of the study and makes recommendations for further research on the topic.

▷ Critically Reading a Research Article

The volume of articles on any single health topic continues to escalate. It is important to be able to evaluate the information for accuracy and saliency from sources of all types. Research articles serve as primary sources of valuable information for health education specialists. Beginning students in the field of health education/promotion are not expected to be able to immediately understand every nuance in a research article. It is essential, however, to begin to frequently read scientific reports and journal articles to become familiar with their style. Often, pre-formulating generic questions suitable for critiquing any study can help when evaluating study results. Following is a sequence of questions found to be of help when such an evaluation is necessary. The list is adapted from *Studying a Study and Testing a Test: How to Read Medical Evidence* (Riegelman, 2005).

1. Were the goals/aims of the study defined in a clear manner?
2. Were the research questions/hypotheses clearly stated?
3. Was the description of the subjects clear? Did the article state how the subjects were recruited?

4. Were the design and location of the study described clearly?

5. Were the data collection instruments described?

6. Were reliability and validity reported for the instruments?

7. Did the results directly address the research questions or hypotheses?

8. Were the conclusions reasonable in light of the research design and data analyses performed?

9. Were the findings extrapolated to a population that is similar to the population studied?

10. Were the study implications meaningful to the population you serve?

The final test comes when students can read an article and begin to view themselves in the position of a reporter who has the task of describing the study, its findings, and its limitations to an audience in no more than five minutes. People who can restate study findings and limitations in their own words have accomplished much in becoming critical consumers of scientific and nonscientific literature as well as better resources for others.

▷ Evaluating the Accuracy of Non-Research-Based Sources

As with journal articles that are research based, it is important to be able to evaluate whether or not the information presented is reliable, regardless of the source. Cottrell (1997) conducted a search for instruments that could assist him in teaching his students to assess the accuracy of information found in almost any type of journal or magazine. The questions that emanated from the results of his search include the following:

1. What are the author's qualifications? Does the person have an academic degree in the field being written about? (A note of caution—a degree does not make someone absolutely qualified, but it provides evidence that *suggests* the person is qualified.)

2. What is the style of presentation? Look for health information written in a scientific style of writing, not a style that uses generalities or testimonials.

3. Are references included? A well-written article provides references to the primary sources used. Be aware when someone is writing about another person's research because that individual may be interpreting the results in a different way than the author did.

4. What is the purpose of the publication? Be aware of publications, news or otherwise, that contain advertisements designed to sell items discussed in the articles.

5. What is the reputation of the publication? Is it refereed? Professional journals are good sources of information. Popular press publications can sometimes have poor information related to health issues.

6. Is the information new? When reading for the first time, be skeptical. Information must be validated over time. New information is newsworthy but may not be valid.

It is important to realize that becoming a skeptical, critical consumer of printed and Web-based health information is an important first step in being seen by others as credible. For the public to use the expertise and training of health education specialists to a greater degree, the health education specialist must develop a reputation for providing accurate and current information.

▷ Writing an Abstract or a Summary

Another valuable skill when reading and interpreting health-related literature of any kind (primary, secondary, tertiary, or popular press) involves learning to write an abstract or a summary of an article (see **Figure 9.2**). Although abstracts and summaries are both short forms of describing a research study, the major differences lie in the extent of the content. Abstracts are short (usually 150–250 words). They are written to identify the purpose of the research, the study questions, the methods used by the researcher, and one or two major findings. Summaries, on the other hand, may be two to three pages in length and include all of the elements of the abstract. In addition, summaries are meant to reveal any secondary findings, to describe study limitations, and to provide a more detailed review of the research-er's conclusions and recommendations from the viewpoint of the summary's author.

It is recommended that beginning health education specialists practice writing both abstracts and summaries of the articles they read. Using this technique sharpens the ability of the health education specialist to discriminate between health-related articles that are of substance and meaning for health education/promotion and those that contain erroneous or misleading claims or information.

▷ Locating Health-Related Information

Health education specialists serve as major health information resource persons for many constituencies. It does not matter if they are employed in the school, the clinic, the work site, or the community setting. In all cases, inquiries from a variety of people wanting to know about a health topic or wanting interpretation of the latest research findings are directed to

▶ **Figure 9.2** Summarizing research articles in small group settings sharpens the ability to correctly interpret research findings.

health education specialists. Therefore, it is essential that the latter be knowledgeable about how to find the information requested. The next section identifies resources that health education specialists can use to locate information on health education/promotion and explains how to access the information.

Journals

As has been previously mentioned, much of the information that health education specialists use to make decisions when planning, implementing, and evaluating health promotion programs can be found in journals that publish primary research articles and position papers about health topics and health programs. The following are examples of journals commonly used by health professionals. The list by no means includes all journals of benefit to the health education specialist.

1. *AIDS Education and Prevention.* An international journal designed to support the efforts of professionals working to prevent HIV and AIDS, *AIDS Education and Prevention* includes scientific articles by leading authorities from many disciplines, research reports on the effectiveness of new strategies and programs, debates about key issues, and reviews of books and video resources. In addition to discussing models of AIDS education and prevention, the journal covers a wide range of public health, psychosocial, ethical, and public policy concerns related to HIV and AIDS.

2. *American Journal of Health Behavior* (formerly *Health Values*). Articles accepted for publication feature research about the impact of personal behavior patterns, practices, and characteristics on health promotion. The journal emphasizes efforts at fostering a better understanding of the multidisciplinary nature of systems and individuals as they interface to impact behavior. Examples of successful multidisciplinary approaches to improving health at the community level are also included. As a note, it has published only online after 2009.

3. *American Journal of Health Promotion.* This journal features original research articles, the testing of health behavioral theory on selected populations, and program evaluation. It is an excellent source of articles related to work-site health promotion.

4. *American Journal of Public Health.* Published by the American Public Health Association, this journal features reports related to health research, program evaluations, and health policy analysis, as well as articles on special topics on the health of selected groups and communities.

5. *Evaluation and the Health Professions.* Articles generally focus on practitioner-friendly research related to the development, implementation, and evaluation of community-based health programs. Healthcare researchers and evaluators are provided with examples of state-of-the-art tools and methods for conducting meaningful evaluations.

6. *Family and Community Health.* Articles contain information and research on nutrition, exercise, health-risk appraisals, and the physical and emotional development of a variety of age groups. The overall goal of this journal is to publish articles that foster the role of self-care, family and community health care, and maintenance in the field of health promotion.

7. *Health Affairs.* This journal is published bimonthly and features health policy–related articles of national concern or interest. Of note is that this publication serves as a major source of primary research concerning healthcare coverage, health economics, health reform, and the impact of policy on the health of the populace.

8. ***The Health Educator: The Journal of Eta Sigma Gamma.*** Published by Eta Sigma Gamma, the health education honor society, this journal includes articles related to most health education/promotion topics in a variety of settings. Many of the studies and commentaries are submitted by undergraduate and graduate students in health education/public health programs.

9. ***The Hastings Center Report.*** This journal focuses on the ethical, social, legal, moral, economic, and religious tenets of health policy and health decisions.

10. ***Health Education & Behavior (formerly Health Education Quarterly).*** The official publication of the Society for Public Health Education, Inc. (SOPHE), its articles center on health behavior and education, case studies in health, program evaluation, and strategies to improve social and behavioral health. Each submission includes a commentary on the application of findings to the practice setting and a "perspectives" section, which presents commentary and insight into the complex world of health behavior.

11. ***Health Education Research.*** Official publication of the International Union for Health Promotion and Education and features articles concerning health promotion program planning, implementation, and evaluation. An effort is made to publish articles that provide a mechanism to assist those in the field to apply the results of the studies.

12. ***Health Promotion International.*** The majority of research studies and commentaries are on issues related to health promotion in schools, clinics, work sites, and communities located outside the United States. To maintain a true international perspective, submissions describing spontaneous activities, organizational change interventions, and social and environmental development are uniquely featured as well.

13. ***Health Promotion Practice.*** A journal that publishes articles devoted to the practical application of health promotion and education in a variety of settings including community, health care, educational, work site, and international. Articles featuring the best practices and their application to health policies that promote health and disease prevention are also a focal point.

14. ***Global Journal for Health Education and Promotion (GJHEP)*** (**formerly** ***The International Electronic Journal of Health Education***). It features articles on nearly every aspect of health education, including school health, community health, work-site health promotion, the ethical implications of health education, and the philosophy of health education. Sagamore Publishing is the new vendor.

15. ***The Journal of American College Health.*** Published by the American College Health Association in cooperation with Heldref Publications, its articles are limited to those that relate to health promotion or health service provision in the college or university environment. This is the *only* journal written by college health professionals for college health professionals.

16. ***Journal of Community Health.*** This is an all-inclusive journal, with articles relating to the practice, teaching, and research of community health; preventive medicine; and analysis of delivery of healthcare services. Many articles focus on projects making an impact on the education of health personnel.

17. ***Journal of Health Communication.*** This peer-reviewed journal is published eight times a year. It presents the latest developments in the field of health communication, including research in risk communication, health literacy, social marketing, communication (from interpersonal to mass media), psychology, government, policy making, and health education around the world.

18. *Journal of Nutrition Education and Behavior.* The official publication of the Society of Nutrition Education and Behavior, this journal publishes articles that are germane to the interface between nutrition education and behavior as practiced worldwide. It serves as a resource for anyone interested in nutrition education or diet and physical behavior.

19. *Journal of Rural Health.* Published for the Rural Health Association, this journal's articles focus on professional practice, research, theory development, and policy issues related to health in the rural setting.

20. *Journal of School Health.* Published for the American School Health Association, all material in this journal is related to the public or private school setting from pre-K through grade 12. Articles generally focus on children's health issues but may include information related to other aspects of coordinated school health programs, such as employee wellness.

21. *Global Health Promotion.* This is an official publication of the International Union for Health Promotion and Education (IUHPE), published by Sage Publications. Most issues are topical in nature (e.g., environmental health, population health, infectious disease prevention) and feature articles related to the application of public health and health promotion in countries around the globe. Articles are published in several languages.

22. *Public Health Reports.* Published by the Association of Schools of Public Health, this journal reports findings from many avenues of research related to health services acquisition, health policy development, and health promotion at the community level.

23. *Health Behavior and Policy Review*. A bi-monthly journal first published in January 2014. The journal, published by Paris Scholar Publishing Ltd, features articles on policy development impacting health behaviors that are population rather than individual focused. Research guiding policy development and prioritizing health policy choices is also a priority.

Indexes and Abstracts

Indexes and **abstracts** provide links to articles from many refereed or peer-reviewed journals, books, and research reports. An index references articles from journals, books, and reports pertaining to topics that fall under the subject headings for which the index was created (e.g., health behavior, physical activity, methamphetamine treatment, or corporate health education/promotion programs). An abstract provides somewhat similar information but also includes short summaries of the article's content to help the researcher determine whether the article contains the information she or he is seeking.

Although some indexes and abstracts can still be found in hard copy, many of them are migrating to online or electronic formats. The cost of publishing paper versions plus the ease of user access to online materials will undoubtedly create a situation in the near future where new editions of paper versions of either indexes or abstracts will no longer be available. *Index Medicus*, an abstract that has been printed for more than a century, is an example of a publication that is no longer available in paper copy because of the high cost of printing the volumes. In its place, the National Library of Medicine and the National Institutes of Health have created a site (http://www.PubMed.gov) that combines the information formerly available in *Index Medicus* with many other sources to create a database that is accessible to anyone with a computer.

Government Documents

The U.S. Government Printing Office (GPO) publishes volumes of materials of use to health education specialists. This section (adapted from the University of Akron library Web site [University of Akron, 2013]) is meant to provide a generic description of the types of documents that can be accessed in the government documents section of an academic library. Because each library has slightly different procedures for finding these documents, students are encouraged to communicate with the government documents librarian at their university for the specifics on locating documents. It should be noted that the U.S. government is shifting away from issuing paper copies and is increasing the number of documents available online.

Government publications range from official documents including laws, court decisions, and records of congressional actions to the results of government-sponsored technical and scientific studies. Information on topics such as obesity, water treatment, or exercise can also be found in a government documents section.

Government documents are not organized under the same classification scheme as a traditional general collection. Instead, they are organized and shelved according to Superintendent of Documents (SuDocs) numbers. The SuDocs number is unique in that it has a colon. For example, A1:1 is an annual report from the Agriculture Department. Numbers of the documents are arranged alphabetically by agency, and the numbers are whole numbers, not decimals (e.g., HE 1.6 comes before HE 1.9). The letter that begins the SuDocs number signifies the publishing agency, as noted:

A	Agriculture Department
C	Census Bureau
D	Department of Defense
E	Department of Energy
HE	Health and Human Services
X–Y	Congress

Government documents contain a storehouse of valuable and current information and should not be overlooked when seeking information on a health topic of interest. Most libraries have online search capabilities for government documents, so as with many traditional sources of information, accessing them has become much less labor intensive.

Electronic Databases

Electronic databases often provide a preferred alternative to manually searching indexes or abstracts (see **Figure 9.3**). As mentioned previously, most, if not all, of the publishers of the hard-copy abstracts and indexes either have converted or are converting their documents to an online format. Much like an index or abstract, each database has a general subject area (e.g., medicine, education, psychology, community health). The electronic database provides access via the Internet. Computer searches using databases are significantly faster than manual searches, and they have the advantage of enabling the user to link several concepts together to provide focus for a search.

For example, if a person wanted to search for articles about "health behavior" and the influence of "health communication" on behavior, an electronic database would allow the

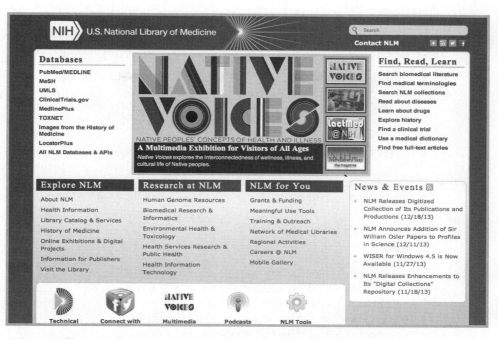

▲ **Figure 9.3** Electronic databases such as the National Library of Medicine (NLM) provide ready access to information on a particular topic.

user to enter both terms into the computer and connect them by placing the word *and* between them. The result will be to eliminate any articles that do not have both *health behavior* and *health communication* as key terms. Other terms can be used to further narrow a search to be as specific as desired. The main concern the computer database user faces is to accurately specify the key terms associated with the information desired, so the resulting list of references that is generated will be of use. Computerized searches require little computer knowledge; however, it is always advisable to seek the assistance of a librarian when beginning to seek information. Users should also know that just because the information is readily available online, it is not free. Academic libraries spend hundreds of thousands of dollars per year to ensure that students and faculty have access to the materials they need using such an expeditious methodology. The databases most used by health education specialists are:

1. ***Educational Resources Information Center (ERIC).*** It includes the *Current Index to Journals in Education (CIJE)* and *Resources in Education* (RIE). ERIC is an information clearinghouse that collects, sorts, classifies, and stores thousands of documents on topics pertaining to education and allied fields of study. An advantage to using ERIC is that many types of documents are contained in the database that are not journal articles—for example, proceedings of meetings, teaching strategies, lesson plans, commentaries, and policy documents.

2. ***MEDLINE.*** This is the premier biomedicine database indexing more than 3,000 journals. It covers the fields of medicine, nursing, dentistry, veterinary medicine, and preclinical sciences.

3. *ScienceDirect.* This is one of the largest full-text scientific databases in the world covering physical sciences, life sciences, health sciences, and engineering material. It indexes more than 2,500 peer-reviewed journals and more than 11,000 books. More than 9.5 million journal articles and book chapters are contained in this database.

4. *Cumulative Index to Nursing and Allied Health Literature (CINAHL).* It contains more than 300,000 citations from 1983 until the present. It references journal articles and book chapters, pamphlets, audiovisuals, educational software, and conference proceedings in the areas of nursing, health education, health services, and healthcare administration.

5. *ETHXWeb.* This database covers the years 1974–2009 and is no longer being updated. Topics include ethical, legal, and public policy issues surrounding health care and biomedical research. Citations are derived from the literature of law, religion, ethics, social sciences, philosophy, the popular media, and the health sciences.

6. *PsycINFO.* This is the largest database of peer-reviewed literature in the areas of mental health and behavior sciences.

7. *Ovid Healthstar.* Ovid Healthstar includes data from the National Library of Medicine's (NLM) MEDLINE and former HealthSTAR databases. As such, it contains citations of the published literature in health services, technology, administration, health policy, health economics, and research. It focuses on both the clinical and nonclinical aspects of healthcare delivery.

8. *PubMed.* A service of the National Library of Medicine that contains more than 17 million citations from MEDLINE and other life science journals for biomedical articles dating back more than a half-century. The database includes links to full text articles and other related resources.

9. *Physical Education Index.* This database includes references to more than 400 periodicals on physical education, health education, dance, physical therapy, and sports medicine.

10. *Google Scholar.* Covers scholarly research from books, theses, dissertations, journal articles, government documents, etc. It indexes professional societies, online repositories, university sites, government Web sites, etc. If you use settings, you can customize it to link to your university library's resources.

▷ The Internet and the World Wide Web

The **World Wide Web** is an interactive information delivery service that includes a repository of resources about almost any subject imaginable including health. The **Internet** consists of a linked global system of computer networks that are connected together through a variety of wireless and other electronic technologies. This linked system enables the user to access information on the World Wide Web (the Web).

To access information on the Web individuals commonly use browsers such as Google, Safari, Mozilla Firefox, and Internet Explorer. Use of the browser involves entering a Web address, which usually starts with the characters *http://* (http stands for **hypertext transfer protocol**). Web addresses are known as URLs, or **Uniform Resource Locators (URL)**, which are unique identifiers for a location on the global Internet much as the mailing address of your home is unique to where you live. The URL is composed of the Internet access protocol, the location, and the file—for example, "http://www.cdc.gov/mmwr/" is the URL for the

home page of the Centers for Disease Control and Prevention (CDC) publication *Morbidity and Mortality Weekly Report* (MMWR). A home page is analogous to a combination of a cover and a table of contents in a book in that it names the site and directs the user to a list of information options available within the site. In the example, the *http://* is the Internet access protocol; the *www.cdc.gov* is the location; and *mmwr/* is the file.

Assume you are looking for information on the seasonal flu vaccine to share in a training session. To find the information at the CDC Web site, you would use your preferred browser and enter CDC in the search function or type in "http://www.cdc.gov" (the URL of the CDC) into the URL bar, and the home page of the CDC will appear.

On the home page of the CDC you can use the search function to find the desired information (see **Figure 9.4**). When looking for information on an organization's home page any word or phrase that turns the cursor into a hand indicates that information has been linked to another section within the site or another site to help the user access additional information about that topic.

Another method for locating information on the Internet involves using a **search engine**. Various search engines are available (e.g., Google, Yahoo, Bing, Ask, and AOL Search). The advantage of using a search engine over typing in a URL (which is specific to one site) is that the search engine allows you to type in the name of the topic you want to find information about, and after a few seconds it identifies and lists multiple sites related to that topic. All the user needs to do to access the information from any of the listed sites is to click the pointer on the name of the site and it will appear. The search engines are usually located on the main search page of the browser or may be accessed by typing in their URL.

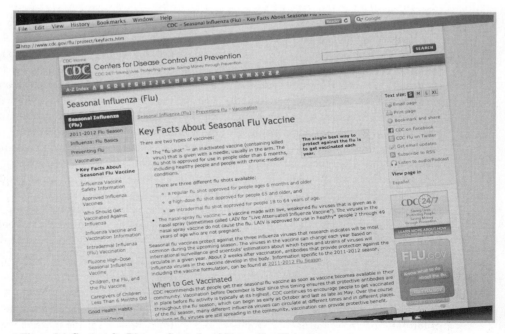

▲ **Figure 9.4** Centers for Disease Control and Prevention Web site

▶ **Figure 9.5** Search engines are valuable tools for research.

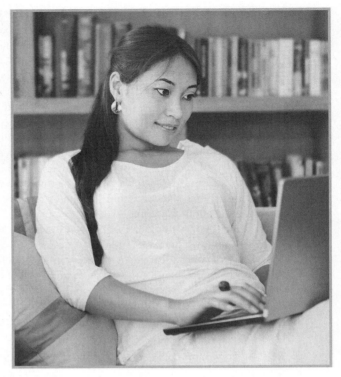

A search engine can be used to research any health-related topic (see **Figure 9.5**). For example, say that you were developing a drug abuse prevention program. In order to research commonly abused drugs, you would enter *methamphetamine* into the search box. Click Search or press the Enter key on the keyboard and a list of relevant sites will appear. Click on any of the sites, and you will be transported to the page and information corresponding to that site.

Sometimes you may want to use a specific search engine to find health information. Just enter the browser name (Google, Yahoo, or Bing) into the URL bar and click Enter. If the term you are searching for has more than one word (such as "sexually transmitted infections"), it is wise to use quotation marks around the term when it is entered into the box marked Search. This will let the search engine know that the exact phrase, as contained in the quotation marks, is to be used when seeking sites that match. If the quotation marks are not used, the search engine will find sites that contain all of the words in the query. However, at least some of the sites might not be relevant to the topic of interest (sexually transmitted infections in this case) because the words can appear in any order and at any place on the sites searched.

▷ Evaluating Information on the Internet

Previously in the chapter, directions were given for evaluating the accuracy and validity of information from journal and popular press sources. Because of the massive amount of information available on the Internet and because nearly anyone can publish on the Web, it is equally imperative that the health education specialist know how to evaluate information obtained via an Internet search. T. J. Madden, a reference specialist in the Albertson Library at Boise State University, suggests using CRAAP test which was originally developed at California State University, Chico (personal communication, April 2013).

Evaluation Criteria

Currency: *The timeliness of the information.*

- When was the information published or posted?
- Has the information been revised or updated?
- Does your topic require current information, or will older sources work as well?
- Are the links functional?

Relevance: *The importance of the information for your needs.*

- Does the information relate to your topic or answer your question?
- Who is the intended audience?
- Is the information at an appropriate level (i.e., not too elementary or advanced for your needs)? Have you looked at a variety of sources before determining this is one you will use?
- Would you be comfortable citing this source in your research paper?

Authority: *The source of the information.*

- Who is the author, publisher, source, or sponsor?
- What are the author's credentials or organizational affiliations?
- Is the author qualified to write on the topic?
- Is there contact information, such as a publisher or e-mail address?
- Does the URL reveal anything about the author or source? examples: .com, .edu, .gov, .org, or .net

Accuracy: *The reliability, truthfulness and correctness of the content.*

- Where does the information come from?
- Is the information supported by evidence?
- Has the information been reviewed or refereed?
- Can you verify any of the information in another source or from personal knowledge?
- Does the language or tone seem unbiased and free of emotion?
- Are there spelling, grammar, or typographical errors?

Purpose: *The reason the information exists.*

- What is the purpose of the information?
- Is it to inform, teach, sell, entertain, or persuade?
- Do the authors or sponsors make their intentions or purpose clear?
- Is the information fact, opinion, or propaganda?
- Does the point of view appear objective and impartial?

Summary

This chapter has presented an overview on accessing and evaluating health-related information. An increasing demand for health information, coupled with the fact that the information is being produced at an ever greater rate, creates added responsibility for health education specialists. Two of the major roles of health education specialists as discussed in Chapter 6 involve being resource people for health information and communicating to others about health education/promotion needs, concerns, and resources. To perform these tasks, the health education specialist must have the skills to find information, must evaluate the source of the information to determine its credibility, and must disseminate the information through the appropriate channels to consumers. In addition, the health education specialist must be able to explain the information effectively. Becoming familiar with the tools found in this chapter is a necessity for all students wanting to enter the field of health education/promotion.

Review Questions

1. Describe the difference between primary, secondary, tertiary, and popular press sources.
2. How do an article abstract and an article summary differ in content?
3. What are the questions you should ask yourself when critiquing a journal article? What are the differences between the questions asked when evaluating a primary research article and those asked when evaluating a secondary source or popular press article?
4. What are five of the most commonly used journals in the field of health education/promotion? What types of information would you expect to find in each of the journals you named?
5. What advantage might the information from a government document have over another source on the same topic?
6. How does one go about evaluating information retrieved from the Internet?
7. In your own words, describe how to access information concerning breast cancer on the Internet. Try using at least two different search engines and compare the results.

Case Study

As a health education/promotion major, you have just finished studying about the Responsibilities and Competencies for Entry-Level Health Education Specialists (found in Appendix B of this text). During this unit the instructor invited a group of practicing health education specialists to the class to participate in a panel discussion on the validity of the various roles in the real-life practice of health education/promotion.

Following the presentation, each of the panelists offered to host two to three students from the class for four hours per week for three weeks at his or her place of work. This opportunity resulted from student questions to the panelists concerning their desire to transfer the classroom learning to the work setting. Several of the students expressed frustration at what they perceived to be the emphasis on theory and the lack of application in their courses and coursework. The panelists readily conceded that the 12-hour block of time each student would spend at the work site with them would not totally solve theory-practical application problems, but they hoped it might help the students to see that, at least in the case of the majority of the responsibilities and competencies, what they studied about in class was what the health education specialist was doing.

After a quick meeting between the instructor and the panel members, placement assignments were made for the students. Because of your interest in becoming a health education specialist in a clinical setting, you were assigned to a community health clinic to shadow a physician to see what kind of health education is given to patients.

On your first day, the physician to whom you are assigned requests that you accompany her into the examination room as she sees patients. During the first two hours, she sees three patients for colds or influenza, two patients for hypertension, one patient for emphysema, one patient for diabetes, one for a broken hand, and two teenage patients for sports physicals. After these appointments, she takes some time to visit with you and discuss your initial perceptions. During the conversation, she asks if you are aware of any good health education/promotion information sites for teens on the Internet. You promise to do some research on this question and bring the information on your next visit. What information do you think would be of benefit to teens? Which two or three sites would you recommend and why?

▷ Critical Thinking Questions

1. Assume that all information about any topic is available on the Web. If that were true, would there be any need for health education specialists? Defend your answer.

2. Make a list of the five greatest advantages and the five greatest disadvantages of the Internet from your perspective. Assuming that your list reflects universal truths about the Internet, how might you persuade a senior citizen who is not a computer user to adopt computer use as a practice?

3. Given that so much information is available online, under what circumstances does it make sense to use the library?

4. If the Internet had been developed in the early 1900s, how might the U.S. healthcare system and the role of health education specialists differ from what they are today?

▷ Activities

1. You are employed as a health education specialist in a district health department and have just received a call from a member of a local coalition wanting to know where to find some peer-reviewed studies that summarize the content and effectiveness of available school-based sexuality education curricula. Use an index to find a reference to an article that meets those criteria.

2. Was the article you located in Activity 1 a primary or secondary source of information? Provide a rationale for your answer.

3. Using a database (CINAHL, MEDLINE, PsycINFO, or ERIC), find a primary research article relating to motorcycle safety (e.g., the use of a helmet, wearing protective gear,

road surfaces). Critique the article by applying the questions found in the "Critically Reading a Research Article" section of this chapter.

4. As a newly employed health education specialist in a hospital outpatient clinic, one of your jobs is to provide information to patients after they have seen the physician. Ms. X has just been diagnosed with coronary artery disease, and the physician has sent her to you to discuss the impact of lifestyle on her condition. Using the Internet, find several sources of information that you could give her to read that might assist you with the education process. Evaluate the accuracy of the information you retrieve.

5. Use your choice of a browser and look up the term *endometriosis*. Then evaluate at least two of the sites that appear using the CRAAP methodology.

▷ Weblinks

EPIDEMIOLOGICAL AND STATISTICAL INFORMATION

1. http://wonder.cdc.gov
   CDC WONDER
   Wide-ranging online data for epidemiologic research—an easy-to-use, menu-driven system that makes the information resources of the CDC available to public health professionals and the public at large. It provides access to a wide array of public health information.

2. http://www.cdc.gov/nchs/
   National Center for Health Statistics (NCHS)
   NCHS is the nation's principal health statistics agency. Their Web site offers access to an extensive collection of health statistics intended to guide those working to improve public health.

3. http://www.cdc.gov/mmwr/
   Morbidity and Mortality Weekly Report (MMWR)
   MMWR is a weekly report prepared by the CDC. State health departments report their findings to MMWR. The site offers access to studies and reports, and also provides useful information on a wide range of diseases.

4. http://www.census.gov
   U.S. Bureau of the Census
   The Web site of the U.S. Census Bureau allows the user to access specific data for his or her state, county, or city. View results from Census 2000 and Census 2010 and access analytical reports on population change, race, age, family structure, and more.

INFECTIOUS DISEASES

5. http://www.cdc.gov/DataStatistics/
   Centers for Disease Control and Prevention—Data and Statistics
   With the mission of preventing illness, disability, and death, the CDC conducts epidemic investigations, laboratory research, and public education programs to attempt to prevent and control diseases and disorders of all types.

CHRONIC DISEASES

6. http://www.cdc.gov/chronicdisease/index.htm

CDC Chronic Disease Prevention and Health Promotion

This section of the CDC is dedicated to chronic diseases and provides links to a variety of helpful sites, including a diabetes public health resource and sites discussing heart disease, nutrition, and physical activity.

7. http://www.nci.nih.gov/

National Cancer Institute (NCI)

The NCI's Web site covers information on a variety of cancer topics, discussing treatment, prevention, research, and much more. The NCI supports prevention and treatment of cancer, rehabilitation, and continued care of cancer patients and their families.

8. http://www.diabetes.org

American Diabetes Association (ADA)

The ADA provides diabetes research, scientific findings, information, and advocacy. The site contains helpful information for people with diabetes, their families, health professionals, and the public.

DISEASE CONTROL AND PREVENTION

9. http://store.samhsa.gov/home

Substance Abuse and Mental Health Services Administration

This site features links to ordering government materials online that focus on professional and research topics, issues in the field of treatment, prevention, and recovery, and information on conditions and disorders.

10. http://www.samhsa.gov/about/csap.aspx

Center for Substance Abuse Prevention (CSAP)

CSAP is funded by the Substance Abuse and Mental Health Services Administration (SAMHSA) and is responsible for improving the access to and quality of substance abuse prevention services to the public. CSAP provides national leadership in the development of policies, programs, and services to prevent the onset of illegal drug use and underage alcohol and tobacco use, and to reduce the negative consequences of using substances.

11. http://www.whitehousedrugpolicy.gov

Office of National Drug Control Policy (ONDCP)

With the goal of reducing illicit drug use, substance abuse-related crimes, drug trafficking, and drug-related health problems, the ONDCP is working to establish a national strategy to fight these dilemmas. The site contains national priorities, annual reports, and a tremendous amount of drug information.

12. http://www.cdc.gov/hiv/aboutDHAP.htm

CDC's Division of HIV/AIDS Prevention

With a mission to prevent HIV infection and reduce the incidence of HIV-related illness, the CDC's Division of HIV/AIDS Prevention Web site provides useful information for those working in the health field. The site includes such topics as prevention tools, research, brochures, and fact sheets.

13. http://www.medmatrix.org

    Medical Matrix

    Medical Matrix is a peer-reviewed site that offers continually updated clinical medicine resources. The information is organized in such a way as to make searching for information more timely and efficient. More than 6,000 medical Web sites are listed.

14. http://www.childrenssafetynetwork.org

    Children's Safety Network

    The Children's Safety Network, funded by the Maternal & Child Health Bureau (MCH) and the U.S. Department of Health and Human Services, provides technical assistance, training, and resources to MCH and other injury prevention professionals in an extensive effort to reduce the burden of injury and violence to our nation's children.

15. http://www.fda.gov/Food/default.htm

    Food and Drug Administration (FDA)

    This site not only outlines national programs intended to increase food safety awareness, but it also contains information concerning the laws enforced by the FDA and provides helpful tips on preventing food-related illness.

16. http://oncolink.com

    OncoLink

    OncoLink, provided by the Abramson Cancer Center of the University of Pennsylvania, is the Web's first cancer resource. The site provides up-to-date cancer news and research. Locate information on the causes of cancer, screening and prevention, clinical trials, and other resources on cancer.

17. http://www.cdc.gov/travel/

    Travelers' Health

    Locate health information for specific destinations, stay up to date on outbreaks throughout the world, and learn how to avoid illness from food and water.

18. http://www.cdc.gov/tb/

    CDC's Division of Tuberculosis Elimination

    With the mission of "preventing, controlling and eventually eliminating tuberculosis from the United States," the Web site of the CDC's Division of Tuberculosis Elimination contains useful information to aid that mission. Learn all there is to know about tuberculosis, locate statistics on its occurrence, and obtain education and training materials on it.

19. http://www.4women.gov

    National Women's Health Information Center

    The National Women's Health Information Center, sponsored by the Department of Health and Human Services Office on Women's Health, provides health information for women across the country. It offers information on heart disease, body image, breastfeeding, screening and immunization schedules, and more.

20. http://www.menshealthnetwork.org

    Men's Health Network

    The Men's Health Network is an informational and educational organization recognizing men's health as a specific social concern.

21. http://www.kidshealth.org/

KidsHealth

KidsHealth is the largest and most visited site on the Web, providing doctor-approved health information about children from before birth through adolescence. Created by the Nemours Foundation's Center for Children's Health Media, the award-winning KidsHealth provides families with accurate, up-to-date, and jargon-free health information they can use.

22. http://www.nsc.org

National Safety Council

The National Safety Council is focused on providing safety and health information to reduce the number of injuries and deaths from preventable accidents. Their Web site contains information on new policies and laws enacted to prevent unintentional injuries. It also provides statistics and helpful tips regarding this health topic.

23. http://ctb.ku.edu

Community Tool Box

The goal of the Community Tool Box is to support work in community health promotion and development. The Tool Box provides multiple pages of practical skill-building information on more than 250 different topics related to community development. Topic sections include step-by-step instruction, examples, checklists, and related resources.

NATIONAL AGENCIES

24. http://www.cdc.gov

CDC—Centers for Disease Control and Prevention

The CDC is recognized as the leading federal agency for protecting the health and safety of the public, providing credible information to enhance health decisions and promote health. The Web site of the CDC includes a variety of helpful health and safety topics. The information covers everything from health promotion to vaccines to traveler's health. Data, statistics, publications, and products are also available.

25. http://www.hhs.gov

USDHHS—Department of Health and Human Services

The Department of Health and Human Services is the U.S. government's principal agency for health protection and the provision of human services. Its site is divided into health topics such as Safety & Wellness, Diseases & Conditions, and Families & Children. Readers can also use the Resource Locator and Reference Collections to find such things as healthcare facilities and publications.

26. http://www.epa.gov

EPA—Environmental Protection Agency

The EPA is focused on protecting human health and the environment by working for a cleaner, healthier environment. The site provides air quality reports, current environmental news stories, and tips on how the public can make the environment healthier. The QuickFinder allows fast and easy access to a variety of environmental topics.

27. http://www.ihs.gov/

IHS—Indian Health Service

Indian Health Service is the Federal Health Program for American Indians and Alaska Natives. IHS is focused on improving the health of these groups while attempting to ensure they have access to culturally acceptable health services.

28. http://www.ama-assn.org

    American Medical Association

    This Web site is divided into a section for physicians and medical students and a section for patients. The patient section allows the user to search for a doctor and obtain health information and resources. The physician section provides information on such topics as medical education, legal issues, and advocacy.

29. http://www.nih.gov

    National Institutes of Health (NIH)

    The Web site of the NIH is loaded with a wide variety of great health information. It contains an A–Z index of health resources, a wealth of grant information, and a section dedicated to scientific resources.

30. http://www.nlm.nih.gov/

    National Library of Medicine (NLM)

    The Web site of the NLM—part of the NIH. Excellent central source of current information on results of health research for the lay person, the practicing health professional, the health researcher, and health librarians. Updated daily.

INTERNATIONAL AGENCIES

31. http://www.who.int/en

    WHO—World Health Organization

    The Web site of WHO is an incredible resource. The site includes a tremendous listing of pages, organized by health and development topics, that contain links to WHO projects, initiatives, activities, information products, and contacts.

32. http://www.paho.org

    PAHO—Pan American Health Organization

    PAHO, affiliated with WHO, focuses on a multitude of public health topics, with the mission of promoting health in the Americas.

WEB-BASED MEDLINE SEARCH SYSTEMS

33. http://www.pubMed.gov/

    PubMed

    PubMed is a service of the NLM. It includes literally millions of citations for biomedical articles going back to the 1950s. The citations are from MEDLINE and additional life science journals. PubMed includes links to many sites providing full-text articles and other related resources.

34. http://www.medscape.com/px/urlinfo

    Medscape from WebMD (free access to MEDLINE)

    Medscape allows the user to register for free access to MEDLINE, continuing medical education (CME) courses, medical journals, medical news, and more. Medline's database of medical abstracts may be searched by title or author.

35. http://www.nlm.nih.gov

    National Library of Medicine (NLM)

    The NLM, on the campus of the NIH in Bethesda, Maryland, is the world's largest medical library. NLM collects materials and provides information and research services in all areas of biomedicine and health care.

36. http://medlineplus.gov

MedlinePlus

Health professionals and the general public alike can easily access information on MedlinePlus that is accurate and up to date. MedlinePlus has extensive information from the National Institutes of Health and other trusted sources on more than 650 diseases and conditions.

PUBLIC HEALTH PRACTICE

37. http://www.cdc.gov/ostlts/index.htm

Office of State, Tribal, Local and Territorial Support (OSTLTS)

This office resulted from a reorganization at the CDC. The priority of the OSTLTS is to improve the capacity and performance of the public health system at all levels. The office works both within CDC and in the field to identify gaps, opportunities for collaboration, and the strategies needed to support growth and enhancement of public health work.

38. http://www.apha.org

American Public Health Association (APHA)

The APHA is the world's largest and oldest organization of public health professionals. Useful sections include Continuing Education, Newsroom, and Science and Programs.

STATE AND LOCAL PUBLIC HEALTH DEPARTMENTS

39. http://www.astho.org/

Association of State and Territorial Health Officials (ASTHO)

ASTHO is the national nonprofit organization representing the public health agencies of the United States, the U.S. Territories, and the District of Columbia, as well as the 120,000 public health professionals these agencies employ. ASTHO members, the chief health officials of these jurisdictions, are dedicated to formulating and influencing sound public health policy and to assuring excellence in state-based public health practice.

40. http://www.healthguideusa.com/index.htm

Health Resource Guide USA

Health Guide USA provides quick reference to a tremendous listing of healthcare-related resources throughout the United States. It provides locations of state and local health departments, as well as medical schools and medical licenses.

GENERAL HEALTH INFORMATION

41. http://www.google.com

Google

Google's keyword search engine is pop-up free and a great tool for finding anything on the Web. Google has several specialized search features Blog Search and Alerts Many people and organizations have a health-related blog and you can use blog search to find these blogs. If you want to receive e-mail updates on various health topics you can set up an Alert and content will be sent directly to your inbox.

42. http://www.myoptumhealth.com/portal

myOptumHealth.com

Provides MD-reviewed information on a variety of health topics. The information is easy to understand and can be used by a health education specialist to research background information related to all aspects of health.

43. http://www.WebMD.com

WebMD

Site devoted to providing current and relevant consumer health information on a variety of topics. Medical facts are reviewed by physicians prior to posting.

44. http://www.yahoo.com/Health/

Yahoo! Health

Get in-depth coverage on a variety of health issues, including a directory of the most popular Web sites related to a particular health topic.

45. http://www.mayoclinic.com

Mayo Clinic

The Mayo Clinic offers a wealth of health information developed and reviewed by more than 2,000 physicians and scientists. The site also allows access to healthy living tools, such as a personal health card, and a first-aid and self-care guide.

46. http://www.berkeleywellness.com

Cal Berkeley Wellness Letter

The Wellness Letter relies on the expertise of the School of Public Health and other researchers at UC Berkeley, as well as other top scientists from around the world. It translates this leading-edge research into practical advice for daily living—at home, at work, while exercising, and in the market or health-food store.

47. http://www.healthfinder.gov

Healthfinder®

Healthfinder, developed by the Department of Health and Human Services, directs the user to various health resources depending on his or her needs. Resources include such things as online publications, clearinghouses, support groups, government agencies, and Web sites.

48. http://www.usa.gov/Citizen/Topics/Health.shtml

USA.gov-Health

The Health and Nutrition section of the U.S. Government's Official Web portal is filled with great health information. The Healthfinder link enables access to the Personal Health Tools link, which features tools for calculating body mass index (BMI) and taking an online checkup. The site also features health topics for population groups and helps the user locate health services in his or her area.

49. http://www.foundationcenter.org

Foundation Center

The Foundation Center has free online grant writing guides and tutorials and fee-based grant writing courses for new and experienced grant writers. The Foundation Finder search is a good way to find funders in your area.

50. http://www.goaskalice.columbia.edu/

Go Ask Alice!

Go Ask Alice's Q&A database houses numerous health-related questions and answers. It is produced by Columbia University's Health Education Program.

51. http://www.health.gov/nhic

National Health Information Center (NHIC)

The NHIC is a health information referral service. NHIC puts health professionals and consumers who have health questions in touch with organizations that are best able to provide answers.

NEWS STORIES

52. http://www.reutershealth.com

Reuters Health Products and Services

Reuters is the premier supplier of health and medical news on the Internet. The Health eLine is a wonderful section for the general public.

53. http://www.usatoday.com/news/health/default.htm

USA Today Health

This section of *USA Today* provides some of the most current news stories related to health.

54. http://www.nlm.nih.gov/medlineplus/newsbydate.html

MedlinePlus—Health News by Date

The news section of MedlinePlus provides current health-related articles from the past 30 days from the New York Times Syndicate, Reuters Health Information, and others.

HEALTH EDUCATION/HEALTH PROMOTION JOBS

55. http://www.hpcareer.net

HPCareer.Net

This is the official career resource site for the American Kinesiotherapy Association (AKTA), the Medical-Fitness Association (MFA), and the National Commission for Health Education Credentialing (NCHEC).

56. http://www.sph.emory.edu/studentservice/career.html

Rollins School of Public Health at Emory—Career Action Center

Includes sections titled Public Health Employment Connection and Public Health Candidate Connection. Career Action Tip Sheets are also available.

HEALTH POLICY

57. http://www.nashp.org

National Academy for State Health Policy

The National Academy for State Health Policy conducts policy analysis; provides training and technical assistance to states; produces informational resources; and convenes state, regional, and national forums. This site enables the user to access these services and the results of policy studies that have been completed.

58. http://www.heritage.org

The Heritage Foundation

This site provides access to well-written and well-documented health policy research and analysis papers in which the conclusions often reflect a more conservative perspective.

59. http://rwjf.org/

    The Robert Wood Johnson Foundation

    The Robert Wood Johnson Foundation has a goal of funding projects that improve the health and health care of all Americans. This site features many of the foundation's policy papers, current and future studies, and projects that the foundation is or will consider funding. The organization is considered nonpartisan.

60. http://kff.org/

    The Henry J. Kaiser Family Foundation

    The Henry J. Kaiser Family Foundation is a nonprofit, privately operating foundation focusing on the major healthcare issues facing the nation. The foundation is an independent voice and source of facts and analysis for policy makers, the media, the healthcare community, and the general public.

61. http://www.commonwealthfund.org/

    The Commonwealth Fund

    This site contains policy briefs and full-text health policy papers that are well written and well documented and are often from a more liberal perspective.

62. http://www.statecoverage.org/

    State Coverage Initiatives (SCI)

    The SCI program is a national initiative of The Robert Wood Johnson Foundation that works with states to plan, execute, and maintain health insurance expansions, as well as to improve the availability and affordability of healthcare coverage. The site includes the results of many states' initiatives to increase health insurance coverage for their residents.

GENERAL

63. http://findarticles.com/p/articles/tn_health

    Find articles

    Provides free access to millions of articles from many top publications.

64. http://www.scholar.google.com

    Google Scholar

    This site provides another alternative to search through scholarly literature across many disciplines and sources, including theses, books, abstracts, and articles.

 ## References

California State University Chico. (2013). Evaluating Information Applying the CRAAP Test. Retrieved May 23, 2013, from http://www.csuchico.edu/lins/handouts/evalsites.html.

Cottrell, R. R. (1997). *A guide to evaluating a journal article.* Unpublished manuscript.

Hibbard, J. H., & Greene, J. (2013). What the evidence shows about patient activation: Better outcomes and health care experiences; fewer data on costs. *Health Affairs, 32* (2), 207–214.

Riegelman, R. K. (2005). *Studying a study and testing a test: How to read medical literature* (5th ed.). Philadelphia: Lippincott, Williams, & Wilkins.

University of Akron. (2013). *Government Documents.* Retrieved on May 27, 2013, from http://www.uakron.edu/libraries/services/services-detail.dot?inode=360659&title=Government%20Documents.

Future Trends in Health Education/Promotion

Chapter Objectives

After reading this chapter and answering the questions at the end, you should be able to:

- Identify two settings in which health education specialists will practice in the next 5 years to a greater degree than they do today.

- Describe four major societal changes that will influence the practice of health education/promotion in the next 10 years.

- Delineate the major implications of credentialing for future health education specialists.

- Compare and contrast the roles of health education specialists in the four practice settings.

- Identify several reasons that health education specialists should be optimistic about future employment opportunities.

- Evaluate the role of the health education specialist in addressing the increasing costs of health care.

It is said that one of the few constants in life is change. Societal trends are having an increasing impact on the profession of health education/promotion. The topic of health is consistently of interest to the populace in the United States. With increasing numbers of citizens interested in health information, spiraling healthcare costs, a reliance on technology for information delivery and acquisition, rapidly changing demographic patterns, a heightened skepticism of the medical establishment and health insurance companies, the passage of the Affordable Care Act, and a more interconnected world, the environment that will confront health education specialists in the next 20 years is quite different from that of only a decade ago. These changes present the health education specialist with enormous opportunities. The focus of this chapter is to explore future developments in the discipline of health education/promotion, and we hope, to create a sense of excitement and anticipation about the challenges that lie ahead.

Imagine that you have just arrived in the United States from another planet. The year is 1990. Assume that the first thing you see is a 1-hour television news program. Based solely on that program and the commercial messages during the station breaks, how would you describe the lives of people on the planet you are visiting? Now, transport yourself ahead to today and repeat the exercise. Although it is not the purpose of this chapter to dwell on comparative history, it is noteworthy that, in a brief, 20-plus year span, the communication methods and patterns in the United States and many other countries have changed dramatically. For example, in the early 1990s there was effectively no online access to information of any sort. In 2010, up to 80 percent of all U.S. adults using the Internet reported using it to seek information about health (Fox, 2011). Several of the aforementioned societal shifts have profound implications for the way health education/promotion will be practiced as the 21st century continues its second decade.

The first section of this chapter discusses changing demographic patterns. Societal trends that are predicted to play a role in the practice of health education/promotion in future decades will be featured. Issues related to credentialing and preparation will follow. Using this information as a foundation, the chapter concludes by postulating about the impact of these changes for the health education specialist in the school, public health, work site, and medical care settings. One caveat is in order before this discussion: Obviously, no one knows exactly what the future will hold. The information presented is meant to stimulate thinking about the role health education specialists will play from now until the years 2020–2030.

▷ Demographic Changes

Over the past 30 years, the population growth rate in the United States has increased at about 1 percent per year. Although this stable growth pattern is probably manageable for the long term, a more in-depth study of the **demographic profile**, the breakdown of the U.S. population by age group, sex, race, and ethnicity, shows a dramatically altered picture from that of just 10 years ago. This consistently changing demographic profile—specifically, a greater percentage of minority residents and an ever aging population—has important implications for the future practice of health education specialists (see **Figure 10.1**).

▶ **Figure 10.1** Health promotion for the elderly will be in increasing demand in the next century.

Minority Population Changes

Clark's (1994) comments, written midway through the last decade of the 20th century, remain cogent today. She states, "We are undergoing a massive change in culture in our society. We are literally looking different as a nation and the conventional majority values and norms are being challenged as we become a more diverse, more ethnic, more integrated culture. Health educators have long prided themselves with working across cultures...The cultural changes are...greater than we have experienced previously" (p. 137).

It seems that the increased racial and ethnic diversity in the United States has several major causes. In the 1800s and early to mid-1900s, the bulk of immigrants to the United States came from Western Europe. Hale (2000) mentions that worsening economic conditions in Mexico and Central America over the decade from 2000 to 2010 are largely responsible for the large number of immigrants from those areas. Gheisar and Clark (2000) write that the refugee populations streaming to the United States from war-ravaged regions of Asia, Africa, and Eastern Europe are presenting new challenges (and opportunities) for the public health community. This wave of new immigration, coupled with the fact that, regardless of country of origin, immigrants have higher rates of fertility than native-born peoples, means that the shifts in culture and the challenges to majority norms alluded to by Clark are likely here to stay.

Statistics from the U.S. Bureau of the Census (2010b) indicate that our country's population grew by 9.7 percent since 2000. The 2010 census found that the U.S. minority population was comprised of 12.4 percent African American, 16.3 percent Hispanic, 5.0 percent Asian or Pacific Islander, and 0.9 percent Native American. **Table 10.1** shows the projected percentage figures for each of these population groups for the years 2010, 2020, 2030, 2040, and 2050 (U.S. Bureau of the Census, 2010b).

From Table 10.1 it is readily apparent that the greatest percentage increase over the next 30 years will come from the Hispanic and Asian/Pacific Islander groups. The projected percentage increase of Hispanics and Asians from 2010 until 2050 is 71 percent and 50 percent, respectively. During this same time period, the percentage of non-Hispanic whites in the population will fall from 63 percent in the year 2010 to about 46 percent in the year 2050, a decrease of about 33 percent.

At least one ramification of these changes, increasing numbers of ethnic minority students in public school, is already being felt in the classrooms of our nation. In 2008, approximately 43 percent of the children in public schools in the United States were minorities. According to the U.S. Census Bureau, in 2012 the majority of children under one year of age in the U.S.

TABLE 10.1 **Projected U.S. population percentages of African Americans, Hispanics, Native Americans, and Asians or Pacific Islanders: 2010, 2020, 2030, 2040, and 2050**

Race	Year				
	2010 (%)	2020 (%)	2030 (%)	2040 (%)	2050 (%)
African American	12.4	12.5	12.7	12.8	13.0
Hispanic	16.3	20.1	22.0	25.0	28.0
Native American	0.9	0.8	0.7	0.7	0.7
Asian/Pacific Islander	5.0	5.6	6.3	7.0	7.6

(U.S. Census Bureau, 2010b)

are minority children (U.S. Census, 2012). From schools in Caldwell, Idaho, with a student population of nearly 60 percent nonwhite, to Chicago, Illinois, with a nonwhite student population of more than 80 percent, the escalating minority population makes an already diverse nation even more so. This trend presents health education specialists with an ever-widening array of opportunities and challenges as the 21st century continues to unfold.

Aging

Another demographic factor that will impact the practice of health education/promotion in the future is the aging population. The U.S. Bureau of the Census (2010b) lists persons age 65 or older as representing 13.0 percent of the U.S. population. Between the years 2010 and 2040, the population older than 65 is expected to grow to equal 23.0 percent of the total. To further illustrate this trend, the median age of the U.S. population in 2010 was 37.2. In the year 2020, it is estimated to be 38.3; and in 2030, it will be nearly 40.

One of the major reasons for the aging trend is that older Americans are living longer than ever before. Other causative factors accentuating changes in age demographics are that married couples in the United States are having fewer children, and the oldest of the baby boomers (those born between 1946 and 1964) are now beginning to retire. This group's massive size causes it to have a dominant effect on U.S. population statistics.

▷ Societal Trends

There probably has not been a time when societal change was as rapid as in the latter decades of the 20th century. For example, since 1960, there have been changes in societal mores and practices, such as more openness to cohabitation, a greater tolerance for premarital sex, more vocal and open gay relationships, a greater number of single-parent households, an increase in child abuse, more violence, an increase in the amount and availability of pornographic materials, massive changes in the number of ethical issues related to medicine, alterations in the way the medical establishment is organized and medical care is delivered, a decreasing respect for authority of any kind, declining support for K–12 public schools and higher education institutions, an infusion of and a reliance on technology, and a distrust of the political establishment in general. All of these factors play a big role in shaping the structure of society in the future. This section discusses several of the major societal trends that experts agree will impact health education/promotion in the new millennium.

Technology

Certainly, the boom in **technology** has affected, if not transformed, the lives of many people around the globe. Many of the advances in communication, transportation, medicine, engineering, and ease of access to information have created an enhanced quality of life for people worldwide. The increased availability and use of technology also creates myriad opportunities for the prospective health education specialist in the planning, design, implementation, and evaluation of programs and materials.

Today, it is impossible to find a campus that does not feature student computer labs in numerous locations and wireless technology in all buildings. In today's environment, many courses and even entire degree programs are offered using Web-based technologies, enabling the student to participate in class sessions in "real time" no matter where he or she resides. The constantly expanding technological capabilities in the field of education have created a learning environment in which information is readily available and lessons can be easily structured to require a greater degree of critical thinking and be more interactive than was possible only a few years ago. An increasing number of journals are published only in electronic form; no printed hard copy is available, and projects are under way to digitize entire collections of books and monographs, making the information contained in those publications not only more readily accessible but also content searchable. There is no doubt that the knowledge explosion trend fueled by new innovations in educational technology will continue and accelerate.

What does this rapid acceleration mean for health education specialists? Gold and Atkinson (2006) offer several intriguing considerations on how the advances in technology can and will revolutionize the delivery of health education/promotion.

- Extending our traditional health education/promotion delivery systems by reaching out across time and space, as well as literacy and language.
- Allowing both synchronous and asynchronous communications in pictures, sounds, movement, and virtual reality.
- Individualizing and personalizing communication and instruction through tailored messages and interventions based on the variables we know are likely to influence interest, ability, readiness, and a host of other relevant variables.
- Extending the way we internalize, understand, individualize, and use massive amounts of data through instant access to even the minutest detail in a large data repository.
- Enhancing opportunities to provide new services and interventions by creating new practices and strategies (p. 46).

The increased use of Web 2.0 and the expanding number and use of social media sites over the past five to eight years have elevated the possibilities for health promotion much as Gold and Atkinson postulated. Research by Thackery and colleagues (2008), Korda and Itani (2013), and Neiger and colleagues (2012) on methods to effectively use social media for health promotion has demonstrated that these media can work to not only inform and change attitudes but to alter behavior. As with most "in person" interventions, however, crafting the messages using behavioral theory and making certain that the message is designed in such a manner that two-way communication is achieved greatly increase the chances of success.

Clearly technology will greatly shape the face of the delivery of health education/promotion into the future. Students of health education/promotion must become familiar with the various media methods available to gather and deliver information including the creation of messages across multiple platforms such as tablets, laptop computers, and phones and, perhaps, in multiple languages. There may be a time in the not too distant future when health education specialists will be able to personalize messages like oncologists will personalize treatments based on DNA tests (D. Zuckerman, personal communication, 2013).

Family Structure

The U.S. family structure has changed dramatically since the 1960s (see **Figure 10.2**). The **traditional family** (two parents and their children) is becoming less and less common because of factors such as high rates of divorce, smaller families, postponed marriage and childbearing, teenage and nonmarital childbearing, stepfamilies, homosexual couples, and

▶ **Figure 10.2** An awareness of different family structures, such as extended families or single parents, is an important consideration when planning prevention messages.

dual-earner marriages (Acock & Demo, 1994). According to the U.S. Census Bureau's American Community Survey (2010a), only 66.7 percent of households fit the bureau's definition of a family with 49.3 percent constituting "family/married couples," and only 30.3 percent of families having children younger than 18 living with them.

In addition, about 33 percent of Americans live alone or in non-family combinations, such as with housemates, friends, or partnerships outside legal marriage. Another 7.3 percent are female-headed families with children, 2.2 percent are male-headed families with children.

In 1970, 85 percent of children younger than the age of 18 lived with both parents, and 18 percent lived with the mother only. In 2012, 64 percent of those younger than 18 lived with both parents, and 24 percent lived with the mother only. Of note is the fact that slightly more than 6 percent of 0- to 17-year-olds in 2012 lived with grandparents, other relatives, or in the homes of nonrelatives (Child Trends Data Bank, 2013).

The impact caused by these new structures is being felt throughout our society. Children are the most affected. Many parents today provide less guidance and support, and many seem to lack the commitment needed to be parents.

Simons-Morton, Greene, and Gottlieb (1995) document other stressful changes in the family. They mention that the high costs of providing for a family today practically require that a family have two incomes. This places a strain even on nuclear families with two parents; affordable daycare services for the children must be obtained. Currently, 71.3 percent of women with children are in the labor force (U.S. Department of Labor, 2011). For many low-income and single-parent families, the choice is no care or supervision at all—a situation that puts children at risk. In addition, fewer employers are offering health insurance, particularly in service-oriented positions that often pay minimum wage and are a major source of employment for many low-skilled workers. As a result, nearly 19 percent of children in the United States are living in poverty. This is the highest rate in the industrialized world (*Kids Count* Data Book, 2010). The linkage between these factors may be a predisposing condition leading to an increased rate of child abuse (McKenzie, Kotecki, & Pinger, 2008). Finally, it is no secret that the economic downturn since 2008 has contributed significantly to increasing the number of families and children under economic stress as a result of job loss or underemployment. Although the number of people employed may soon reach or exceed the number employed before the downturn, the type and often the pay scale of available jobs will be different than before 2008 further exacerbating the problem of economic distress (B. Parrish, personal communication, 2013).

The changes previously noted have significant implications for health education specialists. Family structures will likely remain diverse in the coming years and will probably operate on a new set of norms. In other words, new methods of reaching individuals, families, and communities will need to be created to improve the health of all family members in accordance with their needs.

Political Climate

As was mentioned previously, there remains little doubt that today there is an increasing frustration with politics and politicians in general. Whether a person is a **conservative**, one who generally distrusts governmental regulations and tax-supported programs for addressing social or economic problems; a **moderate**, one who usually acts in a more situationally specific manner in regard to using tax-supported programs to solve societal problems; or a **liberal**, one who generally supports government programs to attack social and economic problems, there seems to be no end to the bickering and infighting among members of various political parties. Many of the political issues considered in Congress relate to health. For example, the landmark agreement between the tobacco industry and the states over the sale and marketing of tobacco products to minors; the addition of prescription drug benefits to Medicare; determination of Medicaid eligibility and Medicaid expansion; the repeal of a motorcycle helmet law in Texas; the passage of a physician-assisted suicide law in Oregon, Washington, Montana, and Vermont; immigration reform and whether to offer healthcare coverage for those undocumented immigrants currently in the United States; climate change; minimum wage; timely physical and mental health care for veterans returning from wars in Iraq and Afghanistan; passage of and stages of implementation of the Affordable Care Act; community health center legislation; gun control; and the debate as to whether to increase spending on school lunches at the expense of food stamp allotments are examples of political issues that directly impact the health of the populace (see **Figure 10.3**).

▶ **Figure 10.3** An awareness of political issues that affect health will be even more crucial in the future.

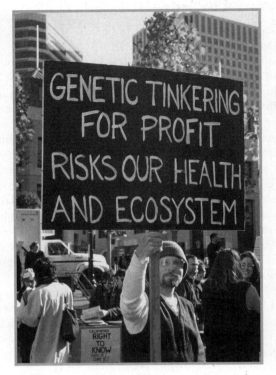

Politics and health seem to be inextricably linked. Some governmental officials and legislators worry that public health professionals infringe on personal autonomy by advocating for seat belt laws, tobacco laws, work site wellness programs, helmet laws, air bags, environmental protection, healthier options in fast foods, gun control laws, and health insurance for all. Others believe that legislation fostering a social climate that enhances the health of the population as a whole is worth the sacrifice of some personal choice and autonomy.

As citizens and professionals, the involvement of health education specialists in the political process is important. O'Rourke (2006) states, "Health education not only seeks to change lifestyles, but to create public understanding of the political issues involved in public health programs" (p. 9). He goes on to challenge all health education specialists to assume a **macrolevel** view of health problems. Using this approach, health education specialists move from a position of assisting behavior change one person at a time to community-based interventions. In implementing the community-based programs, success often depends on the health education specialist's having a working knowledge of the political process and how it impacts every decision. Hunter (2008) supports the fact that public health professionals can no longer be bystanders but must become passionate advocates for healthy change in individuals and communities. He believes that the collective advocacy of all public health practitioners is vital in moving governmental bodies to support and improve health.

There is little doubt that health education specialists must become participants in the political process. O'Rourke (2006) eloquently makes a case for enhancing the effectiveness of health education/promotion through an approach that

> encompasses collective responsibility and community involvement through participation in the political process and service on county health boards, city councils, and school boards. In these capacities, health educators can influence the health of entire communities and not rely on the 'one person at a time' model of improving health through individual responsibility. (p. 8)

To that end, a method for health education specialists to increase their visibility and political clout is advanced by McDermott (2000) when he challenges present and future health education specialists to consider the importance of research in the practice of health education/promotion. For interventions to be effective, health education specialists must use evidence-based practices when these practices are known. Future gains in the effectiveness and scope of prevention programs probably will be made only when health education specialists insist on pushing the research envelope to determine the factors that affect health and cause health disparities in populations, are components of effective intervention programs, and allow for dissemination of these programs across a variety of settings. Including community partners, community-based participatory research, and legislators in these research efforts is a strategy proven to gain trust and allies more welcoming to the benefit of macrolevel initiatives.

Medical Care Establishment and the Affordable Care Act

The healthcare system in the United States continues to be in need of an overhaul. Passage of the Affordable Care Act in early 2010 is a start in the right direction, but the exact impact of that legislation is far from certain as many of the provisions in the plan are set to be enacted from 2014 to 2020. Meanwhile, the cost of care continues to escalate, and the system seems stuck in an unsustainable model of reimbursement for procedures (fee-for-service) instead of a capitated reimbursement structure for helping people stay well. Citizens increasingly desire to be participants in their own care and to be provided with options. Enhancing the quality of life as opposed to simply increasing longevity is becoming a prevalent goal of U.S. healthcare consumers.

There are several reasons for this trend. Although few would deny that our medical care system has been responsible for saving countless lives, clearly health is largely a reflection of the nature of the environments in which a person resides, personal lifestyle choices, and standards of living, and not the medical care system. In the United States, medical care tends to concentrate on secondary and tertiary care and to ignore the value of primary prevention. In the United States, only three cents of every healthcare dollar are spent on prevention and well more than 75 percent of healthcare costs are attributable to preventable disease conditions (Forsberg & Fichtenberg, 2012).

These points are substantiated by Williams, McClellan, and Rivlin (2010) and Goodarz and colleagues (2010) when they state that healthier lives are best fostered in a climate of a culture of health. What seems to be most important in creating and maintaining health are the actions taken by individuals and communities to select and support habits like choosing what food we eat, having healthy relationships, staying physically active, and investing in safe and environmentally friendly neighborhoods. Much of health is tied not to medical intervention but to primary prevention.

The Affordable Care Act has increased the opportunities for health education specialists. Koh and Sebelius (2010) document that this law "promotes wellness in the workplace, providing new health promotion opportunities for employers and employees" (p. 4). In addition, the act strengthens the community role in promoting prevention and serves to enhance partnerships between state and local government and community groups and nonprofits.

Professionals representing the Society for Public Health Education (SOPHE, 2013) have published a "must read" issue brief titled, "Affordable Care Act: Opportunities and Challenges for Health Education Specialists," which discusses the potential expanding roles for health education specialists in both the healthcare and community settings under healthcare reform. This document succinctly captures the positives and barriers inherent as health education specialists strive to become included as members of a health team that seeks to promote health in the whole person.

The Boise, Idaho–based nonprofit corporation, Healthwise, the provider of the Web-based health information found in WebMD and responsible for much of the health education/promotion content disseminated by major insurance companies and hospitals around the country, offers an example of the value of health education/promotion in a clinical arena. Healthwise professionals have developed a health information and education prescription format that is tailored for consumers so that they can obtain the information they need to make choices about their own care. In addition, the information equips them to ask for the care that they need and facilitates their saying no to care that they do not need, Thus, patient autonomy is enhanced.

This approach bodes well for enhanced opportunities for health education specialists who desire to practice in a healthcare setting in large part because of the myriad set of situations, policies, and approaches that seem to have no solution: high pharmaceutical costs, nearly 48 million Americans currently without health insurance (although implementation of provisions in the Affordable Care Act will decrease this number), continuous federal tinkering with both the Medicare and Medicaid systems, lack of oversight for universal quality of care standards, high cost care with limited emphasis on quality, lack of affordability of private pay insurance, inconsistent chronic disease management protocols, and frustration with a lack of emphasis on prevention. Given these circumstances, health education specialists can facilitate patient choice by helping patients understand their options regarding physician choice, healthcare insurance plan, type of care, and intensity of services. In addition, they can assist medical organizations by increasing patient satisfaction through contributing to more one-on-one contact, improving patterns of communication between patient and provider, evaluating outcomes, and enhancing patient compliance with treatment regimens (T. Epperly, personal communication, Family Medicine Residency of Idaho, Boise, May 2013).

▷ Professional Preparation and Credentialing

Although the issues of professional preparation and credentialing were extensively covered in Chapter 6, both have implications for the future practice of health education/promotion. Thus, the reasons why health education/promotion practice might be affected by these issues are of some importance.

Professional Preparation

In this discussion, it is not our intent to provide a list of courses that must be taken to become a "better" health education specialist. Coursework is by nature specific to the institution you are attending. Course titles and descriptions vary widely from one program to another. As you are aware, the coursework you will take in your degree program is interdisciplinary. We attempt to provide some ideas, concepts, and objectives for you to consider as you enter your preparation program.

The social changes previously discussed in this chapter are the challenges driving health education specialists of the future to be proactive in meeting the demands placed on them. What tasks will a health education specialist need to be able to perform to be effective in the decades ahead? Clark (1994) helps answer this question by making several salient points about health education/promotion in the future:

1. The mission will be less providing factual information and more helping people become more analytical thinkers...
2. There will be...stronger partnerships with the medical establishment....
3. Health education specialists will need...Long-term, not short-term, thinking...
4. A greater emphasis will be placed on values clarification....
5. ...Education at the community level will be the focus of most health interventions.
6. There will be an enhanced need for quality research,...
7. Health education specialists must...use technology to help people learn.
8. ...The gap between school and community services will close.
9. Environmental activism will continue to emerge...
10. ...people will judge the success of health education/promotion by whether or not their quality of life has improved.

Several of Clark's thoughts echo those of O'Rourke (2006), who challenges health education specialists to be more macrolevel-oriented. In other words, there is an ever-growing need to facilitate health education/promotion interventions at the community level (as opposed to the individual level, or **microlevel**). Inherent in this charge is that those who reside in the community where the intervention occurs will be totally involved in the planning from the outset. English and Videto (1997) affirm these observations when they state, "Regardless of our place of practice, our ability to identify and meet the needs of our local communities and neighborhoods is likely to be the measure that will determine our success as health educators...successful programs use community involvement" (p. 4).

Three additional documents that provide information about the competencies health education specialists must possess into the future are described next. The first two can be found using the Weblinks at the end of this chapter. The first document features the deliberations by members of the Committee on Educating Public Health Professionals for the 21st Century. The workshop participants who wrote the article "Who Will Keep the Public Healthy? Workshop Summary" (Weblinks #3) identify eight new content areas that should be added to the curricula of individuals studying to practice public health: informatics, genomics, communication, community-based participatory research, global health, health policy, health law, and public health ethics. Although the report is largely directed at universities offering graduate programs, even a cursory glance finds several suggested content areas that are relevant to the practice of health education/promotion. The list also shows the rapidly expanding knowledge base the future health education specialist will need to have to successfully interact with health professionals from a variety of other fields. The more understanding a health education specialist has about the vocabulary and nature of the work of other health providers, the more likely she or he is to be an accepted and valued member of the healthcare community.

The second document presents the results of a study titled "Health Educator Job Analysis 2010." The study was commissioned by the American Association for Health Education (AAHE), the Society for Public Health Education (SOPHE), and the National Commission for Health Education Credentialing (NCHEC). In short, the study describes current health education/promotion practice in the United States and helps set the stage for revisiting competencies for entry-level and advanced practitioners.

The third document, a cogent paper written by McKenzie (2004), cautions that those in charge of health education preparation programs must not assume that it is possible or even advisable to prepare "generic" health education specialists. The four practice settings to which he refers in the quote that follows are discussed later in this chapter. McKenzie states, "...even though the responsibilities and competencies of health educators are similar regardless of the settings, the work is indeed different and the preparation cannot be the same..." (p. 48).

It is apparent that tomorrow's health education specialists must be able to respond rapidly to changes in all avenues of society. When planning, implementing, and evaluating programs and working in multidimensional settings, they must enter into collaborative relationships with healthcare professionals from other disciplines in a spirit of cooperation. Health education specialists who are not afraid to be innovative, who respect but do not fear change, who are not just purveyors of information but community builders and facilitators of learning, who are politically active, who continue to be curious and learn themselves, who have a sense of adventure, and who seek the truth through thoughtful research, study, and dialogue are the individuals who will lead our profession into the next several decades.

Credentialing

The history of and reasons for credentialing were thoroughly covered in Chapter 6. There are, however, several facets of credentialing that need reemphasis because they have profound implications for the future practice of health education/promotion.

The credentialing process as it now stands begins with the candidate's submitting a transcript of coursework in health education to the NCHEC. On verification by NCHEC that the candidate has completed coursework leading to a degree in health education and the coursework has focused on the responsibilities and competencies of an entry-level health education specialist, the applicant is permitted to sit for the certification exam. Exam questions are based on the seven responsibilities and competencies for entry-level health education specialists. Individuals who pass the exam are awarded a Certified Health Education Specialist (CHES) credential. Those individuals must then complete continuing education units on regular basis to maintain their credential.

A question that is often asked is, "should all individuals who seek a CHES certification complete the same process?" As mentioned previously, this tends to skew the credential in favor of creating a generic health education specialist (see McKenzie, 2004).

Some practicing health education specialists argue that the skills needed to teach health in a school setting differ from those needed to conduct a community program at a local American Cancer Society office or to direct health promotion programs at a worksite or clinical healthcare site. For example, school health education specialists often see the need to be content specialists, whereas community health education specialists may be more focused on process and skills.

Health education specialists practice in a variety of settings (e.g., school, work site, community, health care); they may work with different populations (e.g., adults, the aged, children, minorities); they may be process specialists (e.g., program planners, program implementers, program evaluators); or they may be content specialists (e.g., HIV/AIDS, cancer prevention, injury or violence prevention, nutrition). Should there be a generic credential? Perhaps in the future there will be "practice-specific" credentials. A potential important consequence of having a CHES credential is that of eligibility for reimbursement for services rendered. As different care models are advanced with prevention as a focus (thanks to the Affordable Care Act), insurers are limiting the types of providers eligible for reimbursement. Without some external credential or license, it is highly unlikely that any health education services rendered in a medical care setting will be reimbursed (Idaho Blue Shield Human Resources Department, personal communication, June 2008).

The credentialing process is here to stay. The bottom line is that this certification program does "establish a national standard for individual health education specialists. It differs from state and local certifications and registries in that the requirements do not vary from one locale to another" (NCHEC, 2013). The CHES process works well and is endorsed by prevention specialists and organizations nationwide. Potential changes to the credentialing process and necessary competencies that emanate from the study, "Health Educator Job Analysis 2010," referenced in the previous section of this chapter will most likely occur. Students should stay abreast of developments in credentialing by visiting the NCHEC and SOPHE Web sites on a regular basis.

Caile Spear, literally the last president of the now disbanded professional organization, AAHE posits that the joining together of the public health professions that focus on prevention will better make their voice more clearly heard and their message more uniform. She goes on to say that joining of these professions will mimic what funding agencies are doing in that they would be soliciting projects that encompass holistic approaches to addressing health issues. Funding agencies are moving away from providing funds for specific health problems (e.g., substance abuse, child abuse, lack of physical activity, etc.) to funding more global strategies. Similarly, a united group of prevention professionals (including health education specialists), regardless of practice setting, will be more powerful in making a local and national case for the role of prevention in overall health than the current model in which prevention professionals often are members of several different professional organizations (personal communication, May 2013).

As the profession of health education/promotion continues to evolve and health education specialists become more visible partners in the delivery of health services, students considering careers in this field should seriously consider obtaining CHES certification. The CHES credential assists employers in identifying practitioners who have met national standards, and it assures the consumers of health education/promotion services that the health educators with whom they work are competent professionals.

▷ Implications for Practice Settings

Chapter 7 detailed the variety of settings in which health education specialists can practice: the worksite, school, clinical/health care, or public health. Each setting has unique characteristics, and the practice set of skills or competencies may vary from one setting to another. However, the settings also are similar in that the goal of health education/promotion is to create a climate that facilitates the improvement of health status for every member of the population served by each entity. The first part of this chapter described various influences destined to impact the health of the populace into the next century. This section briefly summarizes the future role of the health education specialist in each setting.

School Setting

"Children don't learn as well when they are not healthy" (Seffrin, 1994, p. 397). "Schools are an integral part of the community, and, if we don't have high quality school health education we will pay the price later in higher costs to all of us. Health education specialists regardless of practice setting should support and be champions for well-funded, vigorous and vital school health programs" (Spear, personal communication, August 2010). As the national dialogue over Core Standards for public schools continues, the Coalition of National Health Education Organizations (CNHEO) is advocating for the inclusion of health education as a part of the standards (CNHEO, 2013). These statements characterize the goal and importance of school health education and provide direction for school health education specialists (see **Figure 10.4**). If children's well-being is to be maintained or enhanced, a coordinated approach) to providing health education is needed (Allensworth & Kolbe, 1987). The coordinated school health approach consists of eight components integrated to meet all of the health needs of the children and adolescents attending the school: (1) classroom school health education lessons, (2) the school lunch program, (3) health screenings, (4) physical education, (5) a healthy and safe school environment, (6) the availability of trained school counselors, (7) faculty and staff health promotion, and (8) family and community support

▶ **Figure 10.4** Schools can serve as sites for offering preventive health services and education.

for education and health. Actually implementing this model is a tall order. In their discussion summarizing a study on school health policies and programs, Kolbe and colleagues (1995) note:

> School health policies and programs, particularly at the school level, may not adequately address several of the most serious public health problems today such as violence, unintentional injuries such as motor vehicle crashes, and unintended pregnancies. School health services that do not respond to these problems, classroom instruction that is inadequate in scope and depth, and school health policies that only include punitive rather than remedial responses to violations must be replaced with more responsive programs. (p. 343)

Should you choose to practice health education/promotion in a school setting, what skills and abilities must you possess if schools are to incorporate a coordinated health education/promotion program to address the health needs of children and adolescents, both now and in the future? In light of the information on influences on health in this chapter and that on settings for health education/promotion from Chapter 7, we think that the following skills are imperative. You must be able to:

1. Read and interpret the findings of health research on effective health programs and practices.
2. Create a logical scope and sequence to health content units that incorporate age-appropriate information.
3. Prepare and deliver lessons that are participatory in nature, stress skill development, and foster attitudes necessary for problem solving and informed decision making.
4. Use both qualitative and quantitative strategies to evaluate your lessons, your units, and the district health education/promotion program.
5. Assess the health needs of the students, faculty, and staff.
6. Ensure that health and counseling services are provided for students.
7. Create or coordinate a parent/community health education/promotion advisory council.
8. Actively participate in local, state, regional, and national professional organizations.
9. Use technology and social media to assist in both updating your own skills and delivering health education/promotion messages to your school and community.
10. Learn about the influence of culture on health, cultivate sensitivity toward it, and instill an awareness of it in your teaching.
11. Assist teachers at all grade levels in obtaining age-appropriate health education materials and help coordinate a classroom scope and sequence for all grade levels in your district.
12. Serve as resource person and liaison between the school health setting and other settings in which health education might occur.
13. Acquire sound oral and written communication techniques.
14. Work both independently and as a member of a team.
15. Apply behavior-change strategies and what is known about environmental influences on behavior to the classroom setting.

16. Collaborate with health education specialists practicing in the community, work site, or healthcare setting to coordinate the delivery of disease prevention and health promotion messages and programs.

17. Teach and promote the enhancement of strategies to increase health literacy among the population served to reduce health disparities (Hasnain-Wynia & Wolf, 2010).

School health educators who possess these skills will be well prepared to lead programs that enhance the health of the students, teachers, and staff in their schools.

Work-Site Setting

The workplace of today bears little resemblance to that of only 20 years ago. Because many employers want to attract the best employees and they realize that employee satisfaction is key in productivity and retention, work sites have introduced programs for employees and their families that provide continuing education, recreational opportunities, health promotion, and financial planning. In particular, work sites have become an increasingly important setting for health education/promotion programs. Examples of programs offered include stress management, work-site safety, drug and alcohol abuse prevention, and tobacco cessation. As noted previously in this chapter, the Affordable Care Act also signals the advent of a renewed emphasis on work-site health promotion (Koh & Sebelius, 2010).

The influence of changing demographic patterns on health education/promotion in general was discussed previously. However, another factor must be taken into account when specifically anticipating the future direction of worksite health promotion. The greatest percentage of persons joining the workforce in the decade between 2010 and 2020 will be women and minorities.

The expansion of work-site health promotion programs bodes well for the future of health education/promotion and the concurrent need for an increasing number of trained health education specialists. This truth has broad implications for the future practice of work-site health education/promotion. Together with the information presented both earlier in this chapter and in Chapter 7, the following competencies represent a baseline for the future practice of health education/promotion in worksite settings:

1. Recognize the importance of cultural and demographic influences on individual and group health behavioral choices.

2. Coordinate needs assessments of work-site populace and conduct evaluations of program components.

3. Identify and work with aspects of the corporate organizational climate that facilitate or impede participation.

4. Become familiar with the culture inherent in a business setting.

5. Prepare and conduct prevention presentations to worksite subgroups.

6. Conduct fitness assessments and participate in health screenings.

7. Use up-to-date technology to market programs to work-site supervisors, employees, and their families through newsletters, brochures, Internet chat groups, and social media.

8. Plan and manage a budget.

9. Coordinate employee coalitions and steering committees to maximize employee input into program components.

10. Function as a resource person for health information for employees and their families.

11. Be able to apply behavior-change strategies and what is known about environmental influences on behavior to the work-site setting.

12. Implement programs in a manner consistent with management philosophy.

13. Attain a working knowledge of epidemiological and statistical principles and applications.

14. Acquire sound oral and written communication techniques.

15. Work both independently and as a member of a team.

16. Design and employ evaluation strategies that are outcomes-based to assess program effectiveness.

17. Gain a thorough understanding of current, relevant literature and well-designed research studies that influence health promotion practice in the work-site setting.

18. Teach and promote the enhancement of strategies to increase health literacy among the population served to reduce health disparities (Hasnain-Wynia & Wolf, 2010).

Incorporating competencies such as those listed previously into the professional preparation program will help ensure that you are ready to begin practice as a work-site health education specialist.

Public Health Setting

The community setting (called the *public health setting* in this text) has the greatest variety of options for the practice of health education/promotion. For example, health education specialists are employed in many local, city, state, and federal health departments; in many federal agencies; in county extension agencies; in nonprofit and volunteer health organizations (e.g., American Cancer Society, American Heart Association, American Red Cross); in churches; in homeless shelters; in grassroots community organizations; and in prisons. One reason for the diversity of opportunities is that the mission, goals, and objectives of one community agency may differ dramatically from those of another. Some agencies might have a health education specialist serving as a coordinator of services or as a fund-raiser, whereas in another agency the educator might plan, conduct, and evaluate programs. Another, more obvious reason for increased employment opportunities is that almost every locale in the United States has one of the aforementioned groups.

The purpose of community health organizations is to both monitor and improve the health of the public they serve. Goodman (2000) mentions that when health education specialists combine forces with people from other professional disciplines (e.g., ecologists, economists, anthropologists, communication specialists), the probability of reducing the health risks of populations is heightened. Consequently, collaboration with community organizations and with other professionals to address population health is a skill that all health education specialists must develop. In this era of using health education/promotion to help reduce healthcare costs, and with an increasing need for community-level programs, public health education specialists are well positioned to participate in improving the health of citizens from all regions of the United States.

With employment opportunities for health education specialists in the public setting on the rise, what skills will the public health education specialists of the future need to function effectively? Following is a list of competencies or attributes that will be critical to the effective practice of public health education. They are not in any specific order of importance.

1. Recognize the importance of cultural and demographic influences on individual and group health behavioral choices.

2. Maintain competence in the use of technology and social media to access and deliver health-related information.

3. Learn and use strategies to seek information, guidance, and support from community members regarding their health needs.

4. Assess strengths of communities in building a plan to assist them in meeting their health needs.

5. Apply behavior-change strategies and what is known about environmental influences on behavior to the public health setting.

6. Learn and practice research-based coalition-building strategies.

7. Actively participate in local, state, regional, and national professional organizations.

8. Study and apply the fundamentals of obtaining extramural funding.

9. Use a variety of marketing strategies to reach diverse community constituencies.

10. Learn to be flexible because the job probably will involve changing and varied responsibilities.

11. Learn another language.

12. Advocate policies that enhance the role of prevention and provide for universal access to health services when needed.

13. Foster the ability to work in a multidisciplinary environment.

14. Attain a working knowledge of epidemiological and statistical principles and applications.

15. Acquire excellent oral and written communication techniques.

16. Work independently and as a member of a team.

17. Design and employ evaluation strategies that are outcomes based to assess program effectiveness.

18. Gain a thorough understanding of current, relevant literature and well-designed research studies that influence practice in the community setting (i.e., community-based participatory research).

19. Teach and promote the enhancement of strategies to increase health literacy among the population served to reduce health disparities (Hasnain-Wynia & Wolf, 2010).

A well-trained community health education specialist will undoubtedly make an increased contribution to the health of populations. With the increasing health awareness of U.S. citizens and the multitude of cultural changes in society, community health education specialists have a bright and exciting future.

Clinical or Healthcare Setting

Healthcare settings employ health education specialists in a variety of institutions and a multitude of ways. Health education specialists can be employed in for-profit and public hospitals, health maintenance organizations (HMOs), health insurance corporations, medical care clinics, and home health agencies. They might be involved in conducting one-on-one patient education; planning and implementing education programs for enrollees or other medical providers; coordinating community education programs on a variety of health topics; conducting program evaluations; marketing the health services available through the hospital, clinic, or HMO; conducting health education/promotion activities for the employees; or serving as a member of a community health promotion team.

Epperly (personal communication, May 2013) feels that healthcare providers, insurance companies, and the public in general are becoming more receptive to the notion that accurate and timely health information is an important part of any treatment regimen. Lack of adequate health education/promotion can negate potential positive contributions in the prevention and management of disease. With no end in sight to the skyrocketing costs of health care, the word *prevention* is being incorporated into more care plans than ever before.

Yarnall and colleagues (2003) note that the evidence of preventive services is well established but the rate of the delivery of preventive services by medical providers is severely lacking. Their study of time burdens required to deliver preventive care concluded that the major reason for the lack of delivery is that, to fulfill the U.S. Preventive Health Services Task Force recommendations, a primary care physician with a "normal" practice would have to dedicate nearly 7.5 hours per day solely to the delivery of preventive services. Obviously, this time allocation is impossible because physicians need to spend most their time diagnosing and treating disease. Yarnall's study concludes with the following statement: "Our current system of preventive care delivery—provided by physicians...no longer meets national needs. New methods of preventive care delivery are required, as well as a clearer focus on which services can be best provided, and by whom" (p. 640).

The shift in practice norms by most clinical healthcare professionals requires trained personnel to ensure that education in the healthcare setting meets the needs of both the patient and the provider and motivates the patient to adopt a healthier lifestyle and comply with any treatment regimen. Given the medical community's acceptance of the value of health education/promotion in patient care, the outlook is positive for more employment opportunities for health education specialists in healthcare settings. What skills, competencies, and attributes will be absolutely necessary for the health education specialist of the future who seeks employment in a healthcare setting? Following is a list (in no particular order):

1. Obtain a working knowledge of epidemiological and statistical principles and applications.

2. Maintain competence in the use of technology to access and deliver health-related information.

3. Be able to apply behavior-change strategies and what is known about environmental influences on behavior to the healthcare setting.

4. Recognize the importance of cultural and demographic influences on individual and group health behavioral choices. Health education specialists should be culturally competent.

5. Become familiar with technological innovations to provide better outreach to patients, employees, and their families through a variety of electronic and hard copy newsletters, brochures, Internet chat groups, Web sites, and social media.

6. Provide training in health education/promotion theory to other members of the healthcare team.

7. Become familiar with the clinical disease process.

8. Advocate policies that enhance the role of prevention and provide for universal access to health services when needed.

9. Prepare and deliver lessons that are participatory in nature and research-based, that stress skill development, and that foster attitudes necessary for problem solving and informed decision making.

10. Coordinate interdisciplinary teams or steering committees to maximize input into program components.

11. Learn to be flexible, as the job probably will involve changing and varied responsibilities.

12. Serve as a liaison between the healthcare setting and other settings in which health education might occur.

13. Function as a resource person for health information for patients and their families.

14. Learn another language.

15. Acquire sound oral and written communication techniques.

16. Work independently and as a member of a team.

17. Obtain a working knowledge of the role of informatics in assisting in prevention at all vulnerable points in the causal chains leading to disease, injury, or disability (Davies, Smith, & Gustafson, 2001).

18. Teach and promote the enhancement of strategies to increase health literacy among the population served to reduce health disparities (Hasnain-Wynia & Wolf, 2010).

With rapid changes occurring in medical care delivery today, there is much reason for health education specialists to be optimistic about employment opportunities. As the public demands health education/promotion and disease prevention as a part of their medical care treatment plan, health education specialists will increasingly be identified as the best prepared to assist individuals in adopting healthy lifestyles.

▷ Alternative Settings

Besides the four traditional practice settings previously discussed, there are several other viable alternatives for the practice of health education/promotion into the next century. In this section, we briefly introduce these choices so that individuals who are interested can research them further.

The first alternative is to teach health education/promotion in a **postsecondary institution,** usually defined as an institution that educates people after they graduate from high school. There will continue to be a need for qualified instructors. Minimum standards for obtaining one of these positions is usually a master's degree in health education and two to five years of experience for a community college or vocational school position, and a doctorate and two to five years of experience for a college or university position.

Students who are interested in combining the fields of health education/promotion and journalism can find positions in both the print (traditional print media as well as using blogging, Twitter, and reporting for online sources) and TV media as health reporters for newspapers, magazines, and TV stations. A broad-based knowledge of health issues and a passion for writing or speaking are necessary qualifications.

Because of the increasing interdependence among nations and because there are many areas of the world in which health assistance is badly needed, health education specialist positions will continue to be available in foreign countries. Examples include positions with organizations such as the Peace Corps, Project Hope, the United Nations, the Pan American Health Organization, and the World Health Organization. Many national church organizations also send interdisciplinary health teams to international locations to improve the health of the populace. Often, the health education specialist must have a college degree, some experience, and ability to speak a foreign language.

Medical supply companies, pharmaceutical companies, sports equipment manufacturers, health food stores, and textbook publishers often employ health education specialists in sales positions. A college degree is required. In addition, a willingness to travel, excellent oral and written communication skills, critical thinking, ability to analyze research information (what is "real" and what is "hype") and an ability to work with all types of people are necessary prerequisites.

Because of the aging of the U.S. population, demand for health education specialists in long-term care institutions and retirement communities is escalating. Elders are living longer and want to be active in their retirement years, thus, many employment opportunities are opening up. Usually, a college degree is required. Excellent oral and written communication skills are essential, as is a desire to listen and learn from the wisdom of individuals residing in these communities.

There continues to be an increasing number of opportunities for health education specialists in entrepreneurial and consultant roles. As self-employed persons, these individuals are free to set up their own practice, hiring out as consultants to organizations that temporarily need someone with expertise in grant writing, program planning and evaluation, software development, professional speaking, or technical writing. Other possibilities include contracting with several small businesses to conduct work-site health promotion, freelancing with HMOs and other insurance providers to offer health education/promotion services (reimbursement will be an issue), serving as a content specialist (e.g., stress management, eating disorders, substance abuse) to businesses and corporations, becoming a certified personal trainer, and teaching part-time in colleges, community colleges, or evening community education/promotion programs.

Now that we have explored the differences in the various practice settings, we reemphasize the fact that there are common tasks for health education specialists that transcend the individual practice settings. Dr. John Seffrin, director of the American Cancer Society, eloquently reminds us of the direction health education/promotion must take, no matter what the practice setting, if it is to realize its potential. His scholar's address (Seffrin, 1997), given to members of the AAHE, describes four actions for present and future health education specialists that still ring true today:

1. Look at ourselves as major players in keeping Americans healthy; to that end, work with policy makers to affect legislation that truly promotes health.
2. Collaborate with other health professionals in both the for-profit and the not-for-profit sectors.

3. Strive to exhibit greater professional solidarity; be an advocate for the profession of health education/promotion and the role that trained health education specialists can play as part of the healthcare team.

4. Advocate for those who do not have a voice; be a spokesperson in the political arena, and work to ensure that health services and health education/promotion are available for all.

 ## Summary

This chapter began with the notion of change as a constant. Although no one can actually "see" into the future, it is obvious that flexibility is imperative to adapt to ongoing change. This is an exciting time to become a health education specialist. Opportunities have never been greater, and the future has never looked brighter. The job outlook for health education specialists is anticipated to increase by 37 percent over the next 10 years (Bureau of Labor Statistics, 2013). There is little doubt that health education/promotion will continue to expand in all of the more traditional as well as some of the nontraditional settings. Health education specialists have the training and expertise to make a positive difference in enhancing the quality of life for all people. We wish you success as you begin your journey.

 ## Review Questions

1. Identify three work-site settings in which health education specialists will practice to a greater degree than they currently do.

2. How will each of the societal changes discussed in the chapter impact the practice of health education/promotion in the work-site setting? The clinical/medical care setting? The school setting? The public health setting?

3. What are the implications for health education/promotion graduates who choose not to become credentialed (CHES)?

4. How will changing demographic patterns affect the practice of health education/promotion in nontraditional settings?

5. What is meant by the statement "Health education specialists need to become enhanced advocates for the profession"?

6. How will the passage of the Affordable Care Act impact the practice of health education/promotion?

 ## Case Study

One day, while leaving the health education/promotion office on your campus, you notice an announcement posted on the message board that the health education/promotion program in which you are enrolled is seeking national accreditation. The announcement includes information from the department chair on the reasons for accreditation along with a request for student assistance in working with faculty to prepare the necessary self-study documentation before the visit from an outside review team. Because you are entering the second semester of your junior year, you decide that a great way to learn more about the health education/promotion program and the field of health education/promotion in general would be to volunteer.

You notify the department chair of your willingness to help, and she appoints you to one of the program study committees, specifically the committee dealing with the use of Web-based teaching in delivering the health education/promotion curriculum. You are excited about that committee because you have some opinions on the value of Web-based courses. Although you have never enrolled in a Web-based course yourself, you know people who have, and they seem to have mixed feelings about the courses they have taken. The ambivalence of your classmates has led you to believe that Web-based courses are not as rigorous as courses offered by more traditional methods, and they do not allow for as much interaction between students as do traditionally delivered courses.

At the first meeting of the study committee, the committee chair outlines tasks that will need to be accomplished and suggests a timeline for completion. One of the major tasks is to determine whether the Web-based courses offered by the department are meeting the goals for which they are designed. What key questions would you need to ask to obtain that information? What methods would you use to collect the data? How might the findings be used by health education/promotion programs in planning for the future?

Critical Thinking Questions

1. After reading the chapter and in your opinion, what major demographic trend will most impact the delivery of health education/promotion in the next several decades? Given your answer, describe the health education specialist in the year 2020.

2. Compare and contrast the lists of competencies noted in the chapter for the four major practice settings in which a health education specialist might practice. Use your findings to support or refute the claim made by some professionals that health education specialists will be much more effective if their preparation programs include coursework specific to the settings in which they will practice.

3. Read the report by SOPHE that was referred to in the chapter. Using the information from that report, what duties might you assign to health education specialists desiring to practice in the clinical setting? How might your choices influence the Centers for Disease Control and Prevention goal of eliminating health disparities in the United States within the next 10 years?

4. Assume that it is the year 2045 and you are retiring after many years as a practicing health education specialist. At your retirement banquet, you have been asked to spend five minutes summarizing the accomplishments of your profession. What will you say?

5. What are two ways in which the health education/health promotion community can make the message of prevention more palatable to the public? What are the major barriers you must address? How might you implement your ideas?

Activities

1. Make a list of your five strongest attributes. Make a second list of the five tasks you most like to do. Using these lists and what you know about health education/promotion, write a paragraph describing the "perfect" health education/promotion job for you.

2. Construct and administer a short survey to the health education/promotion faculty at your institution to determine their thoughts on the major factors influencing the current and future practice of health education/promotion. Compile your results.

3. Interview a graduate from your school's health education/promotion program who is now practicing in the field as a certified health education specialist. Try to ascertain his or her feelings about his or her position and the influences he or she feels will impact health education/promotion practice both now and in the future.

4. Write a job description that will be used to advertise for a new public health education specialist position in a work-site setting. In the document be sure to include necessary applicant qualifications and expected duties.

▷ Weblinks

1. **http://www.healthypeople.gov**

   Healthy People 2020

   Web site of the national *Healthy People 2020* documents that describe U.S. goals and objectives for creating a healthier population by 2020.

2. **http://www.kingcounty.gov/healthservices/health.aspx**

   Seattle and King County Public Health Section

   This outstanding Web site was launched by the Seattle King County Health Department to help health education specialists and the public obtain current information on a variety of pertinent public health topics such as bioterrorism preparedness, family planning and reproductive health, diabetes, HIV/AIDS, and others.

3. **http://www.nationalacademies.org**

   "Who Will Keep the Public Healthy?"

   Search the National Academies Web site for a 2003 report from the Institute of Medicine of the National Academies that suggests specific ways to improve public health professionals' capabilities to address new and complex challenges. The report emphasizes that public health professionals in government health departments, other health services, community agencies, and universities have a shared responsibility to prevent illness and injury and keep communities healthy.

4. **http://www.cnheo.org/**

   Coalition of National Health Education Organizations Web site

   Provides a link to the study on Health Educator Job Analysis 2010 that was referenced in the chapter.

5. **http://www.kaiseredu.org**

   The Henry J. Kaiser Family Foundation

   The Kaiser Family Foundation Web site highlights health policy issues and enables the user to access background information on several current health policy topics. Modules and slide tutorials explaining the policy issues are also included.

6. **http://www.rwjf.org/**

   Web site of the Robert Wood Johnson Foundation featuring papers on health policy, health issues analyses, grant opportunities, and research and commentaries on healthcare reform.

7. **http://www.cdc.gov/healthcommunication/**

   CDC Web site on health communications and marketing strategies for health promotion programs. Features examples of programs that have been successful. Also has a portal to the *Health Communication Science Digest* journal.

References

Acock, A. C., & Demo, D. H. (1994). *Family diversity and well-being.* Thousand Oaks, CA: Sage.

Allensworth, D. D., & Kolbe, L. J. (1987). The comprehensive school health program: Exploring an expanded concept. *Journal of School Health, 57* (10), 409–412.

Bureau of Labor Statistics. 2013. U.S. Department of Labor, Occupational Outlook Handbook, Health Educators. 2012–2013 edition. Retrieved on June 3, 2013, from http://www.bls.gov/ooh/community-and-social-service/health-educators.htm.

Child Trends Data Bank. (2013). Family Structure. Retrieved on September 4, 2013, from http://www.childtrendsdatabank.org/.

Clark, N. M. (1994). Health educators and the future: Lead, follow, or get out of the way. *Journal of Health Education, 25* (3), 136–141.

Coalition of National Health Education Organizations (CNHEO). (2013). Improving school health: Elevating health education and physical education. Retrieved on June 3, 2013, from http://www.sophe.org/School%20Health%20Fact%20Sheet-FINAL.pdf.

Davies, J., Smith, G., & Gustafson, D. (2001). Public health informatics transforms the notifiable condition system. *Northwest Public Health, Spring/Summer,* 14–17.

English, G. M., & Videto, D. M. (1997). The future of health education: The knowledge to practice paradox. *Journal of Health Education, 28* (1), 4–8.

Forsberg, V., & Fichtenberg, C. (2012). *The prevention and public health fund: A critical investment in our nation's physical and fiscal health.* American Public Health Association, Center for Public Health Policy Issue Brief, 1–52.

Fox, S. (2011). Health topics: 80% of users look for health information online. Pew Internet and American Life Project. Retrieved May 18, 2013, from http://www.pewinternet.org/Reports/2011/Health Topics.aspx.

Gheisar, R. E., & Clark, C. J. (2000). New immigrant and refugee communities mean new challenges for public health. *Washington Public Health, Fall,* 2. Retrieved August 23, 2013, from http://www.nwpublichealth.org/docs/wph2000/trends.pdf.

Gold, R. S., & Atkinson, N. L. (2006). Imagine this, imagine that. A look into the future of technology for health educators. *The Health Education Monograph Series, 23* (1), 44–48.

Goodarz, D., Rimm, E. B., Oza, S., Kulkarni, S., Murray, C. J. L., et al. (2010). The promise of prevention: The effects of four preventable factors on national life expectancy and life expectancy disparities by race and county in the United States. *PLoS Medicine, 7* (3), 1–13.

Goodman, R. M. (2000). On contemplation at 50: SOPHE Presidential Address. *Health Education and Behavior, 27* (4), 423–429.

Hale, C. (2000). Demographic trends influencing public health practice. *Washington Public Health, Fall,* University of Washington, 1–3.

Hasnain-Wynia, R., & Wolf, M. (2010). Promoting health care equity: Is health literacy a missing link? *Health Services Research, 45* (4), 897–903.

Hunter, D. J. (2008). Health needs more than healthcare: The need for the new paradigm. *European Journal of Public Health, 18* (3), 217–219.

Kids Count Data Book. (2010). New York: Annie E. Casey Foundation. Retrieved on September 9, 2010, from http://www.aecf.org/MajorInitiatives/KIDSCOUNT.aspx.

Koh, H. K., & Sebelius, K. G. (2010). Promoting prevention through the Affordable Care Act. *The New England Journal of Medicine,* 1–5. Retrieved on September 9, 2010, from http://healthpolicyandreform.nejm.org/?p=12171.

Kolbe, L. J., Kann, L., Collins, J. L, Small, M. L., Pateman, B. C., et al. (1995). The School Health Policies and Programs Study (SHPPS): Context, methods, general findings, and future efforts. *Journal of School Health, 65* (8), 339–343.

Korda, H., & Itani, Z. (2013). Harnessing social media for health promotion and behavior change. *Health Promotion Practice 14* (1), 15–23.

McDermott, R. J. (2000). Health education research: Evolution or revolution (or maybe both)? *Journal of Health Education, 31* (5), 264–271.

McKenzie, J. F. (2004). Professional preparation: Is a generic health educator really possible? *American Journal of Health Education, 35* (1), 46–48.

McKenzie, J. F., Kotecki, J. E., & Pinger, R. R. (2008). *An introduction to community health*. Boston, MA: Jones and Bartlett.

National Commission for Health Education Credentialing (NCHEC). (2013). *CHES requirements*. Retrieved on May 21, 2013, from http://www.nchec.org/.

Neiger, B. L., Thackery, R., Van Wagenen, S. A., Hanson, C. L., West, J. H., et al. (2012). Use of social media in health promotion: Purposes, key performance indicators, and evaluation metrics. *Health Promotion Practice, 13* (3), 159–164.

O'Rourke, T. (2006). Philosophical reflections on health education and health promotion: Shifting sands and ebbing tides. *The Health Education Monograph Series, 23* (1), 7–10.

Seffrin, J. R. (1994). America's interest in comprehensive school health education. *Journal of School Health, 64* (10), 397–399.

Seffrin, J. R. (March 1997). *AAHE scholar's address*. St. Louis: American Alliance for Health, Physical Education, Recreation, and Dance Convention.

Simons-Morton, B.G., Greene, W.H., & Gottlieb, N.H. (1995). Introduction to health education and health promotion (2nd ed.). Prospect Heights, IL: Waveland Press.

Society for Public Health Education (SOPHE). (2013). Affordable Care Act: Opportunities and Challenges for Health Education Specialists. Retrieved on May 22, 2013, from http://www.sophe.org/Sophe/PDF/ACA-Opportunities-and-Challenges-for-Health-Educators-FINAL.pdf.

Thackery, R., Neiger, B. L., Hanson, C. L., & McKenzie, J. F. (2008). Enhancing promotional strategies within social marketing programs: Use of web 2.0 social media. *Health Promotion Practice, 9*(4), 338–343.

U.S. Census Bureau. (2010a). American Community Survey. Retrieved May 18, 2013, from http://factfinder2.census.gov.

U.S. Census Bureau. (2010b). American Factfinder. Retrieved May 17, 2013, from http://factfinder2.census.gov.

U.S. Census Bureau. (2012). Most children younger than 1 are minorities. Retrieved June 2, 2013, from http://www.census.gov/newsroom/releases/archives/population/cb12-90.html.

U.S. Department of Labor, Bureau of Labor Statistics. (2011). Women in the labor force: A databook (2010 edition). Retrieved May 27, 2013, from http://www.bls.gov/cps/wlf-databook-2011.pdf.

Williams, D. R., McClellan, M. B., & Rivlin, A. M. (2010). Beyond the Affordable Care Act: Achieving real improvements in American's health. *Health Affairs, 29* (8), 1481–1488.

Yarnall, K. S. H., Pollack, K. I., Østbye, T., Krause, K. M., & Michener L. (2003). Primary care: Is there enough time for prevention? *American Journal of Public Health, 93* (4), 635–641.

DEVELOPMENT OF A UNIFIED CODE OF
ETHICS FOR THE HEALTH EDUCATION
PROFESSION[1]

The earliest code of ethics for health educators appears to be the 1976 Society for Public Health Education (SOPHE) Code of Ethics, which was developed to guide professional behaviors toward the highest standards of practice for the profession. Following member input, Ethics Committee Chair Elizabeth Bernheimer and Paul Mico refined the code in 1978. Between 1980 and 1983 renewed attention to the code of ethics resulted in a revision that was to be reviewed by SOPHE chapters and, if accepted, then submitted to other health education professional associations to serve as a guide for the profession (Bloom, 1999). The 1983 SOPHE Code of Ethics was a combination of standards and principles but no specific rules of conduct at that time (Taub, Kreuter, Parcel, & Vitello, 1987).

Following the previous recommendation of SOPHE president, Lawrence Green, that SOPHE, the American Association for Health Education (AAHE), and the Public Health Education section of APHA consider appointing joint committees, a SOPHE–AAHE Joint Committee was appointed by then-AAHE president Peter Cortese and then-SOPHE president Ruth Richards in 1984. This committee was charged with developing a profession-wide code of ethics (Bloom, 1999). Between August 1984 and November 1985 the committee, chaired by Alyson Taub, carried out its charge to (1) identify and use all existing health education ethics statements, (2) determine the appropriate relationship between the code of ethics and the role delineation guidelines, including recommendations for enforcement, and (3) to prepare an ethics document for approval as a profession-wide code of ethics. The joint committee found that the only health education organization to work on ethics, other than SOPHE, was the American College Health Association, which included a section on ethics in their *Recommended Standards and Practices for a College Health Education Program*. The committee concluded that it was premature to describe how the code might relate to the role delineation guidelines and further recommended that individual responsibility for adhering to the Code of Ethics be the method of enforcement. Finally, the joint committee recommended that, in the absence of resources to retain expert consultation in development of ethical codes of conduct, the 1983 SOPHE Code of Ethics be adopted profession-wide and serve as a basis for the next step involving development of rules of conduct (Taub et al., 1987). Although SOPHE accepted the joint committee's recommendation, there was no similar action by AAHE (Bloom, 1999). The AAHE board chose not to accept the suggestion of adopting the SOPHE code on behalf of the profession because they realized that the membership of AAHE needed to be more completely involved in discussing and formulating

---

[1] This introduction was prepared through the joint efforts of Ellen Capwell (SOPHE), Becky Smith (AAHE), Janet Shirreffs (AAHE), and Larry K. Olsen (ASHA). Prepared 11/14/99.

a Code of Ethics before the AAHE board could adequately represent the interests and needs of AAHE members in collaborative work on ethics with other professional societies.

In September of 1991, an ad hoc AAHE ethics committee, chaired by Janet Shirreffs, was charged by president Thomas O'Rourke to develop a code of ethics that represented the professional needs of the variety of health education professionals in the membership of AAHE. They were to review the literature, including other professional codes of ethics, and conduct in-depth surveys of AAHE members. For the next two years, the AAHE ethics committee executed its charge through a variety of venues, including correspondence, surveys, face-to-face meetings, presentations, and discussion sessions at the national conventions of the American Association for Health Education (AAHE), The American School Health Association (ASHA), and the Americans Public Health Association (APHA), and through conducting focus group sessions at strategic locations around the country. Based on the work of this committee, an AAHE Code of Ethics was adopted by the AAHE Board of Directors in April 1993 (AAHE, 1994). Subsequently, both AAHE and SOPHE continued to focus on ethical issues. SOPHE has promoted programming in ethics through its annual and midyear meetings. In December 1992, a summary of the 1983 SOPHE Code of Ethics was prepared by Sarah Olson and distributed as a promotional piece. The SOPHE Board of Trustees supported the summary Code of Ethics in 1994. Since 1993, AAHE has had a standing committee on ethics that recently proposed convention programming and publications in the area of ethics. Recognizing the need to work with other organizations toward a profession-wide code of ethics, the SOPHE Board requested that the Coalition of National Health Education Organizations (CNHEO) propose a strategy for accomplishing this goal. In July 1994, the board adopted a motion that SOPHE support a profession-wide code of ethics based on ethical principles and that AAHE should be contacted for support in the effort (Bloom, 1999).

In 1995, the National Commission for Health Education Credentialing, Inc. (NCHEC) and CNHEO cosponsored a conference, The Health Education Profession in the Twenty-First Century: Setting the Stage (Brown, Cissell, DuShaw, Goodhart, McDermott, et al., 1996). During that conference, it was recommended that efforts be expanded to develop a profession-wide code of ethics.

Shortly thereafter, delegates to the CNHEO pledged to work toward development of a profession-wide code of ethics using the existing SOPHE and AAHE codes as a starting point (Bloom, 1999). A National Ethics Task Force was subsequently developed, with representatives from the various organizations represented on the coalition. It was decided that the coalition delegates would not be the task force. As a result, the various member organizations of the coalition were asked to recommend individuals for inclusion on this important task force.

During the November 1996 APHA meeting, Larry Olsen, who was the coordinator of the CNHEO and delegate to the coalition from ASHA, William Livingood (SOPHE), and Beverly Mahoney (AAHE) led a session on ethics sponsored by the CNHEO. At that meeting, the basic conceptual plan that had been developed by the coalition's Ethics Task Force was presented. Those attending the session were asked to provide input, both for the process and the content of the "new" code of ethics. Those in attendance were strong in their support for the importance of having a code of ethics for the profession that would provide an ethical framework for health educators, regardless of the setting in which health education was practiced.

The Ethics Task Force of the coalition reviewed the two existing codes (SOPHE and AAHE) along with the supporting documents for both and decided that they would enlist the support of a consultant to assist in the unification process. Claire Stiles of Eckerd College was subsequently retained to offer comments about the proposals of the task force, as well as the various drafts that would be developed.

A presentation on behalf of the Ethics Task Force was made in November 1997 at the national APHA meeting in Indianapolis, and the first draft of the Unified Code of Ethics was presented. Attendees were asked to comment about the draft document and were asked to take copies of the draft document to distribute among their constituencies. Comments from professionals in the field were returned to and considered by the task force.

A second (revised) draft of the Unified Code was presented during the March 1998 AAHE meeting in Reno. Comments received from the APHA Indianapolis meeting and field distribution had been incorporated into the document. In addition, the AAHE Ethics Committee had the opportunity to comment about the new document. During the presentation in Reno, participants were put into small groups to discuss and comment on each of the articles included in the draft document. These comments were subsequently incorporated into the document and the stage was set for a series of meetings designed to elicit commentary from professionals in the field, as well as those who attended the meetings of national professional health education organizations.

Following yet another revision of the emerging code, presentations on behalf of the task force were made in San Antonio in May 1998 at the joint SOPHE/ASTDHPPHE meeting; in San Diego in June 1998 at the national meeting of the American College Health Association ACHA; and in Colorado Springs in October 1998 at the national meeting of ASHA. Throughout this process, comments and suggestions about the code were received and examined by the task force. Throughout this process of revision and refinement, care was taken to retain the context and concepts present in the original SOPHE and AAHE documents.

The first final draft of the Unified Code of Ethics was presented in Washington, D.C., at the November 1998 meeting of the APHA. The coalition also met in conjunction with APHA, and it was decided that the final draft of the Unified Code would be prepared for presentation to the field in 1999.

In April 1999 the Unified Code of Ethics was presented in Boston at the national AAHE meeting. During that meeting the coalition also met and it was decided that all delegates to the coalition, as well as the task force members, would examine closely the work that had been done and offer comments and suggestions. It was further decided that coalition delegates would be sent a copy of the entire document (both the long and short forms), so that the documents could be discussed during the coalition's May 1999 conference call. During that conference call, the delegates voted to present the Code of Ethics to their respective organizations, for ratification during the remainder of 1999.

On November 8, 1999, the coalition delegates met in Chicago in conjunction with the APHA's annual meeting. At that meeting, the Code of Ethics was a topic of discussion. Letters had been received from all the delegate organizations indicating that they had approved the document. It was moved and seconded that the Code of Ethics be approved and distributed to the profession. There being no further comments by the CNHEO delegates, the Code of Ethics was approved unanimously as a Code of Ethics for the profession of Health Education.

The Code of Ethics that has evolved from this long and arduous process is not seen as a completed project. Rather, it is envisioned as a living document that will continue to evolve as the practice of Health Education changes to meet the challenges of the new millennium.

▷ References

Association for the Advancement of Health Education (AAHE). (1994). Code of ethics for health educators. *Journal of Health Education, 25* (4), 197–200.

Bloom, F. K. (1999). The Society for Public Health Education: Its development and contributions: 1976–1996. Unpublished doctoral dissertation, Columbia University.

Brown, K. M., Cissell, W., DuShaw, M., Goodhart, F., McDermott, R., Middleton, K., Tappe, M., & Welsh, V. (1996). The health education profession in the twenty-first century: Setting the stage. *Journal of Health Education, 27* (6), 357–364.

Taub, A., Kreuter, M., Parcel, G., & Vitello, E. (1987). Report from the AAHE/SOPHE Joint Committee on Ethics. *Health Education Quarterly, 14* (1), 79–90.

Members of the Ethics Task Force

Mal Goldsmith (ASHA)

Alyson Taub (SHES Section, APHA)

June Gorski (SOPHE)

Ken McLeroy (PHEHP Section, APHA)

Larry K. Olsen (ASHA), Committee Chair

Wanda Jubb (SSDHPER)

CODE OF ETHICS FOR THE HEALTH EDUCATION PROFESSION

Long Version[2]

Preamble

The health education profession is dedicated to excellence in the practice of promoting individual, family, organizational, and community health. Guided by common ideals, health educators are responsible for upholding the integrity and ethics of the profession as they face the daily challenges of making decisions. By acknowledging the value of diversity in society and embracing a cross-cultural approach, health educators support the worth, dignity, potential, and uniqueness of all people.

The Code of Ethics provides a framework of shared values within which health education is practiced. The Code of Ethics is grounded in fundamental ethical principles that underlie all health care services: respect for autonomy, promotion of social justice, active promotion of good, and avoidance of harm. The responsibility of each health educator is to aspire to the highest possible standards of conduct and to encourage the ethical behavior of all those with whom they work.

Regardless of job title, professional affiliation, work setting, or population served, health educators abide by these guidelines when making professional decisions.

---

[2] Used with the permission of the Coalition of National Health Education Organizations.

Article I: Responsibility to the Public

A health educator's ultimate responsibility is to educate people for the purpose of promoting, maintaining, and improving individual, family, and community health. When a conflict of issues arises among individuals, groups, organizations, agencies, or institutions, health educators must consider all issues and give priority to those that promote wellness and quality of living through principles of self-determination and freedom of choice for the individual.

Section 1

Health educators support the right of individuals to make informed decisions regarding health, as long as such decisions pose no threat to the health of others.

Section 2

Health educators encourage actions and social policies that support and facilitate the best balance of benefits over harm for all affected parties.

Section 3

Health educators accurately communicate the potential benefits and consequences of the services and programs with which they are associated.

Section 4

Health educators accept the responsibility to act on issues that can adversely affect the health of individuals, families, and communities.

Section 5

Health educators are truthful about their qualifications and the limitations of their expertise and provide services consistent with their competencies.

Section 6

Health educators protect the privacy and dignity of individuals.

Section 7

Health educators actively involve individuals, groups, and communities in the entire educational process so that all aspects of the process are clearly understood by those who may be affected.

Section 8

Health educators respect and acknowledge the rights of others to hold diverse values, attitudes, and opinions.

Section 9

Health educators provide services equitably to all people.

Article II: Responsibility to the Profession

Health educators are responsible for their professional behavior, for the reputation of their profession, and for promoting ethical conduct among their colleagues.

Section 1

Health educators maintain, improve, and expand their professional competence through continued study and education; membership, participation, and leadership in professional organizations; and involvement in issues related to the health of the public.

Section 2

Health educators model and encourage nondiscriminatory standards of behavior in their interactions with others.

Section 3

Health educators encourage and accept responsible critical discourse to protect and enhance the profession.

Section 4

Health educators contribute to the development of the profession by sharing the processes and outcomes of their work.

Section 5

Health educators are aware of possible professional conflicts of interest, exercise integrity in conflict situations, and do not manipulate or violate the rights of others.

Section 6

Health educators give appropriate recognition to others for their professional contributions and achievements.

Article III: Responsibility to Employers

Health educators recognize the boundaries of their professional competence and are accountable for their professional activities and actions.

Section 1

Health educators accurately represent their qualifications and the qualifications of others whom they recommend.

Section 2

Health educators use appropriate standards, theories, and guidelines as criteria when carrying out their professional responsibilities.

Section 3

Health educators accurately represent potential service and program outcomes to employers.

Section 4

Health educators anticipate and disclose competing commitments, conflicts of interest, and endorsement of products.

Section 5

Health educators openly communicate to employers expectations of job-related assignments that conflict with their professional ethics.

Section 6

Health educators maintain competence in their areas of professional practice.

Article IV: Responsibility in the Delivery of Health Education

Health educators promote integrity in the delivery of health education. They respect the rights, dignity, confidentiality, and worth of all people by adapting strategies and methods to meet the needs of diverse populations and communities.

Section 1

Health educators are sensitive to social and cultural diversity and are in accord with the law when planning and implementing programs.

Section 2

Health educators are informed of the latest advances in theory, research, and practice, and use strategies and methods that are grounded in and contribute to development of professional standards, theories, guidelines, statistics, and experience.

Section 3

Health educators are committed to rigorous evaluation of both program effectiveness and the methods used to achieve results.

Section 4

Health educators empower individuals to adopt healthy lifestyles through informed choice rather than by coercion or intimidation.

Section 5

Health educators communicate the potential outcomes of proposed services, strategies, and pending decisions to all individuals who will be affected.

Article V: Responsibility in Research and Evaluation

Health educators contribute to the health of the population and to the profession through research and evaluation activities. When planning and conducting research or evaluation, health educators do so in accordance with federal and state laws and regulations, organizational and institutional policies, and professional standards.

Section 1

Health educators support principles and practices of research and evaluation that do no harm to individuals, groups, society, or the environment.

Section 2

Health educators ensure that participation in research is voluntary and is based upon the informed consent of the participants.

Section 3

Health educators respect the privacy, rights, and dignity of research participants, and honor commitments made to those participants.

Section 4

Health educators treat all information obtained from participants as confidential unless otherwise required by law.

Section 5

Health educators take credit, including authorship, only for work they have actually performed and give credit to the contributions of others.

Section 6

Health educators who serve as research or evaluation consultants discuss their results only with those to whom they are providing service, unless maintaining such confidentiality would jeopardize the health or safety of others.

Section 7

Health educators report the results of their research and evaluation objectively, accurately, and in a timely fashion.

Article VI: Responsibility in Professional Preparation

Those involved in the preparation and training of health educators have an obligation to accord learners the same respect and treatment given other groups by providing quality education that benefits the profession and the public.

Section 1

Health educators select students for professional preparation programs based upon equal opportunity for all, and the individual's academic performance, abilities, and potential contribution to the profession and the public's health.

Section 2

Health educators strive to make the educational environment and culture conducive to the health of all involved, and free from sexual harassment and all forms of discrimination.

Section 3

Health educators involved in professional preparation and professional development engage in careful preparation; present material that is accurate, up-to-date, and timely; provide reasonable and timely feedback; state clear and reasonable expectations; and conduct fair assessments and evaluations of learners.

Section 4

Health educators provide objective and accurate counseling to learners about career opportunities, development, and advancement, and assist learners to secure professional employment.

Section 5

Health educators provide adequate supervision and meaningful opportunities for the professional development of learners.

CODE OF ETHICS FOR THE HEALTH EDUCATION PROFESSION

Short Version[3]

Preamble

The health education profession is dedicated to excellence in the practice of promoting individual, family, organizational, and community health. The Code of Ethics provides a framework of shared values within which health education is practiced. The responsibility of each health educator is to aspire to the highest possible standards of conduct and to encourage the ethical behavior of all those with whom they work.

Article I: Responsibility to the Public

A health educator's ultimate responsibility is to educate people for the purpose of promoting, maintaining, and improving individual, family, and community health. When a conflict of issues arises among individuals, groups, organizations, agencies, or institutions, health educators must consider all issues and give priority to those that promote wellness and quality of living through principles of self-determination and freedom of choice for the individual.

Article II: Responsibility to the Profession

Health educators are responsible for their professional behavior, for the reputation of their profession, and for promoting ethical conduct among their colleagues.

Article III: Responsibility to Employers

Health educators recognize the boundaries of their professional competence and are accountable for their professional activities and actions.

Article IV: Responsibility in the Delivery of Health Education

Health educators promote integrity in the delivery of health education. They respect the rights, dignity, confidentiality, and worth of all people by adapting strategies and methods to meet the needs of diverse populations and communities.

Article V: Responsibility in Research and Evaluation

Health educators contribute to the health of the population and to the profession through research and evaluation activities. When planning and conducting research or evaluation, health educators do so in accordance with federal and state laws and regulations, organizational and institutional policies, and professional standards.

Article VI: Responsibility in Professional Preparation

Those involved in the preparation and training of health educators have an obligation to accord learners the same respect and treatment given other groups by providing quality education that benefits the profession and the public.

---

[3] Used with the permission of the Coalition of National Health Education Organizations.

The Seven Areas of Responsibility are a comprehensive set of competencies and sub-competencies defining the role of the health education specialist. These responsibilities were verified through the 2010 Health Educator Job Analysis Project and serve as the basis of the Certified Health Education Specialist (CHES) exam beginning in April 2011 and the Master Certified Health Education Specialist (MCHES) exam in October 2011. The sub-competencies shaded are advanced-level only and were not included in the entry-level CHES examination. However the advanced-level sub-competences were included in the October 2011 MCHES examination.

AREA OF RESPONSIBILITY I

Assess Needs, Assets, and Capacity for Health Education

Competency 1.1:   Plan Assessment Process

1.1.1. Identify existing and needed resources to conduct assessments

1.1.2. Identify stakeholders to participate in the assessment process

1.1.3. Apply theories and models to develop assessment strategies

1.1.4. Develop plans for data collection, analysis, and interpretation

1.1.5. Engage stakeholders to participate in the assessment process

1.1.6. Integrate research designs, methods, and instruments into assessment plan

Competency 1.2:   Access Existing Information and Data Related to Health

1.2.1. Identify sources of data related to health

1.2.2. Critique sources of health information using theory and evidence from the literature

1.2.3. Select valid sources of information about health

1.2.4. Identify gaps in data using theories and assessment models

1.2.5. Establish collaborative relationships and agreements that facilitate access to data

1.2.6. Conduct searches of existing databases for specific health-related data

Competency 1.3:   Collect Quantitative and/or Qualitative Data Related to Health

1.3.1. Collect primary and/or secondary data

1.3.2. Integrate primary data with secondary data

1.3.3. Identify data collection instruments and methods

1.3.4. Develop data collection instruments and methods

1.3.5. Train personnel and stakeholders regarding data collection

1.3.6. Use data collection instruments and methods

1.3.7. Employ ethical standards when collecting data

Competency 1.4: *Examine Relationships Among Behavioral, Environmental, and Genetic Factors That Enhance or Compromise Health*

1.4.1. Identify factors that influence health behaviors

1.4.2. Analyze factors that influence health behaviors

1.4.3. Identify factors that enhance or compromise health

1.4.4. Analyze factors that enhance or compromise health

Competency 1.5: *Examine Factors That Influence the Learning Process*

1.5.1. Identify factors that foster or hinder the learning process

1.5.2. Analyze factors that foster or hinder the learning process

1.5.3. Identify factors that foster or hinder attitudes and belief

1.5.4. Analyze factors that foster or hinder attitudes and beliefs

1.5.5. Identify factors that foster or hinder skill building

1.5.6. Analyze factors that foster or hinder skill building

Competency 1.6: *Examine Factors That Enhance or Compromise the Process of Health Education*

1.6.1. Determine the extent of available health education programs, interventions, and policies

1.6.2. Assess the quality of available health education programs, interventions, and policies

1.6.3. Identify existing and potential partners for the provision of health education

1.6.4. Assess social, environmental, and political conditions that may impact health education

1.6.5. Analyze the capacity for developing needed health education

1.6.6. Assess the need for resources to foster health education

Competency 1.7: *Infer Needs for Health Education Based on Assessment Findings*

1.7.1. Analyze assessment findings

1.7.2. Synthesize assessment findings

1.7.3. Prioritize health education needs

1.7.4. Identify emerging health education needs

1.7.5. Report assessment findings

AREA OF RESPONSIBILITY II

Plan Health Education

Competency 2.1: *Involve Priority Populations and Other Stakeholders in the Planning Process*

2.1.1. Incorporate principles of community organization

2.1.2. Identify priority populations and other stakeholders

2.1.3. Communicate need for health education to priority populations and other stakeholders

2.1.4. Develop collaborative efforts among priority populations and other stakeholders

2.1.5. Elicit input from priority populations and other stakeholders

2.1.6. Obtain commitments from priority populations and other stakeholders

Competency 2.2:   Develop Goals and Objectives

2.2.1. Use assessment results to inform the planning process

2.2.2. Identify desired outcomes utilizing the needs assessment results

2.2.3. Select planning model(s) for health education

2.2.4. Develop goal statements

2.2.5. Formulate specific, measurable, attainable, realistic, and time-sensitive objectives

2.2.6. Assess resources needed to achieve objectives

Competency 2.3:   Select or Design Strategies and Interventions

2.3.1. Assess efficacy of various strategies to ensure consistency with objectives

2.3.2. Design theory-based strategies and interventions to achieve stated objectives

2.3.3. Select a variety of strategies and interventions to achieve stated objectives

2.3.4. Comply with legal and ethical principles in designing strategies and interventions

2.3.5. Apply principles of cultural competence in selecting and designing strategies and interventions

2.3.6. Pilot test strategies and interventions

Competency 2.4:   Develop a Scope and Sequence for the Delivery of Health Education

2.4.1. Determine the range of health education needed to achieve goals and objectives

2.4.2. Select resources required to implement health education

2.4.3. Use logic models to guide the planning process

2.4.4. Organize health education into a logical sequence

2.4.5. Develop a timeline for the delivery of health education

2.4.6. Analyze the opportunity for integrating health education into other programs

2.4.7. Develop a process for integrating health education into other programs

Competency 2.5:   Address Factors That Affect Implementation

2.5.1. Identify factors that foster or hinder implementation

2.5.2. Analyze factors that foster or hinder implementation

2.5.3. Use findings of pilot to refine implementation plans as needed

2.5.4. Develop a conducive learning environment

AREA OF RESPONSIBILITY III

Implement Health Education

Competency 3.1:   Implement a Plan of Action

3.1.1. Assess readiness for implementation

3.1.2. Collect baseline data

3.1.3. Use strategies to ensure cultural competence in implementing health education plans

3.1.4. Use a variety of strategies to deliver a plan of action

3.1.5. Promote plan of action

3.1.6. Apply theories and models of implementation

3.1.7. Launch plan of action

Competency 3.2:   Monitor Implementation of Health Education

3.2.1. Monitor progress in accordance with timeline

3.2.2. Assess progress in achieving objectives

3.2.3. Modify plan of action as needed

3.2.4. Monitor use of resources

3.2.5. Monitor compliance with legal and ethical principles

Competency 3.3:   Train Individuals Involved in Implementation of Health Education

3.3.1. Select training participants needed for implementation

3.3.2. Identify training needs

3.3.3. Develop training objectives

3.3.4. Create training using best practices

3.3.5. Demonstrate a wide range of training strategies

3.3.6. Deliver training

3.3.7. Evaluate training

3.3.8. Use evaluation findings to plan future training

AREA OF RESPONSIBILITY IV

Conduct Evaluation and Research Related to Health Education

Competency 4.1:   Develop Evaluation/Research Plan

4.1.1. Create purpose statement

4.1.2. Develop evaluation/research questions

4.1.3. Assess feasibility of conducting evaluation/research

4.1.4. Critique evaluation and research methods and findings found in the related literature

4.1.5. Synthesize information found in the literature

4.1.6. Assess the merits and limitations of qualitative and quantitative data collection for evaluation

4.1.7. Assess the merits and limitations of qualitative and quantitative data collection for research

4.1.8. Identify existing data collection instruments

4.1.9. Critique existing data collection instruments for evaluation

4.1.10. Critique existing data collection instruments for research

4.1.11. Create a logic model to guide the evaluation process

4.1.12. Develop data analysis plan for evaluation

4.1.13. Develop data analysis plan for research

4.1.14. Apply ethical standards in developing the evaluation/research plan

Competency 4.2: Design Instruments to Collect

4.2.1. Identify useable questions from existing instruments

4.2.2. Write new items to be used in data collection for evaluation

4.2.3. Write new items to be used in data collection for research

4.2.4. Establish validity of data collection instruments

4.2.5. Establish reliability of data collection instruments

Competency 4.3: Collect and Analyze Evaluation/Research Data

4.3.1. Collect data based on the evaluation/research plan

4.3.2. Monitor data collection and management

4.3.3. Analyze data using descriptive statistics

4.3.4. Analyze data using inferential and/or other advanced statistical methods

4.3.5. Analyze data using qualitative methods

4.3.6. Apply ethical standards in collecting and analyzing data

Competency 4.4: Interpret Results of the Evaluation/Research

4.4.1. Compare results to evaluation/research questions

4.4.2. Compare results to other findings

4.4.3. Propose possible explanations of findings

4.4.4. Identify possible limitations of findings

4.4.5. Develop recommendations based on results

Competency 4.5: Apply Findings from Evaluation/Research

4.5.1. Communicate findings to stakeholders

4.5.2. Evaluate feasibility of implementing recommendations from evaluation

4.5.3. Apply evaluation findings in policy analysis and program development

4.5.4. Disseminate research findings through professional conference presentations

AREA OF RESPONSIBILITY V

Administer and Manage Health Education

Competency 5.1: Manage Fiscal Resources

5.1.1. Identify fiscal and other resources

5.1.2. Prepare requests/proposals to obtain fiscal resources

5.1.3. Develop budgets to support health education efforts

5.1.4. Manage program budgets

5.1.5. Prepare budget reports

5.1.6. Demonstrate ethical behavior in managing fiscal resources

Competency 5.2: Obtain Acceptance and Support for Programs

5.2.1. Use communication strategies to obtain program support

5.2.2. Facilitate cooperation among stakeholders responsible for health education

5.2.3. Prepare reports to obtain and/or maintain program support

5.2.4. Synthesize data for purposes of reporting

5.2.5. Provide support for individuals who deliver professional development opportunities

5.2.6. Explain how program goals align with organizational structure, mission, and goals

Competency 5.3: Demonstrate Leadership

5.3.1. Conduct strategic planning

5.3.2. Analyze an organization's culture in relationship to health education goals

5.3.3. Promote collaboration among stakeholders

5.3.4. Develop strategies to reinforce or change organizational culture to achieve health education goals

5.3.5. Comply with existing laws and regulations

5.3.6. Adhere to ethical standards of the profession

5.3.7. Facilitate efforts to achieve organizational mission

5.3.8. Analyze the need for a systems approach to change

5.3.9. Facilitate needed changes to organizational cultures

Competency 5.4: Manage Human Resources

5.4.1. Develop volunteer opportunities

5.4.2. Demonstrate leadership skills in managing human resources

5.4.3. Apply human resource policies consistent with relevant laws and regulations

5.4.4. Evaluate qualifications of staff and volunteers needed for programs

5.4.5. Recruit volunteers and staff

5.4.6. Employ conflict resolution strategies

5.4.7. Apply appropriate methods for team development

5.4.8. Model professional practices and ethical behavior

5.4.9. Develop strategies to enhance staff and volunteers' career development

5.4.10. Implement strategies to enhance staff and volunteers' career development

5.4.11. Evaluate performance of staff and volunteers

Competency 5.5: Facilitate Partnerships in Support of Health Education

5.5.1. Identify potential partner(s)

5.5.2. Assess capacity of potential partner(s) to meet program goals

5.5.3. Facilitate partner relationship(s)

5.5.4. Elicit feedback from partner(s)

5.5.5. Evaluate feasibility of continuing partnership

AREA OF RESPONSIBILITY VI

Serve as a Health Education Resource Person

Competency 6.1: Obtain and Disseminate Health-Related Information

6.1.1. Assess information needs

6.1.2. Identify valid information resources

6.1.3. Critique resource materials for accuracy, relevance, and timeliness

6.1.4. Convey health-related information to priority populations

6.1.5. Convey health-related information to key stakeholders

Competency 6.2: Provide Training

6.2.1. Analyze requests for training

6.2.2. Prioritize requests for training

6.2.3. Identify priority populations

6.2.4. Assess needs for training

6.2.5. Identify existing resources that meet training needs

6.2.6. Use learning theory to develop or adapt training programs

6.2.7. Develop training plan

6.2.8. Implement training sessions and programs

6.2.9. Use a variety of resources and strategies

6.2.10. Evaluate impact of training programs

Competency 6.3: Serve as a Health Education Consultant

6.3.1. Assess needs for assistance

6.3.2. Prioritize requests for assistance

6.3.3. Define parameters of effective consultative relationships

6.3.4. Establish consultative relationships

6.3.5. Provide expert assistance

6.3.6. Facilitate collaborative efforts to achieve program goals

6.3.7. Evaluate the effectiveness of the expert assistance provided

6.3.8. Apply ethical principles in consultative relationships

AREA OF RESPONSIBILITY VII

Communicate and Advocate for Health and Health Education

Competency 7.1: Assess and Prioritize Health Information and Advocacy Needs

7.1.1. Identify current and emerging issues that may influence health and health education

7.1.2. Access accurate resources related to identified issues

7.1.3. Analyze the impact of existing and proposed policies on health

7.1.4. Analyze factors that influence decision-makers

Competency 7.2:   Identify and Develop a Variety of Communication Strategies, Methods, and Techniques

7.2.1. Create messages using communication theories and models

7.2.2. Tailor messages to priority populations

7.2.3. Incorporate images to enhance messages

7.2.4. Select effective methods or channels for communicating to priority populations

7.2.5. Pilot test messages and delivery methods with priority populations

7.2.6. Revise messages based on pilot feedback

Competency 7.3:   Deliver Messages Using a Variety of Strategies, Methods, and Techniques

7.3.1. Use techniques that empower individuals and communities to improve their health

7.3.2. Employ technology to communicate to priority populations

7.3.3. Evaluate the delivery of communication strategies, methods, and techniques

Competency 7.4:   Engage in Health Education Advocacy

7.4.1. Engage stakeholders in advocacy

7.4.2. Develop an advocacy plan in compliance with local, state, and/or federal policies and procedures

7.4.3. Comply with organizational policies related to participating in advocacy

7.4.4. Communicate the impact of health and health education on organizational and socio-ecological factors

7.4.5. Use data to support advocacy messages

7.4.6. Implement advocacy plans

7.4.7. Incorporate media and technology in advocacy

7.4.8. Participate in advocacy initiatives

7.4.9. Lead advocacy initiatives

7.4.10. Evaluate advocacy efforts

Competency 7.5:   Influence Policy to Promote Health

7.5.1. Use evaluation and research findings in policy analysis

7.5.2. Identify the significance and implications of health policy for individuals, groups, and communities

7.5.3. Advocate for health-related policies, regulations, laws, or rules

7.5.4. Use evidence-based research to develop policies to promote health

7.5.5. Employ policy and media advocacy techniques to influence decision-makers

Competency 7.6:   Promote the Health Education Profession

7.6.1. Develop a personal plan for professional growth and service

7.6.2. Describe state-of-the-art health education practice

7.6.3. Explain the major responsibilities of the health education specialist in the practice of health education

7.6.4. Explain the role of health education associations in advancing the profession

7.6.5. Explain the benefits of participating in professional organizations

7.6.6. Facilitate professional growth of self and others

7.6.7. Explain the history of the health education profession and its current and future implications for professional practice

7.6.8. Explain the role of credentialing in the promotion of the health education profession

7.6.9. Engage in professional development activities

7.6.10. Serve as a mentor to others

7.6.11. Develop materials that contribute to the professional literature

7.6.12. Engage in service to advance the health education profession

Source: From The National Commission for Health Education Credentialing, Inc. http://www.nchec.org. Used by permission of NCHEC.

A New Perspective on the Health of Canadians
the Canadian publication that presented the epidemiological evidence supporting the importance of lifestyle and environmental factors on health and sickness and called for numerous national health promotion strategies to encourage Canadians to become more responsible for their own health.

abstracts short summaries of research studies that have appeared in selected journals.

accreditation the status of public recognition that an accrediting agency grants to an education institution or program that meets the agency's standards or requirements" (National Transition Task Force on Accreditation in Health Education, 2013) (Chapter 6).

action stage a stage of the Transtheoretical Model in which a person is overtly making changes.

actual behavioral control having the "the skills, resources, and other prerequisites needed to perform a given behavior" (Ajzen, 2006) (Chapter 4).

adjusted rate a rate that is statistically adjusted for a certain characteristic, such as age, expressed for a total population.

administrative and policy assessment is "an analysis of the policies, resources, and circumstances prevailing in an organizational situation to facilitate or hinder the development of the health program" (Green & Kreuter, 2005, p. G-1) (Chapter 4).

advocacy "the actions or endeavors individuals or groups engage in in order to alter public opinion in favor or in opposition to a certain policy" (Pinzon-Perez & Perez, 1999, p. 29) (Chapter 1).

Affordable Care Act (ACA) the official title of healthcare reform legislation that was passed by Congress in March 2010. All of the provisions of the ACA will be fully implemented by 2020.

American Academy of Health Behavior (AAHB) society of researchers and scholars in the areas of human behavior, health education, and health promotion.

American Alliance for Health, Physical Education, Recreation and Dance (AAHPERD) is the largest organization of professionals involved in physical education, physical activity, dance, school health and sport—all specialties related to achieving an active, healthy lifestyle.

American Association for Health Education (AAHE) was a professional association within AAHPERD. As of May 1, 2013, the AAHE was formally retired.

American College Health Association (ACHA) a professional association comprising mostly individuals who work in colleges and universities.

American Public Health Association (APHA) a professional association for those individuals working in the fields of public health.

American Red Cross (ARC) a quasi-governmental organization.

American School Health Association (ASHA) a professional association comprising individuals interested in coordinated school health.

anonymity exists when no one, including those conducting the program, can relate a participant's identity to any information pertaining to the program.

Asclepiads a brotherhood of men associated with the Asclepian temples who first began the practice of medicine based on a more rational basis.

Asclepius the Greek god of medicine, for whom many temples were built.

assessment the estimation of the relative magnitude, importance, or value of objects observed.

attitude toward the behavior an attitude about a certain behavior; a construct of the theory of planned behavior.

bacteriological period of public health the period of 1875 to 1900, during which great advancements in the study of bacteria occurred.

behavioral capability the knowledge and skills necessary to perform a behavior.

behavior change philosophy involves a health education specialist using behavioral contracts, goal setting, and self-monitoring to help foster and motivate the modification of an unhealthy habit in an individual with whom the health education specialist is working.

beneficence "simply doing good" (Balog et al., 1985, p. 91) (Chapter 5).

benevolence see *beneficence*.

caduceus the serpent and staff symbol of medicine, which was the symbol of the Asclepian Temples.

capacity "refers to both individual and collective resources that can be brought to bear for health enhancement" (Gilmore & Campbell, 2005, p. 7) (Chapter 6).

CDCynergy (or Cynergy) a health communication planning model developed by the Office of Communication at the Centers for Disease Control and Prevention.

certification "a process by which a professional organization grants recognition to an individual who, upon completion of a competency-based curriculum, can demonstrate a predetermined standard of performance" (Cleary, 1995, p. 39) (Chapter 6).

Certified Health Education Specialist (CHES) a health education specialist who has met all necessary requirements and has been certified by the National Commission for Health Education Credentialing, Inc.

chain of infection a model used to help explain the spread of a communicable disease from one host to another.

Coalition of National Health Education Organizations, USA (CNHEO) a coalition made up of representatives from eight professional associations, of which health education specialists are members.

code of ethics "document that maps the dimensions of the profession's collective social responsibility and acknowledges the obligations individual practitioners share in meeting the profession's responsibilities" (Feeney & Freeman, 1999, p. 6) (Chapter 5).

Code of Hammurabi the earliest written record concerning public health.

cognitive-based philosophy a philosophy that focuses on the acquisition of content and factual information to increase knowledge so a person is better equipped to make health-related decisions.

communicable disease model a model used to help explain the spread of a communicable disease from one host to another via the elements of agent, host, and environment.

communicable diseases those diseases for which biological agents or their products are the cause and that are transmissible from one individual to another (McKenzie et al., 2012) (Chapter 1).

community empowerment "the process by which people gain control over the factors and decisions that shape their lives. It is the process by which they increase their assets and attributes and build capacities to gain access, partners, networks and/or a voice, in order to gain control" (World Health Organization, 2013) (Chapter 6).

community health "the health status of a defined group of people and the actions and conditions to promote, protect and preserve their health" (Joint Committee, 2012, p. 15) (Chapter 1).

community health education health education/ promotion programs conducted in departments of health, voluntary agencies, hospitals, religious organizations, and so on.

competencies "reflects the ability of the student to understand, know, etc." (National Commission for Health Education Credentialing, Inc., 1996, p. 12) (Chapter 6).

Competencies Update Project (CUP) a project to review and update both entry-level and advanced-level health education/promotion competencies.

comprehensive school health instruction the development, delivery, and evaluation of a planned curriculum, preschool through grade 12, with goals, objectives, content sequence, and specific classroom lessons that include, but are not limited to, the following major content areas: community health, consumer health, environmental health, family life, mental and emotional health, injury prevention and safety, nutrition, personal health, prevention and control of disease, and substance use and abuse (Joint Committee on Health Education Terminology, 1991a, p. 102) (Chapter 2).

concepts the primary elements, building blocks, or major components of theories.

confidentiality exists when only those responsible for conducting a program can link information about a participant with that person and have promised not to reveal such to others.

consequentialism see *teleological theories*.

conservative a person who generally distrusts governmental regulations and tax-supported programs for addressing social or economic problems.

construct a concept that has been developed, created, or adopted for use with a specific theory.

contemplation stage a stage of the Transtheoretical Model in which a person is seriously thinking about change in the next six months.

continuum theories those behavior change theories that identify variables that influence actions and combine them into a single equation that predicts the likelihood of action (Weinstein, Rothman, & Sutton, 1998; Weinstein, Sandman, & Blalock, 2008) (Chapter 4).

coordinated school health "an organized set of policies, procedures, and activities designed to protect, promote, and improve the health and well-being of pre-K through 12 students and staff, thus improving a student's ability to learn. It includes, but is not limited to, comprehensive school health education; school health services; a healthy school environment; school counseling; psychological and social services; physical education; school nutrition services; family and community involvement in school health; and school-site health promotion for staff" (Joint Terminology Committee, 2012, p. 16) (Chapter 1).

credentialing a process whereby an individual or a professional preparation program meets the specified standards established by the credentialing body and is thus recognized for having done so.

crude rate the rate expressed for a total population.

cue to action a construct of the health belief model that motivates a person to act.

cultural competence "a developmental process defined as a set of values, principles, behaviors, attitudes, and policies that enable health professionals to work effectively across racial, ethnic, and linguistically diverse populations." (Joint Committee, 2012, p. 16) (Chapter 1).

death rates the number of deaths per 100,000 resident population, sometimes referred to as mortality or fatality rates.

decision-making philosophy the belief that the use of scenarios, case studies, and simulated problems is the best method to motivate persons to adopt positive health behaviors.

demographic profile a statistical breakdown of the population of a country, region, state, or city by age group, sex, race, and ethnicity.

deontological theories (or formalism or nonconsequentialism) "are those that claim that certain actions are inherently right or wrong, or good or bad, without regard for their consequences" (Reamer, 2006, p. 65) (Chapter 5).

determinants of health include genetics, health behaviors, social circumstances, environmental conditions, and access to health services.

Diffusion Theory a theory that provides an explanation for the movement of an innovation through a population.

Directors of Health Promotion and Education (DHPE) a professional association composed of individuals who, by position, head their state or territory public health education/promotion efforts.

disability-adjusted life years (DALYs) a measure of health that takes into effect the severity of the health condition, age, and impact on the future.

disease prevention "the process of reducing risks and alleviating disease to promote, preserve, and restore health and minimize suffering and distress" (Joint Terminology Committee, 2001, p. 99) (Chapter 1).

distributive justice deals with the allocation of resources (Summers, 2009) (Chapter 5).

early adopters a group of people who are interested in innovation, but who do not want to be the first involved.

early majority a group of people who may be interested in an innovation but will need some external motivation to get involved.

eclectic health education/promotion philosophy a philosophical approach held by health education specialists that no one philosophy is "right" for all times and circumstances and that the best philosophy involves blending the various philosophical approaches or using different approaches depending on the setting (school, community, work site).

ecological approaches see *socio-ecological approach*.

ecological assessment is "a systematic assessment of factors in the social and physical environment that interact with behavior to produce health effects or quality-of-life outcomes" (Green & Kreuter, 2005, p. G-3) (Chapter 4).

ecological perspective see *socio-ecological approach*.

educational assessment is "the delineation of factors that predispose, enable, and reinforce a specific behavior, or through behavior, environmental changes" (Green & Kreuter, 2005, p. G-3) (Chapter 4).

elaboration the amount of cognitive processing (i.e., thought) that a person puts into receiving messages (Petty, Barden, & Wheeler) (Chapter 4).

electronic database computerized storage disks containing a large compilation of references; each database is specific to a general subject area (e.g., education, medicine) and provides access to the cumulative information found in several index or abstract sources on that subject area.

emotional-coping response to learn, a person must be able to deal with the sources of anxiety that surround a behavior.

empowerment "social action process for people to gain mastery over their lives and the lives of their communities" (Minkler, Wallerstein, & Wilson, 2008, p. 294) (Chapter 1).

enabling factor "any characteristic of the environment that facilitates action and any skill or resource required to attain a specific behavior" (Green & Kreuter, 1999, p. 505) (Chapter 4).

endemic occurs regularly in a population as a matter of course.

environment "all those matters related to health which are external to the human body and over which the individual has little or no control" (Lalonde, 1974, p. 32) (Chapter 1).

environmental assessment "a systematic assessment of factors in the social and physical environment that interact with behavior to produce health effects or quality-of-life outcomes. Also referred to as *ecological assessment*" (Green & Kreuter, 1999, p. 505) (Chapter 4).

epidemic an unexpectedly large number of cases of an illness, specific health-related behavior, or health-related event in a population.

epidemiological assessment "the delineation of the extent, distribution, and causes of a health problem in a defined population" (Green & Kreuter, 2005, p. G-3) (Chapter 4).

epidemiological data information gathered when measuring health and ill health.

epidemiology "the study of the distribution and determinants of health-related states or events in specific populations, and the application of this study to control health problems" (Dictionary of Epidemiology as cited in Last, 2007, p. iii) (Chapter 1).

epistemology the study of knowledge (Thiroux, 1995) (Chapter 5).

Eta Sigma Gamma (ESG) the national health education honorary society.

ethical good/bad and right/wrong.

ethical dilemma "a situation that forces a decision that involves breaking some ethical norm or contradicting some ethical value" (Pozgar, 2013, p. 534) (Chapter 5).

ethics "the study of morality, one of the three major areas of philosophy, also referred to as moral philosophy" (Thiroux, 1995) (Chapter 5).

evidence a body of data that can be used to make decisions about planning.

evidence-based practice the process of systematically finding, appraising, and using evidence as the basis for decision making when planning health education/promotion programs (Cottrell & McKenzie, 2011) (Chapter 1).

expectancies values people place on expected outcomes.

expectations beliefs about the likely outcomes of certain behaviors.

formalism see *deontological theories*.

freeing or functioning philosophy proponents of this philosophy help the person make the best health choices possible for that person, based on the individual's needs and interests, not on societal expectations.

generalized model a planning model that includes the five major steps in developing a program.

global health "health problems, issues, and concerns that transcend national boundaries and are beyond the control of individual nations, and are best addressed by cooperative actions and solutions" (Joint Committee, 2012, p. 17) (Chapter 1).

goodness (rightness) a state or quality of being good; one of the five principles of common moral ground.

government documents unclassified publications authored and disseminated by federal, state, or local agencies intended for public use.

governmental health agencies agencies designated as having authority for certain specific duties or tasks outlined by the governmental bodies that oversee them.

graduate research assistantship an award given a graduate student who works closely with one or more faculty members on a research project; the student is usually granted tuition assistance and a stipend in return for the work.

graduate teaching assistantship an award given a graduate student who teaches for the program and in return is usually granted tuition assistance and a stipend.

hard money funds used to support health education/promotion positions and programs that are part of the regular budget of an employer.

health "is a dynamic state or condition that is multidimensional (i.e., physical, emotional, social, intellectual, spiritual, and occupational) a resource for living, and results from a person's interactions with and adaptation to the environment" (Joint Committee, 2012, p. 10) (Chapter 1).

health-adjusted life expectancy (HALE) the number of years of healthy life expected, on average, in a given population.

health advocacy "the processes by which the actions of individuals or groups attempt to bring about social, environmental and/or organizational change on behalf of a particular health goal, program, interest, or population" (Joint Committee, 2012, p. 17) (Chapter 1).

health behavior see *lifestyle*.

Health Belief Model an intrapersonal theory that "addresses a person's perceptions of the threat of a health problem and the accompanying appraisal of a recommended behavior for preventing or managing the problem" (Glanz & Rimer, 1995, p. 17) (Chapter 4).

healthcare organization "consists of the quantity, quality, arrangement, nature and relationships of people and resources in the provision of health care" (Lalonde, 1974, p. 32), also referred to as the health care system.

healthcare settings locations for health education/promotion programs, including public and for-profit hospitals, free-standing medical care clinics, home health agencies, and physician organizations such as health maintenance organizations (HMOs) and preferred provider organizations (PPOs).

health disparity the difference in health between different populations often caused by two health inequities—lack of access to care and lack of quality care (McKenzie et al., 2012) (Chapter 1).

health education "any combination of planned learning experiences using evidence based practices and/or sound theories that provide the opportunity to acquire knowledge, attitudes, and skills needed adopt and maintain healthy behaviors" (Joint Committee, 2012, p. 17) (Chapter 1).

health education research "a systematic investigation involving the analysis of collected information or data that ultimately is used to enhance health education knowledge or practice, and answers one or more questions about a health-related theory, behavior or phenomenon" (Cottrell & McKenzie, 2011, p. 2) (Chapter 6).

health education specialist "an individual who has met, at a minimum, baccalaureate-level required health education academic preparation qualifications, who serves in a variety of settings, and is able to use appropriate educational strategies and methods to facilitate the development of policies, procedures, interventions, and systems conducive to the health of individuals, groups, and communities" (Joint Committee, 2012, p. 18) (Chapter 1).

health field a term that includes all matters that affect health; far more encompassing than the healthcare system.

Health Field Concept a framework that was developed in Canada to study health; it has four elements: human biology, environment, lifestyle, and healthcare organization.

health literacy the capacity of individuals to access, interpret, and understand basic health information and services and the skills to use the information and services to promote health.

health promotion "any planned combination of educational, political, environmental, regulatory, or organizational mechanisms that support actions and conditions of living conducive to the health of individuals, groups, and communities" (Joint Committee, 2012, p. 17) (Chapter 1).

Healthy People the first major U.S. government document recognizing the importance of lifestyle in promoting health and well-being.

Healthy People 2000: National Health Promotion and Disease Prevention Objectives a document that contains the health objectives for the United States during the 1990s.

Healthy People 2010: Understanding and Improving Health a document that contains the health objectives for the United States during the 2000s.

Healthy People 2020 the latest listing of National Health Objectives for the United States through the year 2020.

health-related quality of life (HRQOL) "those aspects of overall quality of life that can be clearly shown to affect health—either physical or mental" (CDC, 2011b, ¶ 3) (Chapter 1).

Hippocrates a Greek physician from the Asclepian tradition who eventually became known as the father of medicine.

holistic philosophy the philosophy that the mind and body blend into a single unit; the person is a unified being.

home page analogous to a combination of a cover and table of contents in a book, a home page names a specific Web site and directs the user to options within that site.

human biology "all those aspects of health, both physical and mental, which are developed within the human body as a consequence of the basic biology of man [sic] and the organic make-up of an individual" (Lalonde, 1974, p. 31) (Chapter 1).

Hygeia the daughter of Asclepios granted the power to prevent disease.

hypertext transfer protocol the protocol for exchanging hypertext documents between sites on the Web.

impact evaluation "the assessment of program effects on intermediate objectives including changes in predisposing, enabling, and reinforcing factors, behavioral and environmental changes, and possibly health and social outcomes" (Green & Kreuter, 2005, p. G-5) (Chapter 4).

implementation "the act of converting program objectives into actions through policy changes, regulation and organization" (Green & Kreuter, 2005, G-5) (Chapter 4).

indexes reference books that provide links to articles from many refereed journals, books, and selected reports; each index is written to target specific subject headings, so one index is not all-encompassing for all subjects.

individual freedom (equality principle, or principle of autonomy) people, being individuals with individual differences, must have the freedom to choose their own ways and means of being moral within the framework of value of life, goodness, justice, and truth-telling (Thiroux, 1995) (Chapter 5).

informed consent requires: (a) disclosure of relevant information to prospective participants about the program; (b) their comprehension of the information; and (c) their voluntary agreement, free from coercion and undue influence, to participate (OHSR, 2006) (Chapter 5).

innovators the first people to adopt an innovation.

intention "is an indication of a person's readiness to perform a given behavior, and it is considered to be the immediate antecedent of behavior" (Ajzen, 2006) (Chapter 4).

International Union for Health Promotion and Education (IUHPE) a professional association open to individuals who are interested in health education/promotion worldwide.

Internet an integrated network of computers that spans the entire world; the computers can transfer data to one another via phone lines, microwaves, fiber optics, and satellites (Kittleson, 1997) (Chapter 9).

intervention alignment matching appropriate strategies and interventions with projected changes and outcomes.

intervention mapping a six-phase program planning model guided by diagrams and matrices that incorporate outputs of the assessment process with relevant theory to help develop appropriate interventions for priority populations.

justice (fairness) "human beings should treat other human beings fairly and justly in distributing goodness and badness among them" (Thiroux, 1995, p. 184) (Chapter 5); a basic principle of ethics.

laggards the last group of people to get involved in an innovation, if they get involved at all.

late majority a group of people who are skeptical and will not adopt an innovation until most people in the social system have done so.

liberal generally, a person who favors governmental programs to address perceived social and economic inequities between segments of society.

licensure "a process by which an agency or government (usually a state) grants permission to individuals to practice a given profession by certifying that those licensed have attained specific standards of competence" (Cleary, 1995, p. 39) (Chapter 6).

life expectancy "the average number of years of life remaining to a person at a particular age and based on a given set of age-specific death rates—generally the mortality conditions existing in the period mentioned. Life expectancy may be determined by race, sex, or other characteristics using age-specific death rates for the population with that characteristic" (NCHS, 2013, p. 452) (Chapter 1).

lifestyle "an aggregation of decisions by individuals which affect their health and over which they more or less have control" (Lalonde, 1974, p. 32) (Chapter 1).

likelihood of taking action chances that a person will behave in a particular way; a construct of the health belief model.

local health department (LHD) a governmental organization that is located in a city or county.

locus of control one's perception of the center of control over reinforcement.

macrolevel having health education/promotion interventions targeted to the community as a whole, instead of to individuals.

maintenance stage the stage of the Transtheoretical Model in which a person is taking steps to sustain change and resist temptation to relapse.

Master Certified Health Education Specialist (MCHES) an advanced level of certification available for health education specialists who health education or a master's degree in a related field along with at least 25 semester hours of health education coursework. The MCHES exam must be taken and passed to receive this credential.

MAPP is the acronym for the planning model titled Mobilizing for Action through Planning and Partnerships created by the National Association of County and City Health Officials.

MATCH an acronym for Multilevel Approach To Community Health.

M.A., M.Ed., M.H.S., M.P.H., M.S., M.S.P.H. degree designations available to master's-level health education/promotion students, depending on the institution they attend and their area of emphasis.

Medicaid government health insurance for the poor.

Medicare government health insurance for the elderly and disabled.

metaphysics the study of the nature of reality (Thiroux, 1995) (Chapter 5).

miasmas theory a belief that vapors, or miasmas, rising from rotting refuse could travel through the air for great distances and result in disease when inhaled.

microlevel targeting health education/promotion interventions to individuals.

model "is a composite, a mixture of ideas or concepts taken from any number of theories and used together" (Hayden, 2009, p. 1) (Chapter 4).

moderate a person who acts in a more situationally specific manner in regard to using tax-supported programs to solve social problems.

modifiable risk factors changeable or controllable risk factors.

moral good/bad and right/wrong.

moral philosophy see *ethics*.

moral sensitivity being aware that an ethical problem exists and having an understanding of what impact different courses of action may have on the people involved (Rest et al., 1999) (Chapter 5).

multicausation disease model a model that explains the onset of disease caused by more than one factor.

multitasking the skill of coordinating and completing multiple health education/promotion projects at the same time.

National Commission for Health Education Credentialing, Inc. (NCHEC) the organization that oversees the health education certification process.

National Task Force on the Preparation and Practice of Health Educators the group that oversaw development of the roles and responsibilities of health education specialists and ultimately the CHES credentialing system.

National Wellness Institute, Inc. (NWI) a professional association for those interested in wellness programs.

needs assessment a process that helps program planners determine what health problems might exist in any given group of people, what assets are available in the community to address the health problems, and the overall capacity of the community to address the health issues (McKenzie et al., 2009) (Chapter 6).

networking establishing and maintaining a wide range of contacts in the field that may be of help when looking for a job and in carrying out one's job responsibilities once hired.

noncommunicable diseases those that cannot be transmitted from an infected person to a susceptible, healthy one (McKenzie et al., 2012) (Chapter 1).

nonconsequential see *deontological theories*.

nongovernmental health agencies those that operate, for the most part, free from governmental interference as long as they comply with the Internal Revenue Service's guidelines for their tax status (McKenzie et al., 2012) (Chapter 8).

nonmaleficence "the non-infliction of harm to others" (Balog et al., 1985, p. 91) (Chapter 5).

nonmodifiable risk factors nonchangeable or non-controllable risk factors.

objective statement describing specific, measurable cognitive or affective changes in the learner. An objective establishes a performance standard for the learner.

open access journals are journals that are available to the reader online without restriction to cost, membership, or legal barriers with the exception that the reader must be able to access the Internet.

outcome evaluation "assessment of the effects of a program on its ultimate objectives, including changes in health and social benefits or quality of life" (Green & Kreuter, 2005, p. G-6) (Chapter 4).

ownership a feeling of responsibility for program outcomes.

Panacea the daughter of Asclepios granted the power to treat disease.

pandemic an outbreak over a wide geographical area, such as a continent.

participation the active involvement of those in the priority population in helping identify, plan, and implement programs to address the health problems they face.

perceived barriers the cost of engaging in a health behavior; a construct of the Health Belief Model.

perceived behavioral control a belief held by people that they have control over a behavior; a construct of the theory of planned behavior.

perceived benefits a belief that a particular health recommendation would be beneficial in reducing a perceived threat; a construct of the Health Belief Model.

perceived seriousness/severity a belief that a health problem is serious; a construct of the Health Belief Model.

perceived susceptibility a belief that one is vulnerable to a health problem; a construct of the Health Belief Model.

perceived threat a belief that one is vulnerable to a serious health problem or to the sequelae of that illness or condition; a construct of the Health Belief Model.

philanthropic foundation "endowed institution that donates money for the good of humankind" (McKenzie et al., 2012, p. 57) (Chapter 8).

philodoxy literally means "the love of opinion" but often is used in the context of letting opinion define reality.

philosophy a statement summarizing the attitudes, principles, beliefs, values, and concepts held by an individual or a group.

philosophy of symmetry a philosophy of health with physical, emotional, spiritual, and social components of health.

popular press publications publications ranging from weekly summary magazines (e.g., *Newsweek*) to monthly magazines (e.g., *Better Homes and Gardens*); often, articles include editorials; information from these sources should be heavily scrutinized before using.

population-based approaches community health methods that are used to help change behavior in groups of people. Examples include policy development, policy advocacy, organizational change, community development, empowerment of individuals, and economic supports.

population health "the health status of people who are not organized and have no identity as a group or locality and the actions and conditions to promote, protect, and preserve their health" (McKenzie et al., 2012, p. 7) (Chapter 1).

portfolio a collection of evidence that enables students to demonstrate mastery of desired course or program outcomes.

postsecondary institution in the United States, an institution that provides further education after high school.

PRECEDE-PROCEED an acronym for a theory of implementation that stands for Predisposing, Reinforcing, and Enabling Constructs in Educational/Environmental Diagnosis and Evaluation and Policy, Regulatory, and Organizational Constructs in Educational and Environmental Development.

precontemplation stage the stage of the Transtheoretical Model in which a person is not thinking about change in the next six months.

predisposing factor "any characteristic of a person or population that motivates behavior prior to the occurrence of the behavior" (Green & Kreuter, 2005, p. G-6) (Chapter 4).

preparation stage the stage of the Transtheoretical Model in which a person is actively planning change.

prevention the planning for and measures taken to forestall the onset of, limit the spread of, and rehabilitate after pathogenesis or other health problems.

primary data original data gathered by the health education specialist as part of a needs assessment; this includes data gathered from telephone surveys, focus groups, and interviews.

primary prevention preventive measures that forestall the onset of illness or injury during the prepathogenesis period.

primary sources published studies or eyewitness accounts written by the person(s) who actually conducted the study or observed the event.

privacy "the claim of individuals, groups, or institutions to determine for themselves when, how, and to what extent information about them is communicated to others" (Westin, 1968, p. 7) (Chapter 5).

procedural justice deals with whether or not fair procedures were in place and whether those procedures were followed (Summers, 2009) (Chapter 5).

process evaluation "the assessment of policies, materials, personnel, performance, quality of practice or services, and other inputs and implementation experiences" (Green & Kreuter, 2005, p. G-6) (Chapter 4).

professional ethics "actions that are right and wrong in the workplace and are of public matter. Professional moral principles are not statements of taste or preference; they tell practitioners what they ought to do and what they ought not to do" (Feeney & Freeman, 1999, p. 6) (Chapter 5).

professional health associations/organizations organizations that promote the high standards of professional practice for their respective professions, thereby improving the health of society by improving the people in the professions (McKenzie et al., 2012) (Chapter 8).

Promoting Health/Preventing Disease: Objectives for the Nation a document containing 226 health objectives for the United States to be accomplished during the 1980s.

public health "is the science and the art of protecting and improving the health of communities through education, promotion of healthy lifestyles, and research for disease and injury prevention" (Association of Schools of Public Health, n. d., ¶ 1) (Chapter 1).

public health agencies also called "official governmental health agencies"; agencies usually financed through public tax monies and typically offering health promotion and education programs.

quality assurance "The planned and systematic activities necessary to provide adequate confidence that the product or service will meet given requirements" (Quality Assurance Solutions, 2010) (Chapter 6).

quasi-governmental health agencies agencies that possess some of the characteristics of a governmental health agency but also possess some of the characteristics of nongovernmental agencies.

rate "a measure of some event, disease, or condition in relation to a unit of population, along with some specification of time" (NCHS, 2013, p. 468) (Chapter 1).

reciprocal determinism "behavior changes result from an interaction between the person and the environment; change is bidirectional" (Glanz & Rimer, 1995) (Chapter 4).

reduction of threat a belief that a particular health recommendation would be beneficial in reducing a threat at a subjectively acceptable cost; a construct of the health belief model.

refereed or peer reviewed journal a journal that publishes original manuscripts only after they have been read and critiqued by a panel of experts in the field.

reinforcement a response to behavior that increases the chance of recurrence.

reinforcing factor "any reward or punishment following or anticipated as a consequence of a behavior, serving to strengthen the motivation for the behavior after it occurs" (Green & Kreuter, 2005, G-7) (Chapter 4).

research ethics "comprises principles and standards that, along with underlying values, guide appropriate conduct relevant to research decisions" (Kimmel, 2007, p. 6) (Chapter 5).

responsibilities the seven major responsibilities of all entry-level health education specialists.

risk factors those inherited, environmental, and behavioral influences "which are known (or thought) to increase the likelihood of physical or mental problems" (Slee et al., 2008, p. 510) (Chapter 1).

role delineation the process of identifying the specific responsibilities, competencies, and subcompetencies associated with the practice of health education/promotion.

Rule of Sufficiency the programs, strategies, initiatives, methods implemented must be sufficiently robust, or effective enough, that the stated objectives will have a reasonable chance of being met.

School Health Advisory Council (SHAC) community members such as parents; medical, health, and safety professionals; and political, religious, and corporate or business leaders who assist with the planning and promotion of school health initiatives.

school health education/promotion health education programs that instruct school-age children about health and health-related behaviors.

School Health Education Evaluation Study a landmark study that examined the entire health program of selected schools in the Los Angeles area.

School Health Education Study a nationwide study that examined the status of health education and resulted in the development of an important curriculum.

search engine site on the World Wide Web specifically designed to search for all links associated with a word or phrase that the user wants information on; the search engines greatly decrease the time it takes to search for information on the Web; examples are Google, Yahoo®, and Bing.

secondary data preexisting data used by a health education specialist in a needs assessment.

secondary prevention preventive measures that lead to early diagnosis and prompt treatment of a disease or an injury to limit disability, impairment, or dependency and to prevent more severe pathogenesis.

secondary sources articles that often provide an overview or a summary of several related studies or that chronicle the history of several related events, written by someone who did not conduct the study or observe firsthand the event that is written about.

self-control (self-regulation) gaining control over one's own behavior by monitoring and adjusting it.

self-efficacy people's confidence in their ability to perform a certain desired task or function.

septicemia "the presence of bacteria in the blood (bacteremia), often associated with severe disease" (NLM & NIH, 2003, p. 1).

service learning course credit for students to work with a community agency to meet an identified community need.

situational analysis is "the combination of social and epidemiological assessments of conditions, trends, and priorities with a preliminary scan of determinants, relevant policies, resources, organizational support, and regulations that might anticipate or permit action in advance of a more complete assessment of behavioral, environmental, educational, ecological, and administrative factors" (Green & Kreuter, 2005, p. G-7 & 8) (Chapter 4).

SMART is an acronym for a social marketing planning model titled the Social Marketing Assessment and Response Tool.

Smith Papyri the oldest written document related to health, which describes various surgical techniques and dates back to 1600 B.C.

social assessment "the assessment in both objective and subjective terms of high-priority problems or aspirations for the common good, defined for a population by economic and social indicators and by individuals in terms of their quality of life" (Green & Kreuter, 1999, p. 509) (Chapter 4).

social capital "the relationships and structures within a community, such as civic participation, networks, norms of reciprocity, and trust, that promote cooperation of mutual benefit" (Putnam, 1995, p. 66) (Chapter 4).

social change philosophy a philosophy emphasizing the role of health education/promotion in creating social, economic, and political change that benefits the health of individuals and groups.

social determinants of health "conditions in the environments in which people are born, live, learn, work, play, worship, and age that affect a wide range of health, functioning, and quality-of-life outcomes and risk" (USDHHS, 2013, ¶4) (Chapter 1).

social ecology an approach to health education/promotion that goes beyond individual behavior change to examine and modify the social, political, and economic factors impacting health behavior decisions.

social marketing "the application of commercial marketing technologies to the analysis, planning, execution, and evaluation of programs designed to influence the voluntary behavior of target audiences in order to improve their personal welfare and that of their society" (Andreasen, 1995, p. 7) (Chapter 4).

social media "media that used the Internet and other technologies to allow for social interaction" (McKenzie et al., 2012, p. 448) (Chapter 1).

social network "web of social relationships that surround people" (Heaney & Israel, 2008, p. 190) (Chapter 4).

social networking connecting to other individuals (or organizations) that are tied (connected) by one or more specific types of interdependency, such as friendship, kinship, common interest, financial exchange, occupational or professional interests, or beliefs. Facebook, Myspace, LinkedIn, Twitter, YouTube, and Instagram are just a few examples of social networking sites that may be of value to health education specialists.

social norms "what are perceived to be true and acceptable" (Simons-Morton et al., 2012, p. 158) (Chapter 4).

Society for Public Health Education, Inc. (SOPHE) a professional association for health education specialists.

Society of State Leaders of Health and Physical Education a professional association composed of individuals who, by position in a state or territorial department of education, represent their state or territory.

socio-ecological approach behavior has multiple levels of influences.

soft money funds to support health education/promotion positions and programs secured through grants or contracts, which may be discontinued at the end of a designated period.

specific rate a rate for a particular population subgroup, such as for a particular disease (i.e., disease-specific) or for a particular age of people.

stage theories those behavior change theories that comprise an ordered set of categories into which people can be classified and for which factors could be identified that could induce movement from one category to the next (Weinstein & Sandman, 2002) (Chapter 4).

sub-competencies "reflects the ability of the student to list, describe, etc." (National Commission for Health Education Credentialing, Inc. 1996, p. 12) (Chapter 6).

subjective norm a belief held by people that others (individuals or groups) think they should do something and that they care about what others think; a construct of the theory of planned behavior.

technology any device used by society to increase access to or opportunity for people to be exposed to that device—for example, computers and television have increased educational access and opportunities for many people; thus, they are examples of technology.

teleological theories (or **consequentialism**) evaluate the moral status of an act by the goodness of the consequences (Reamer, 2006) (Chapter 5).

termination zero chance of relapse.

tertiary prevention preventive measures aimed at rehabilitation following significant pathogenesis.

tertiary sources publications such as pamphlets, handbooks, or brochures containing information collected from primary or secondary sources.

theories/models of implementation theories and models used in planning, implementing, and evaluating health education/promotion programs.

theory "a set of interrelated concepts, definitions, and propositions that presents a systematic view of events or situations by specifying relations among variables in order to explain and predict the events of the situations" (Glanz et al., 2008b, p. 25) (Chapter 4).

Theory of Planned Behavior an intrapersonal theory that addresses individuals' intentions to perform a given behavior as a function of their attitude toward performing the behavior, their beliefs about what is relevant, what others think they should do, and their perception of the ease or difficulty in performing the behavior.

traditional family a family having two parents and their children.

Transtheoretical Model of Change also known as the stages of change model, it is an intrapersonal theory that addresses an "individual's readiness to change or attempt to change toward healthy behaviors" (Glanz & Rimer, 1995, p. 17) (Chapter 4).

truth telling (honesty) to tell the truth; one of the five principles of common moral ground.

Uniform Resource Locator (URL) identifier for a site on the World Wide Web; specifies locations, or addresses.

value of life a basic principle of ethics: no life should be ended without strong justification.

variable the operational (practical use) form of a construct.

voluntary health agencies "organizations that are created by concerned citizens to deal with health needs not met by governmental agencies" (McKenzie et al., 2012) (Chapters 7 and 8); these organizations rely heavily on volunteer help and donations to function.

wellness "an approach to health that focuses on balancing the many aspects, or dimensions, of a person's life through increasing the adoption of health enhancing conditions and behaviors rather than attempting to minimize conditions of illness" (Joint Committee, 2012, p. 10) (Chapter 1).

worksite health promotion health education/promotion programs offered by business and industry entities for their employees.

World Wide Web an interactive information delivery service that includes a repository of resources about most subjects; documents are related by subject area and linked together, thus creating a "web" (Madden, 2010) (Chapter 9).

years of potential life lost (YPLL) a measure of premature mortality calculated by subtracting a person's age at death from 75 years (NCHS, 2013) (Chapter 1).

Chapter 1

P. 7: Jaime Harding;   p. 19: Fritz Hoffmann/The Image Works.

Chapter 2

P. 37: Image copyright © The Metropolitan Museum of Art. Image source: Art Resource, NY; p. 39: Richard Ashworth/Robert Harding Picture Library Ltd/Alamy;   p. 40: Alinari/Art Resource, NY;   p. 41: Garry Gay/Alamy;   p. 42: Mrakor/Fotolia;   p. 43: stevanzz/Fotolia; p. 49: Robert Harding World Imagery;   p. 52: Library of Congress;   p. 53: M&N/Alamy; p. 55: James Gathany, Centers for Disease Control and Prevention;   p. 61: Library of Congress Prints and Photographs Division Washington [LC-DIG-nclc-02986];   p. 65: Exactostock/ SuperStock.

Chapter 3

P. 78: James T. Girvan;   p. 81: Surgeon General/U.S. Department of Health & Human Services; p. 82: Tao Associates/The Image Bank/Getty Images;   p. 89: Travis Leyva.

Chapter 4

P. 103: Kevin Schafer/Photo Library/Getty images;   p. 106: Image Source/SuperStock;   p. 116: AP Photo/Ron Edmonds; p 119: Trevor Newby.

Chapter 5

P. 145: (left) Bettmann/CORBIS, (right) Kitty/Fotolia;   p. 148: Janine Wiedel Photolibrary/ Alamy;   p. 152: Spencer Grant/PhotoEdit.

Chapter 6

p. 169: Dr. Helen P. Cleary;   p. 172: Lauren Clark;   p. 175: Gary D. Gilmore, MPH, Ph.D., CHES Professor and Director Graduate Community Health Programs University of Wisconsin - La Crosse;   p. 184: Lucky winner/Alamy;   p. 192: Jovanni Reyes.

Chapter 7

P. 206: David Buffington/Getty Images;   p. 208: Carolyn Conley;   p. 211: Raymond Boyd/Getty Images;   p. 212: Jennifer O'Donell;   p. 217: Patricia Stewart;   p. 221: iofoto/Shutterstock;   p. 223: Nicole Gaudette;   p. 227: Robert Clay/Alamy;   p. 228: Carrie Wilcox;   p. 233: Jodi Brawley; p. 235: Emily Miller;   p. 239: Nicole Nichols;   p. 242: Melinda Hershey;   p. 246: Copyright held by, and used with permission of, The University of Texas M. D. Anderson Cancer Center.

Chapter 8

P. 255: James F. McKenzie;   p. 264: U.S. Public Health Service;   p. 265: Will & Deni McIntrye/ Science Source;   p. 267: Leslie Gray;   p. 272: Janet Kamini.

Chapter 9

P. 287: Stephanie Wheeler;   p. 288: ACE STOCK LIMITED/Alamy;   p. 292: Mark Richards/ PhotoEdit;   p. 297: NIH Library of Medicine;   p. 299: NetPhotos/Alamy;   p. 300: Creativa/ Fotolia.

Chapter 10

P. 314: Robert Kneschke/Fotolia;   p. 318: (top) Siberia/Fotolia, (bottom) Richard Lord/The Image Works;   p. 320: Rachel Epstein/PhotoEdit;   p. 326: Bob Daemmrich /The Image Works.